Study Guide and Skills Performance Checklists

to Accompany

POTTER * PERRY
Fundamentals of Nursing

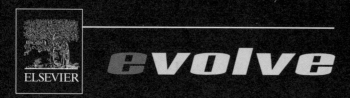

- **Student Learning Activities** include Crosswords, Hangman, Match Its, Picture Its, Case Studies, and Short Answer Questions.

- **Review Questions** include answers and rationales.

- **Concept Map Exercises** challenge you to recognize the association amo multiple nursing diagnoses and their relationship to medical diagnosis.

- **Critical Thinking Exercises** challenge you to recognize how nursing process and critical thinking come together to help you provide the best care for clients.

- **Animations** include exciting images related to various chapters in the textbo

- **Video Clips** demonstrate important steps in various nursing skills throughout textbook.

- **WebLinks** are an exciting resource that lets you link to hundreds of websites carefully chosen to supplement the content of the textbook.

- **Content Updates** include the latest information from the authors of the text book to keep you current with recent developments in this area of study.

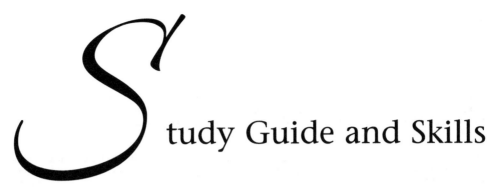

Study Guide and Skills

Performance Checklists

to Accompany
POTTER * PERRY
Fundamentals of Nursing

Geralyn Ochs, RN, MSN, BC-ACNP, ANP
Assistant Professor in Adult Nursing
St. Louis University School of Nursing

Performance Checklists by
Patricia Castaldi, BSN, MSN
Director, Practical Nursing Program
Union County College
Plainfield, New Jersey

6th edition

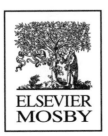

ELSEVIER
MOSBY

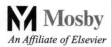
Mosby
An Affiliate of Elsevier

11830 Westline Industrial Drive
St. Louis, MO 63146

STUDY GUIDE AND SKILLS PERFORMANCE CHECKLISTS
TO ACCOMPANY FUNDAMENTALS OF NURSING, 6TH EDITION
Copyright 2005, 2001, 1997 by Mosby, Inc. All rights reserved.

Permissions may be sought directly from Elsevier's Health Sciences Rights
Department in Philadelphia, PA, USA: phone: (+1) 215 239 3804, fax: (+1) 215 239 3805,
e-mail: healthpermissions@elsevier.com. You may also complete your request on-line
via the Elsevier homepage (http://www.elsevier.com), by selecting 'Customer Support'
and then 'Obtaining Permissions'.

Notice

Nursing is an ever-changing field. Standard safety precautions must be followed but as new research and clinical experience broaden our knowledge, changes in treatment and drug therapy may become necessary or appropriate. Readers are advised to check the most current product information provided by the manufacturer of each drug to be administered to verify the recommended dose, the method and duration of administration, and contraindications. It is the responsibility of the treating physician, relying on experience and knowledge of the patient, to determine dosages and the best treatment for each individual patient. Neither the Publisher nor the author assumes any liability for any injury and/or damage to persons or property arising from this publication.

The Publisher

ISBN-13: 978-0-323-02585-0
ISBN-10: 0-323-02585-4

Executive Editor: Susan R. Epstein
Senior Developmental Editor: Maria Broeker
Publishing Services Manager: Gayle May

Printed in the United States of America

06 07 08   6 5 4

To my husband,
Jim,
for his unending support,
love and friendship.

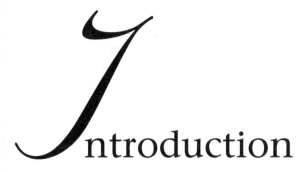

Introduction

The *Study Guide to accompany Fundamentals of Nursing*, sixth edition, has been developed to encourage independent learning for beginning nursing students. As you begin to read the text, you may note a difference in style and format from other books you've used in the past. The terms are new, and the focus of the content is different. You may be wondering, "How will I possibly learn all of the material in this chapter?" The essential objective of this study guide is to assist you in this endeavor—to help you learn *what* you need to know and then self-test with hundreds of review questions.

This study guide follows the text chapter for chapter. Whatever chapter your instructor assigns, you will use the same chapter number in this study guide. The outline format was designed to help you learn to read nursing content more effectively and with greater understanding. Each chapter of this study guide has the following sections to assist you to comprehend and recall.

The *Preliminary Reading* section is designed to teach prereading strategies. You need to become familiar with the chapter by first reading the chapter title, the key concepts and key terms (found at the end of each chapter), and all headings, as well as review all photographs, drawings, tables, and boxes. This can be done rather quickly and will give you an overall idea of the content of the chapter.

The *Comprehensive Understanding* section is next and is in outline format. This will prove to be a very valuable tool not only as you first read the chapter but also as you review for tests. This outline identifies the topics and main ideas of each chapter as an aid to concentration, comprehension, and retaining textbook information. By completing this outline you will learn to "pull-out" key information in the chapter. As you write the answers in the study guide, you will be reinforcing that content. Once completed, this outline will serve as a review tool for exams.

The Review Questions in each chapter provide a valuable means of testing and reinforcing your knowledge of the material read and the answers written in the outline. Each question is multiple choice and written in the NCLEX®-style format. As a further aid for independent learning, each answer requires a rationale (the reason *why* the option you selected is correct). After you have completed the review questions, you can check the answers in the back of the study guide.

NCLEX is a registered trademark of the National Council of State Boards of Nursing, Inc.

The clinical chapters, Chapters 26 to 30 and 36 to 49, include exercises based on the care plans found in the text. These exercises provide practice in synthesizing the nursing process and critical thinking as you, the nurse, care for clients. Taking one aspect of the nursing process, you will be asked to imagine you are the nurse in the case study and to think about what knowledge, experiences, standards, and attitudes might be used in caring for the client. Write your answers in the approprite boxes and check them against the answer key.

When you finish answering the review questions and synthesis exercises, take a few minutes for self-evaluation. If you answered a question incorrectly, begin to analyze the thoughts that led you to the wrong answer:

- Did you miss the key word or phrase?
- Did you read into something that wasn't stated?
- Did you not understand the subject matter?
- Did you use an incorrect rationale for selecting your response?

Each incorrect response is an opportunity to learn. Go back to the text and reread any content that is still unclear. In the long run, it will be a time-saving activity.

A performance checklist is provided for each of the s presented in the text. The checklists may be used by instructors to evaluate your competence in performing the techniques. You may need to adapt these s in order to meet a client's special needs or follow the particular policy of an institution.

The learning activities presented in this study guide will assist you in completing the semester with a firm understanding of nursing concepts and processes that you can rely on all of your professional career.

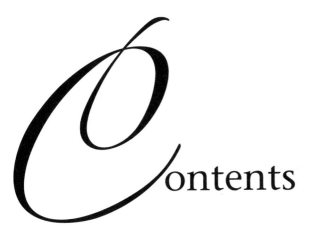

ontents

Procedure Performance Checklists

Study Guide and Skills Performance Checklists

to Accompany

POTTER * PERRY
Fundamentals of Nursing

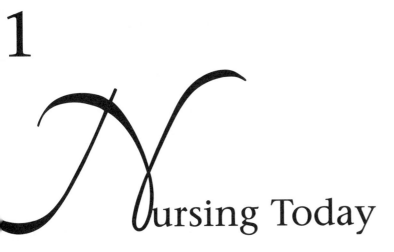

1

Nursing Today

Preliminary Reading

Chapter 1, pp. 1-19

Comprehensive Understanding

- Define *nursing* (according to the International Council of Nurses). _____ _____

Historical Perspective Highlights

- Nursing continues to respond to the needs of the client. Identify some of the times that nursing has responded.

    _____

    _____

- Nurses are active in social policy and political arenas. Give an example.

    _____

    _____

- Briefly explain how each of the following have influenced nursing.

    a. Florence Nightingale: _____

    b. Civil War: _____

    c. Twentieth century: _____

    d. Twenty-first century: _____

Societal Influences on Nursing

- Briefly explain the following external forces that have affected nursing practice.

  a. Demographic changes: _____

  _____

  b. Women's health care issues: _____

  _____

  c. Human rights movement: _____

  _____

  d. Medically underserved: _____

  _____

  e. Threat of bioterrorism: _____

  _____

Needs of the Consumer

- Briefly explain.

  a. Cultural diversity: _____

  _____

  _____

  b. Health promotion and wellness: _____

  _____

  _____

Influence of Today's Health Care Delivery System

- Briefly explain each of the following.

  a. Rising health care costs: _____

  _____

  b. Evidence-based practice: _____

  _____

  c. Nursing and biomedical research: _____

  _____

  d. Nursing shortage: _____

  _____

Nursing as a Profession

Professionalism
- List the five primary characteristics of a profession.

  a. _____

  b. _____

  c. _____

  d. _____

  e. _____

- Describe standards of professional performance. _____

  _____

  _____

- Describe standards of care. _____

  _____

  _____

- Describe code of Ethics. _____

  _____

  _____

Educational Preparation

Professional Registered Nurse Education
- As the profession of nursing grew, various educational routes for becoming an RN were developed. Briefly explain the following.

  a. Associate degree education: _____

  _____

  b. Baccalaureate education: _____

  _____

- Explain the two advanced educational preparations that a nurse may seek.

  a. Master's: _____

  _____

  b. Doctorate: _____

  _____

- Describe what continuing education and in-service education consist of. _____

_____

_____

Nursing Practice
- Nurse Practice Acts: _____

_____

_____

- Licensure: _____

_____

_____

- Certification: _____

_____

_____

- Science and art of nursing practice: _____

_____

_____

Accreditation
- To be accredited, nursing programs must meet certain criteria established by the National League for Nursing (NLN). Briefly explain the purpose of accreditation.

_____

_____

_____

Licensure
- In the United States, RN candidates must pass the National Council Licensure Examination for Registered Nurses (NCLEX-RN). This provides a standardized minimum knowledge base for the client population nurses serve.

Certification
- The nurse may choose to work toward certification in a specific area of nursing practice. Minimal requirements are set based on the specific certification.

Continuing and In-Service Education
- The goals of continuing education are to: ____

_____

_____

- An in-service education program is: _____

_____

_____

Professional Responsibilities and Roles

- The contemporary nurse functions in the following roles. Briefly explain each.

  a. Autonomy: _____

  _____

  b. Accountability: _____

  _____

  c. Caregiver: _____

  _____

  d. Advocate: _____

  _____

  e. Educator: _____

  _____

  f. Communicator: _____

  _____

  g. Manager: _____

  _____

Career Development

- Explain each of the following career roles and functions.

  a. Clinician: _____

  _____

  b. Advanced practice nurse: _____

  _____

  c. Clinical nurse specialist: _____

  _____

  d. Nurse practitioner: _____

  _____

e. Certified nurse-midwife: _____

_____

f. Certified registered nurse anesthetist: _____

_____

g. Nurse educator: _____

_____

h. Nurse administrator: _____

_____

i. Nurse researcher: _____

_____

Professional Nursing Organizations

- Briefly identify the issues with which the following organizations deal.

    a. ANA: _____

    _____

    b. NLN:_____

    _____

    c. NSNA: _____

    _____

Trends in Nursing

- Briefly explain the following trends.

    a. Expansion of employment opportunities:

    _____

    _____

    b. Nursing's public perception: _____

    _____

    _____

    c. Nursing's impact on politics and health policy: _____

    _____

- *Healthy People 2010* is a document for:

_____

_____

Review Questions

The student should select the appropriate answer and cite the rationale for choosing that particular answer.

1. The factor that best advanced the practice of nursing in the first century was:
   a. Teachings of Christianity
   b. Growth of cities
   c. Better education of nurses
   d. Improved conditions for women

   Answer: _____ Rationale: _____

   _____

   _____

2. Nursing education programs may seek voluntary accreditation by the appropriate council of the:
   a. American Nurses Association
   b. International Council of Nurses
   c. Congress for Nursing Practice
   d. National League for Nursing

   Answer: _____ Rationale: _____

   _____

   _____

3. The graduate nurse must pass a licensure examination administered by the:
   a. Accredited school of nursing
   b. American Nurses Association
   c. State boards of nursing
   d. National League for Nursing

   Answer: _____ Rationale: _____

   _____

   _____

4. When Mr. Jones had his leg amputated, the nurse assisted him as he learned to cope with the artificial limb and new routine. The nurse's primary role at this time was:
   a. Rehabilitator
   b. Manager
   c. Friend
   d. Advisor

Answer: _____ Rationale: _____

_____

_____

5. A group that lobbies at the state and federal levels for advancement of the nurse's role, economic interest, and health care is the:
   a. American Nurses Association
   b. State boards of nursing
   c. National Student Nurses' Association
   d. American Hospital Association

Answer: _____ Rationale: _____

_____

_____

2

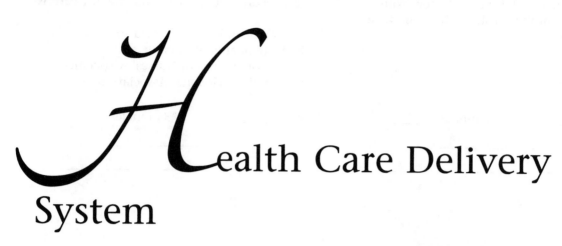

Health Care Delivery System

*P*reliminary Reading

Chapter 2, pp. 26-45

*C*omprehensive Understanding

Health Care Regulation and Competition

- Briefly explain the following regulatory or government interventions that attempt to control health care spending.

    a. Professional standards review organizations (PSROs): _____

    _____

    _____

    b. Prospective payment systems (PPS): _____

    _____

    _____

    c. Utilization review (UR): _____

    _____

    _____

    d. Diagnosis-related groups (DRGs): _____

    _____

    _____

    e. Capitation: _____

    _____

    _____

f. Resource utilization groups (RUGs): _____

_____

_____

g. Managed care: _____

_____

_____

Nursing Implications

- Briefly explain how these regulatory and competitive approaches affect the nursing profession and the quality of care. _____

_____

Levels of Health Care

- The health care industry is moving toward health care practices that emphasize managing health rather than managing illness.

- A wellness perspective focuses on the health of populations rather than individuals. With this perspective, health care systems are moving toward integrated delivery networks (IDNs). Briefly explain this system.

_____

_____

_____

Preventive and Primary Health Care Services

- Define *primary care*. _____

_____

_____

- The Institute of Medicine describes six core attributes of primary care:

a. _____

b. _____

c. _____

d. _____

e. _____

f. _____

- The focus of health promotion is: _____

_____

_____

- Explain the focus of the following levels of care and the nurse's role in each.

a. Health promotion services: _____

_____

_____

b. Preventive care: _____

_____

_____

c. School health services: _____

_____

_____

d. Occupational health services: _____

_____

_____

e. Physician's offices _____

_____

_____

f. Clinics: _____

_____

_____

g. Nursing centers: _____

_____

_____

h. Block and parish nursing: _____

_____

_____

i. Volunteer agencies: _____

_____

_____

- Primary health care is an approach for: _____

_____

_____

- The primary health care model focuses on collaboration of: _____
  _____
  _____

Secondary and Tertiary Care

- Explain the focus of the services of acute care nurses in the hospital. _____
  _____
  _____

- Explain the case management model of care.
  _____
  _____
  _____

- Explain the purpose of discharge planning.
  _____
  _____
  _____

- A critical pathway is: _____
  _____
  _____

- Tips on making the referral process successful include:
  a. _____
  b. _____
  c. _____
  d. _____

- JCAHO requires the following instruction before clients leave health care facilities:
  a. _____
  b. _____
  c. _____
  d. _____
  e. _____
  f. _____
  g. _____

- Briefly explain the purpose of the following areas in a hospital.
  a. Intensive care unit (ICU): _____
  _____
  b. Psychiatric facilities: _____
  _____

- Briefly explain the differences between a rural and an urban hospital. _____
  _____
  _____

Restorative Care

- The goal of restorative care is: _____
  _____
  _____

- Explain the function of the restorative care team. _____
  _____
  _____

- Briefly define *home care*. _____
  _____
  _____

- Home care agencies provide: _____
  _____
  _____

- Rehabilitation services include: _____
  _____
  _____

- Extended care facilities include the following. Briefly explain each.
  a. Intermediate care: _____
  _____
  b. Skilled nursing facilities: _____
  _____

8   Chapter 2: Health Care Delivery System

Continuing Care

- Continuing care/long-term care offer services for: _____
_____
_____

- List the reasons why the need for continuing health care services is growing. _____
_____
_____
_____

- Briefly explain the services provided in nursing facilities. _____
_____
_____

- Describe the purpose of AAA. _____
_____
_____

- Identify the types of services provided by the OAA and AAA. _____
_____
_____

- A nursing center is: _____
_____
_____

- The OBRA's resident bill of rights states that:
_____
_____
_____

- Interdisciplinary functional assessment is the cornerstone of clinical practice within nursing facilities. The focus is: _____
_____
_____

- Describe the Resident Assessment Instrument (RAI). _____
_____
_____

- Assisted living is: _____
_____
_____

- Define *respite care*. _____
_____
_____

- Identify the services provided by adult day care centers. _____
_____
_____

- Hospice is a system designed to: _____
_____
_____

- The focus of hospice care is: _____
_____
_____

Issues in Health Care Delivery

- Consumers of health care want to access appropriate, cost-effective, quality health care.

- Define *evidence-based practice*. _____
_____
_____

- List four websites for evidence-based nursing.
_____
_____
_____
_____

- The Pew Health Professions Commission (1991) identified six critical competencies needed for health professions. Identify them.

  a. _____

  b. _____

  c. _____

  d. _____

  e. _____

  f. _____

Knowing Clients

- Tanner describes five aspects of knowing clients.

  a. _____

  b. _____

  c. _____

  d. _____

  e. _____

- List and briefly explain the working habits of knowing your clients.

  a. _____

  b. _____

  c. _____

  d. _____

  e. _____

  f. _____

  g. _____

- Briefly explain the following.

  a. Unlicensed assistive personnel (UAP): _____

  _____

  _____

  b. Delegation: _____

  _____

  _____

Quality Health Care

- Quality health care is difficult to define. Health care providers are trying to define and measure quality in terms of outcomes. _____

  _____

  _____

- Examples of outcomes are: _____

  _____

  _____

- Health Plan Employer Data and Information Set (HEDIS) is a database of: _____

  _____

  _____

- The Picker/Commonwealth Program for Patient-Centered Care identified seven dimensions of care that affect a client's experiences with health care. Name them.

  a. _____

  b. _____

  c. _____

  d. _____

  e. _____

  f. _____

  g. _____

Review Questions

The student should select the appropriate answer and cite the rationale for choosing that particular answer.

1. The federal law allowing nurse practitioners to deliver primary health care in underserved areas is the:
   a. Rural Health Clinics Act
   b. Hill-Burton Act
   c. National Health Planning and Resources Development Act
   d. Social Security Amendment Act of 1972

Answer: _____ Rationale: _____

_____

_____

2. Health promotion activities are designed to help clients:
   a. Reduce the risk of illness
   b. Maintain maximal function
   c. Promote habits related to health care
   d. All of the above

Answer: _____ Rationale: _____

_____

_____

3. Rehabilitation services begin:
   a. When the client enters the health care system
   b. After the client requests rehabilitation services
   c. After the client's physical condition stabilizes
   d. When the client is discharged from the hospital

Answer: _____ Rationale: _____

_____

_____

4. An example of an extended care facility is a:
   a. Home health agency
   b. Suicide prevention center
   c. State-owned psychiatric hospital
   d. Nursing facility

Answer: _____ Rationale: _____

_____

_____

5. A client and his or her family facing the end stages of a terminal illness might best be served by a:
   a. Rehabilitation center
   b. Extended care facility
   c. Hospice
   d. Crisis intervention center

Answer: _____ Rationale: _____

_____

_____

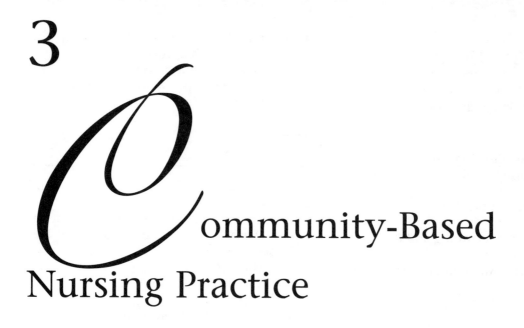

3

Community-Based Nursing Practice

Preliminary Reading

Chapter 3, pp. 46-59

Comprehensive Understanding

Community-Based Health Care

- Community-based nursing involves: _____

  _____

  _____

Achieving Healthy Populations and Communities

- Give an example of assessment. _____

  _____

  _____

- Give an example of each of the levels of the health services pyramid.

  a. Population-based health care: _____

  _____

  b. Clinical preventive services: _____

  _____

  c. Primary health care: _____

  _____

  d. Secondary health care: _____

  _____

e. Tertiary health care: _____

_____

Community Health Nursing

- Briefly describe the differences between:

    a. Public health focus: _____

    _____

    b. Community health nursing: _____

    _____

Nursing Practice in Community Health

- Briefly explain the nursing focus in community health nursing. _____

_____

_____

_____

Community-Based Nursing

- Community based nursing involves the _____ and _____ care of indi

  viduals and families that enhance _____.

- The philosophical foundation is: _____

_____

_____

- Briefly explain the focus of the community-based nurse. _____

_____

_____

Vulnerable Populations

- Vulnerable populations are: _____

_____

_____

- Explain how a nurse becomes culturally competent. _____

_____

_____

_____

- List some of the reasons why vulnerable populations typically experience poorer out comes. _____

_____

_____

_____

- Briefly describe the following vulnerable groups and identify their risk factors.

    a. Poor and homeless: _____

    _____

    _____

    b. Abused clients: _____

    _____

    _____

    c. Substance abusers: _____

    _____

    _____

    d. Severely mentally ill: _____

    _____

    _____

    e. Older adults: _____

    _____

    _____

Competency in Community-Based Nursing

- A nurse in a community-based practice must have a variety of skills and talents in assisting clients within the community. Briefly explain the competencies the nurse needs in the following roles.

    a. Case manager: _____

    _____

    _____

    b. Collaborator: _____

    _____

    _____

    c. Educator: _____

    _____

    _____

d. Counselor: _____

_____

e. Client advocate: _____

_____

f. Change agent: _____

_____

Community Assessment

- The community is viewed as having three components. Briefly explain each one.

a. Structure: _____

_____

b. Population: _____

_____

c. Social system: _____

_____

Changing Clients' Health

- The challenge is how to promote and protect a client's health within the context of the community.

- The most important theme to consider in order to be an effective community-based nurse is to:

_____

_____

- Identify some factors that nurses must consider in community-based practice.

_____

_____

_____

_____

Review Questions

The student should select the appropriate answer and cite the rationale for choosing that particular answer.

1. Which of the following is not an example of a primary care setting?
   a. Elementary school
   b. Hospital
   c. Business
   d. Neighborhood health center

   Answer: _____ Rationale: _____

   _____

   _____

2. Among the communication skills needed to provide nursing care to community clients is the ability to:
   a. Clarify client values and care expectations
   b. Follow medical prescriptions in many settings
   c. Manage generational interfamilial conflict
   d. Speak the client's language or dialects

   Answer: _____ Rationale: _____

   _____

   _____

3. Which of the following is an example of an intrinsic risk factor for homelessness?
   a. Living below the poverty line
   b. Psychotic mental disorders
   c. Severe anxiety disorders
   d. Progressive chronic alcoholism

   Answer: _____ Rationale: _____

   _____

   _____

4. When the community health nurse refers clients to appropriate resources and monitors and coordinates the extent and adequacy of services to meet family health care needs, the nurse is functioning in the role of:
   a. Collaborator
   b. Advocate
   c. Counselor
   d. Case manager

Answer: _____ Rationale: _____

_____

_____

5. The first step in community assessment is determining the community's:
   a. Set factors
   b. Goals
   c. Boundaries
   d. Throughputs

Answer: _____ Rationale: _____

_____

_____

4

Theoretical Foundations of Nursing Practice

Preliminary Readings

Chapter 4, pp. 60-72

Comprehensive Understanding

- The domain of nursing: _____
    - a. Domain: _____
    - b. Paradigm: _____

- Briefly explain the four linkages of interest in the nursing paradigm.
    - a. Person: _____
      _____
    - b. Health: _____
      _____
    - c. Environment/situation: _____
      _____
    - d. Nursing: _____
      _____

Theory

- Define nursing theory. _____

- Theory provides nurses with a perspective to view client situations and a method to analyze and interpret information.

Components of a Theory
- Explain the following components of a theory.

  a. Concepts: _____

  _____

  b. Definitions: _____

  _____

  c. Assumptions: _____

  _____

  d. Phenomena: _____

  _____

Types of Theory
- Briefly explain the following classifications of theories.

  a. Grand theories: _____

  _____

  _____

  b. Middle-range theories: _____

  _____

  _____

  c. Descriptive theories: _____

  _____

  _____

  d. Prescriptive theories: _____

  _____

  _____

Theoretical Models
- A theoretical model refers to: _____

  _____

  _____

Relationship of Theory to the Nursing Process and Client Needs

- Historically, nursing theories were studied in an isolated academic environment independent of nursing practice. The move now is toward nursing science or evidence-based practice.

Interdisciplinary Theories

- An interdisciplinary theory is: _____

  _____

  _____

Systems Theory
- A system is: _____

  _____

- Define *input.* _____

  _____

- Define *output.* _____

  _____

- Define *feedback.* _____

  _____

Basic Human Needs
- List the five levels of the hierarchy of human needs.

  a. _____

  b. _____

  c. _____

  d. _____

  e. _____

Health and Wellness Models
- Health and wellness models are designed to:

  _____

  _____

  _____

Stress and Adaptation
- The models that explain the stress response are: _____

  _____

  _____

Developmental Theories
- The developmental theories explain the:

  _____

  _____

Psychosocial Theories

- Give some examples of psychosocial theories.

_____

_____

_____

Selected Nursing Theories

- Briefly summarize the basic concepts relevant to the following nursing theories.

   a. Nightingale: _____

   _____

   _____

   _____

   _____

   b. Peplau: _____

   _____

   _____

   _____

   _____

   c. Henderson: _____

   _____

   _____

   _____

   _____

   d. Abdellah: _____

   _____

   _____

   _____

   _____

   e. Johnson: _____

   _____

   _____

   _____

   _____

   e. Roger: _____

   _____

   _____

   _____

   _____

   f. Orem: _____

   _____

   _____

   _____

   _____

   g. Neuman: _____

   _____

   _____

   _____

   _____

   h. Leininger: _____

   _____

   _____

   _____

   i. King: _____

   _____

   _____

   _____

   j. Roy: _____

   _____

   _____

   _____

   _____

   k. Watson: _____

   _____

   _____

   _____

   _____

   l. Benner and Wrubel: _____

   _____

   _____

   _____

   _____

The Link Between Theory and Knowledge Development in Nursing

- Differentiate between theoretical knowledge and practical knowledge.

  a. Theoretical knowledge: _____

  _____

  _____

  _____

  b. Practical knowledge: _____

  _____

  _____

  _____

- Briefly explain each of the following.

  a. Theory-generating research: _____

  _____

  b. Theory-testing research: _____

  _____

Review Questions

The student should select the appropriate answer and cite the rationale for choosing that particular answer.

1. Which of the following is a borrowed theory that has been applied to nursing?
   a. Orem's model of self-care
   b. Erickson's theory of psychosocial development
   c. Roger's theory of integrality
   d. Roy's adaptation model

Answer: _____ Rationale: _____

_____

_____

2. Which of the following conceptual models views the person and the environment as energy fields coextensive with the universe?
   a. King's model of personal, interpersonal, and social systems
   b. Orem's model of self-care
   c. Roy's adaptation model
   d. Roger's life process interactive person-environmental model

Answer: _____ Rationale: _____

_____

_____

3. Who is considered to have been the first nursing theorist?
   a. Florence Nightingale
   b. Virginia Henderson
   c. Adelaide Nutting
   d. Linda Richards

Answer: _____ Rationale: _____

_____

_____

4. How would you distinguish between theories and assumptions?
   a. Assumptions are tested, and theories are not.
   b. Assumptions are assumed to be true, but theories are not.
   c. Theories organize reality, but assumptions are not real.
   d. Theories test hypotheses, but assumptions need no scientific proof.

Answer: _____ Rationale: _____

_____

_____

5. The development of nursing knowledge depends on:
   a. Science and philosophy
   b. Logic and reasoning
   c. Observation and verification
   d. Definitions and hypothesis

Answer: _____ Rationale: _____

_____

_____

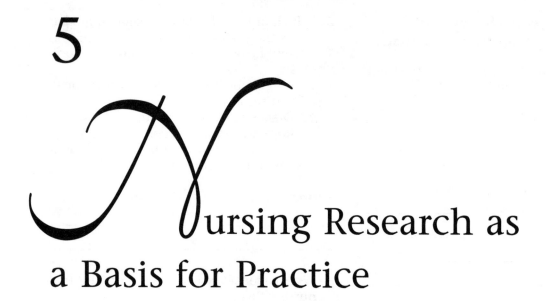

5

Nursing Research as a Basis for Practice

Preliminary Reading

Chapter 5, pp. 73-88

Comprehensive Understanding

- Nursing research involves: _____

  _____

Historical Perspective

- Briefly explain the significance of each of the following.

  a. Florence Nightingale: _____

  _____

  b. Goldmark report: _____

  _____

  c. 1950: _____

  _____

  d. 1960: _____

  _____

  e. 1970: _____

  _____

f. 1981: _____

_____

_____

- Identify the priorities for nursing research as identified by the National Institute of Nursing Research Priorities. _____

_____

_____

- Define *outcomes research.* _____

_____

Scientific Research in Nursing

Knowledge Acquisition

- Knowledge is acquired in many ways. Scientific research is the most reliable and objective of all methods of gaining knowledge.

- The following are ways an individual acquires knowledge. Briefly explain each one.

a. Tradition: _____

_____

b. Information seeking: _____

_____

c. Experience: _____

_____

d. Problem solving: _____

_____

e. Critical thinking: _____

_____

Scientific Method

- Define *scientific method.* _____

_____

- List the five characteristics of scientific research.

a. _____

b. _____

c. _____

d. _____

e. _____

Nursing and the Scientific Approach

- The purpose of the scientific approach is to:

_____

_____

_____

- Research provides a way for nursing questions and problems to be studied in greater depth within the context of nursing.

- Briefly describe the methods used to study clinical problems.

a. Historical: _____

_____

b. Exploratory: _____

_____

c. Evaluation: _____

_____

d. Descriptive: _____

_____

e. Experimental: _____

_____

f. Correlational: _____

_____

Research Methods

- The two broad approaches to research are

_____ and _____.

Quantitative Research

- Quantitative nursing research is: _____

_____

- Briefly explain the following quantitative approaches to answer research questions.

    a. Experimental study: _____

    _____

    _____

    b. Surveys: _____

    _____

    _____

    c. Evaluation: _____

    _____

    _____

Qualitative Research

- Qualitative research is: _____

_____

- Define the following design strategies that are used with qualitative research.

    a. Ethnography: _____

    _____

    _____

    b. Phenomenology: _____

    _____

    c. Grounded theory: _____

    _____

Research Process

- The research process consists of phases or steps. Briefly explain each of the following.

    a. Problem identification: _____

    _____

    b. Study design: _____

    _____

    c. Conducting the study: _____

    _____

    d. Data analysis: _____

    _____

    e. Use of the findings: _____

    _____

Conducting Nursing Research

- Briefly explain the 1997 American Nurses Association (ANA) position statement of nursing research. _____

    _____

- Briefly explain the expectations of the following levels of nursing preparation with clinical nursing research.

    a. Associate degree: _____

    _____

    b. Baccalaureate degree: _____

    _____

    c. Master's degree: _____

    _____

    d. Doctorally prepared: _____

    _____

Ethical Issues in Research

Rights of Human Subjects

- Informed consent means that research subjects:

    a. _____

    b. _____

    c. _____

    d. _____

- Confidentiality is: _____

    _____

- Anonymity is: _____

    _____

- Briefly explain the responsibilities of the Institutional Review Board (IRB). _____

_____

_____

_____

- Health Insurance Portability and Accountability Act of 1996 (HIPAA) requires health care institutions to: _____

_____

Applying Research to Nursing Practice

- Biomedical research is: _____

_____

_____

Research Report Versus Clinical Article

- The typical research report has the following parts. Briefly explain each section.

  a. Abstract: _____

  _____

  b. Introduction: _____

  _____

  c. Methods section: _____

  _____

  d. Results section: _____

  _____

  e. Discussion section: _____

  _____

  f. Reference list: _____

  _____

- Explain the difference between a primary and secondary source. _____

_____

- Identify some common sources of research studies. _____

_____

_____

_____

Organizing Information from a Research Report

- Define *citations*. _____

_____

_____

Identifying Clinical Nursing Problems

- List three characteristics of a clinical nursing problem with the potential to be researched.

  a. _____

  b. _____

  c. _____

Research Utilization

- To use findings in clinical practice, the nurse must be aware of the problems already studied.

- List four criteria used to determine if research findings should be applied to nursing practice.

  a. _____

  b. _____

  c. _____

  d. _____

- Define *research utilization*. _____

_____

_____

- Identify barriers to using research in clinical settings. _____

_____

_____

$\mathcal{R}$eview Questions

The student should select the appropriate answer and cite the rationale for choosing that particular answer.

1. The researcher's refusal to disclose the names of subjects is:
   a. Confidentiality
   b. Anonymity
   c. Informed consent
   d. Protection of clients

Answer: _____ Rationale: _____

_____

_____

2. The purpose of an institutional review board is to:
   a. Ensure that federal funds are equitably appropriated
   b. Conduct research benefiting the public
   c. Determine the risk status of clients in research projects
   d. Ensure that ethical principles are observed in human-subject research

Answer: _____ Rationale: _____

_____

_____

3. Research studies can most easily be identified by:
   a. Looking for the word "research" in the title of the report
   b. Looking for the study only in research journals
   c. Examining the contents of the report
   d. Reading the abstract and conclusion of the report

Answer: _____ Rationale: _____

_____

_____

4. Which statement concerning research reports is accurate?
   a. Nursing textbooks are primary sources of information.
   b. Primary sources are those written by one of the researchers in the study.
   c. The fact that a report is a primary source guarantees its accuracy.
   d. Secondary sources are the best source of information about the research study.

Answer: _____ Rationale: _____

_____

_____

5. A research report includes all of the following except:
   a. A summary of literature used to identify the research problem
   b. The researcher's interpretation of the study results
   c. A summary of other research studies with the same results
   d. A description of methods used to conduct the study

Answer: _____ Rationale: _____

_____

_____

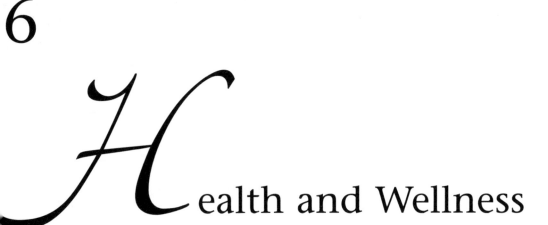

6

Health and Wellness

Preliminary Reading

Chapter 6, pp. 89-105

Comprehensive Understanding

- Define *illness behavior*. _____

Healthy People Documents

- Goals for *Healthy People 2010* include:

    a. _____

    b. _____

- The four focus areas of *Healthy People 2010* are:

    a. _____

    b. _____

    c. _____

    d. _____

Definition of Health

- Define *health*. _____

_____

- Pender defines *health* as: _____

  a. _____

  b. _____

  c. _____

  d. _____

  e. _____

Models of Health and Illness

- A model is: _____

- Health beliefs are a person's _____,

  _____, and _____

  about health and illness.

- Health beliefs can impact health behavior, and they can positively or negatively affect a person's health. Identify some practices of each health behavior.

  a. Positive health behavior: _____

  _____

  _____

  b. Negative health behavior: _____

  _____

  _____

Health Belief Model
- Describe the health belief model. _____

  _____

  _____

- Central to the health belief model are three components. Identify them.

  a. _____

  b. _____

  c. _____

Health Promotion Model
- The focus of this model is to explain why individuals engage in health promotion activities. Identify the three functions on which the health promotion model focuses.

  a. _____

  b. _____

  c. _____

Basic Human Needs Model
- List in order the five levels of Maslow's hierarchy of needs.

  a. _____

  b. _____

  c. _____

  d. _____

  e. _____

Holistic Health Models
- Define the main concepts of the holistic health

  model. _____

  _____

  _____

- Clients use alternative therapies because: _____

  _____

  _____

Variables Influencing Health and Health Beliefs and Practices

- Internal and external variables can influence how a person thinks and acts. Understanding the way in which these variables affect a client allows the nurse to plan and deliver individualized care.

Internal Variables
- Internal variables include a person's developmental stage, intellectual background, perception of personal functioning, and emotional and spiritual factors. Identify and cite a personal example of how each of the following internal variables affects the client's health belief and practices.

  a. Developmental stage: _____

  _____

  _____

  _____

  b. Intellectual background: _____

  _____

  _____

  _____

c. Perception of functioning: _____

_____

_____

_____

d. Emotional factors: _____

_____

_____

_____

e. Spiritual factors: _____

_____

_____

_____

External Variables

• External variables influence a person's health beliefs and practices, including family practices, socioeconomic factors, and cultural variables. Identify and cite a personal example of how each of the following external variables affects the client's health beliefs and practices.

   a. Family practices: _____

_____

_____

   b. Socioeconomic factors: _____

_____

_____

   c. Cultural background: _____

_____

_____

Health Promotion, Wellness, and Illness Prevention

• The concepts of health promotion, wellness, and illness prevention are closely related, and in practice overlap to some extent. All are focused on the future; the difference between them involves motivations and goals. Briefly explain each one.

   a. Health promotion: _____

_____

b. Wellness: _____

_____

c. Illness prevention: _____

_____

• There are passive and active strategies for health promotion. Give two examples of each.

   a. Passive strategies: _____

_____

_____

   b. Active strategies: _____

_____

_____

Levels of Preventive Care

• Identify the health activities of each of the following levels of preventive care.

   a. Primary: _____

_____

_____

   b. Secondary: _____

_____

_____

   c. Tertiary: _____

_____

Risk Factors

• Define *risk factor*. _____

_____

_____

• Identify at least two risk factors for each of the following categories.

   a. Genetic and physiological factors: _____

_____

_____

   b. Age: _____

_____

_____

c. Environment: _____

_____

_____

d. Lifestyle: _____

_____

_____

- The goal of risk factor identification is: _____

_____

_____

Risk Factor Modification and Changing Health Behaviors

- Risk factor modification, health promotion, illness prevention activities, or any program that attempts to change unhealthy lifestyle behaviors can be considered a wellness strategy.

- Briefly explain the five stages of health behavior change.

    a. Precontemplation: _____

    _____

    _____

    b. Contemplation: _____

    _____

    _____

    c. Preparation: _____

    _____

    _____

    d. Action: _____

    _____

    _____

    e. Maintenance: _____

    _____

Illness

- Define *illness*. _____

_____

_____

Acute Illness and Chronic Illness

- Explain the two general classifications of illness.

    a. Acute illness: _____

    _____

    _____

    b. Chronic illness: _____

    _____

    _____

Illness Behavior

- _____, _____, _____, and _____ can all affect illness behavior.

Variables Influencing Illness and Illness Behavior

- Give examples of the following.

    a. Internal variables: _____

    _____

    _____

    b. External variables: _____

    _____

    _____

Impact of Illness on the Client and Family

- Illness is never an isolated event. The client and family commonly experience the following. Briefly explain each one.

    a. Behavioral and emotional changes: _____

    _____

    _____

    b. Impact on body image: _____

    _____

    _____

    c. Impact on self-concept: _____

    _____

    _____

    d. Impact on family roles: _____

    _____

    _____

e. Impact on family dynamics: _____

_____

_____

*R*eview Questions

The student should select the appropriate answer and cite the rationale for choosing that particular answer.

1. Internal variables influencing health beliefs and practices include:
   a. Family practices and cultural background
   b. Socioeconomic factors and intellectual background
   c. Spiritual factors and developmental stage
   d. Cultural background and perception of functioning

Answer: _____   Rationale: _____

_____

_____

2. Any variable increasing the vulnerability of an individual or a group to an illness or accident is a (an):
   a. Illness behavior
   b. Risk factor
   c. Negative health behavior
   d. Lifestyle determinant

Answer: _____   Rationale: _____

_____

_____

3. All of the following characterize illness behavior except:
   a. Calling a physician
   b. Ignoring a physical symptom
   c. Interpreting physical symptoms
   d. Withdrawing from work activities

Answer: _____   Rationale: _____

_____

_____

4. The term high-level wellness is best defined as:
   a. Being free from chronic disease
   b. Surviving beyond one's life expectancy
   c. Fluctuating on a wellness-illness continuum within the health spectrum
   d. Functioning at one's best biophysical level

Answer: _____   Rationale: _____

_____

_____

5. Marsha states, "My chubby size runs in our family. It's a glandular condition. Exercise and diet won't change things much." The nurse determines that this is an example of Marsha's:
   a. Acute situation
   b. Active strategy
   c. Positive health behavior
   d. Health beliefs

Answer: _____   Rationale: _____

_____

_____

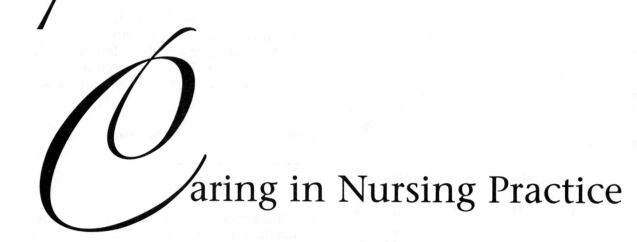

7

Caring in Nursing Practice

Preliminary Reading

Chapter 7, pp. 106-117

Comprehensive Understanding

Theoretical Views on Caring

- Caring is a universal phenomenon that influences the ways in which people _____,

  _____, and _____ in relation to one another.

- Caring in nursing has been studied from a variety of philosophical and ethical perspectives.

Caring Is Primary
- Dr. Patricia Benner does not try to predict or control phenomena but attempts to give nurses a rich,

  holistic understanding of nursing practice and caring through the interpretation of _____.

- Briefly summarize how Benner describes the relationship among health, illness, and disease. _____

  _____

  _____

  _____

The Essence of Nursing and Health
- Explain Leininger's concept of care from a transcultural perspective. _____

  _____

  _____

  _____

- Define *acts of caring* according to Leininger.

  _____

  _____

  _____

- Caring, according to Leininger, is a universal phenomenon, but the expressions, processes, and patterns of caring vary among cultures.

  _____

  _____

  _____

Transpersonal Caring

- Summarize Watson's transpersonal caring theory (transformative model). _____

  _____

  _____

  _____

Swanson's Theory of Caring

- Swanson's theory of caring consists of five categories. Explain each.

  a. Knowing: _____

  _____

  _____

  b. Being with: _____

  _____

  _____

  c. Doing for: _____

  _____

  _____

  d. Enabling: _____

  _____

  _____

  e. Maintaining belief: _____

  _____

  _____

Summary of Theoretical Views

- Identify the common themes among the many nursing theorists. _____

  _____

  _____

  _____

Clients' Perceptions of Caring

- Establishing a _____, _____, and _____ are recurrent caring behaviors that researchers have identified.

- When clients sense that health care providers are interested in them as people, clients will be more willing to follow recommendations and therapeutic plans.

- The nurse needs to consider how clients perceive caring and the best approaches to providing care.

Ethics of Care

- Caring is interpreted by many as being a moral imperative.

- In any client encounter, a nurse must know what behavior is ethically appropriate.

- Define *ethics of care*. _____

  _____

  _____

Caring in Nursing Practice

- As nurses deal with health and illness in their practice, they grow in their ability to care.

- Nurse behaviors that have been shown to be related to caring include: _____

  _____

  _____

Providing Presence
- Summarize the concept of *presence*. _____

  _____

  _____

- Identify ways a nurse can establish presence with his or her clients. _____

_____

_____

Touch

- The use of touch is one comforting approach whereby the nurse reaches out to clients to communicate concern and support.

- Give some examples of protective and task-oriented touch. _____

_____

_____

Listening

- Listening conveys the nurse's full attention and interest. Listening to the meaning of what a client says helps create a mutual relationship.

- A nurse must be able to give clients his or her full, focused attention as their stories are told.

- When an ill person chooses to tell his or her story, it involves reaching out to another human being.

- Briefly summarize Frank's view of the clinical relationship the nurse and client share. _____

_____

_____

- Describe what listening involves. _____

_____

_____

Knowing the Client

- To know a client means that the nurse _____, _____, and _____.

- Knowing the client is at the core of the process by which nurses make clinical decisions. By establishing a caring relationship, the mutuality that develops helps the nurse to better know the client as an individual and to then choose the most appropriate and efficacious nursing therapies.

- Describe the following nurses and how they differ in knowing their clients.

    a. Expert nurse: _____

    _____

    _____

    b. Novice nurse: _____

    _____

    _____

Spiritual Caring

- Spiritual health is achieved when: _____

_____

_____

- Spirituality offers a sense of _____, _____, and _____.

- When a caring relationship is established, the client and nurse come to know one another so that both move toward a healing relationship by:

    a. _____

    b. _____

    c. _____

Family Care

- Success with nursing interventions often depends on the family's willingness to

_____,

_____,

_____,

and _____.

- List the 10 caring behaviors that are perceived as most hopeful by families of cancer clients.

    a. _____

    b. _____

    c. _____

    d. _____

    e. _____

f. _____

g. _____

h. _____

i. _____

j. _____

The Challenge of Caring

- The nursing professionals, unlike medical professionals, can care for and assist people without medical diagnoses or new technologies and treatments.

- Caring motivates people to become nurses, and it becomes a source of satisfaction when we know we have made a difference in our clients' lives.

- Summarize the challenges facing nursing in today's health care system.

_____

_____

Review Questions

The student should select the appropriate answer and cite the rationale for choosing that particular answer.

1. Leininger's care theory states that the client's caring values and behaviors are derived largely from:
   a. Experience
   b. Gender
   c. Culture
   d. Religious beliefs

Answer: _____ Rationale: _____

_____

_____

2. The central common theme of the caring theories is:
   a. Pathophysiology and self-care abilities
   b. Compensation for client disabilities
   c. The nurse-client relationship and psychosocial aspects of care
   d. Maintenance of client homeostasis

Answer: _____ Rationale: _____

_____

_____

3. In order for the nurse to effectively listen to the client, he or she needs to:
   a. Sit with the legs crossed
   b. Lean back in the chair
   c. Respond quickly with appropriate answers to the client
   d. Maintain good eye contact

Answer: _____ Rationale: _____

_____

_____

4. The nurse demonstrates caring by:
   a. Helping family members become active participants in the care of the client
   b. Doing all the necessary tasks for the client
   c. Following all of the physician's orders accurately
   d. Maintaining professionalism at all costs

Answer: _____ Rationale: _____

_____

_____

5. According to Benner, the major characteristic that separates a "proficient" nurse from a "novice" nurse is:
   a. The ability to understand situations holistically
   b. An advanced educational preparation
   c. An intuitive understanding of situations
   d. Performance that is competitive

Answer: _____ Rationale: _____

_____

_____

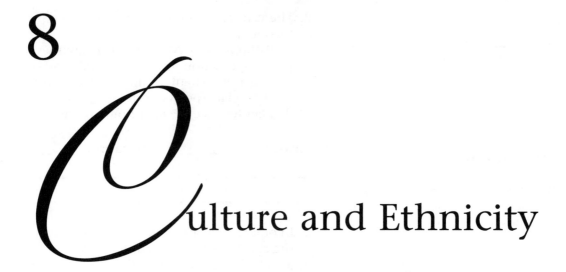

8 Culture and Ethnicity

Preliminary Reading

Chapter 8, pp. 118-138

Comprehensive Understanding

Important Definitions

- To provide culturally competent care, the nurse must understand cultural concepts. Briefly explain each of the following.

  a. Culture: _____

  _____

  b. Dominant culture: _____

  _____

  c. Subcultures: _____

  _____

  d. Ethnicity: _____

  _____

  e. Race: _____

  _____

  f. Enculturation: _____

  _____

  g. Acculturation: _____

  _____

  h. Assimilation: _____

  _____

i. Biculturalism: _____

_____

j. Cultural backlash: _____

_____

k. Stereotypes: _____

_____

Culturally Congruent Care

- Define *transcultural nursing.* _____

_____

_____

- State the goal of culturally congruent care. ___

_____

_____

- Define *culturally competent care.* _____

_____

_____

- Cultural competence has five interlocking components. Briefly explain each one.

  a. _____

  b. _____

  c. _____

  d. _____

  e. _____

Cultural Conflicts

- Define the following terms.

  a. *Ethnocentrism:* _____

  _____

  b. *Discrimination:* _____

  _____

  c. *Cultural imposition:* _____

  _____

Cultural Context of Health and Caring

- Culture is the context by which groups interpret and define their experiences relevant to life transitions.
- Culture is the framework used in defining social phenomena.

- Briefly explain the difference between western and non-western cultures. _____

_____

_____

Cultural Healing Modalities and Healers

- Health care systems have evolved into the following. Explain each one.

  a. Externalizing systems: _____

  _____

  _____

  b. Internalizing systems: _____

  _____

  _____

- Foster identified two distinct categories of cross-cultural healers. Explain each one.

  a. Naturalistic practitioners: _____

  _____

  b. Personalistic practitioners: _____

  _____

  _____

Culture Bound Syndrome

- Define *culture bound syndrome.* _____

_____

_____

Culture and Life Transitions

- Define *rites of passage.* _____

_____

_____

- Briefly explain the following phases of life and the cultural differences that apply to each.

  a. Pregnancy: _____

  _____

  _____

  b. Childbirth: _____

  _____

  _____

c. Newborn: _____

_____

_____

d. Postpartum: _____

_____

_____

e. Grief and loss: _____

_____

_____

- Culture strongly influences pain expression and the need for pain medication.

Cultural Assessment

- _____ is a systematic and comprehensive examination of the cultural care values, beliefs, and practices.

_____

_____

- The goal of a cultural assessment is: _____

_____

_____

- Briefly explain each part of the cultural assessment.

  a. Census data: _____

  _____

  _____

  b. Asking questions: _____

  _____

  _____

  c. Establish relationship: _____

  _____

  _____

  d. Impression management: _____

  _____

  _____

Selected Components of Cultural Assessment

- Explain the following components of a cultural assessment.

  a. Ethnic heritage and ethnohistory: _____

  _____

  _____

  b. Biocultural history: _____

  _____

  _____

  c. Social organization: _____

  _____

  _____

  d. Religious and spiritual: _____

  _____

  _____

  e. Communication patterns: _____

  _____

  _____

  f. Time orientation: _____

  _____

  _____

  g. Caring beliefs and practices: _____

  _____

  _____

- List the recurrent caring constructs identified in both western and non-western cultures.

  a. _____
  b. _____
  c. _____
  d. _____
  e. _____
  f. _____
  g. _____
  h. _____
  i. _____
  j. _____

- Briefly explain the three nursing decision and action modes to achieve culturally congruent care.

  a. Cultural care preservation or maintenance:

  _____

  _____

  b. Cultural care accommodation or negotiation: _____

  _____

  c. Cultural care repatterning or restructuring:

  _____

  _____

$\mathcal{R}$eview Questions

The student should select the appropriate answer and cite the rationale for choosing that particular answer.

1. Which of the following is not included in evaluating the degree of heritage consistency in a client?
   a. Gender
   b. Culture
   c. Ethnicity
   d. Religion

   Answer: _____ Rationale: _____

   _____

   _____

2. When providing care to clients with varied cultural backgrounds, it is imperative for the nurse to recognize that:
   a. Cultural considerations must be put aside if basic needs are in jeopardy
   b. Generalizations about the behavior of a particular group may be inaccurate
   c. Current health standards should determine the acceptability of cultural practices
   d. Similar reactions to stress will occur when individuals have the same cultural background

   Answer: _____ Rationale: _____

   _____

   _____

3. To respect a client's personal space and territoriality, the nurse:
   a. Avoids the use of touch
   b. Explains nursing care and procedures
   c. Keeps the curtains pulled around the client's bed
   d. Stands 8 feet away from the bed, if possible

   Answer: _____ Rationale: _____

   _____

   _____

4. To be effective in meeting various ethnic needs, the nurse should:
   a. Treat all clients alike
   b. Be aware of clients' cultural differences
   c. Act as if he or she is comfortable with the client's behavior
   d. Avoid asking questions about the client's cultural background

   Answer: _____ Rationale: _____

   _____

   _____

5. The most important factor in providing nursing care to clients in a specific ethnic group is:
   a. Communication
   b. Time orientation
   c. Biological variation
   d. Environmental control

   Answer: _____ Rationale: _____

   _____

   _____

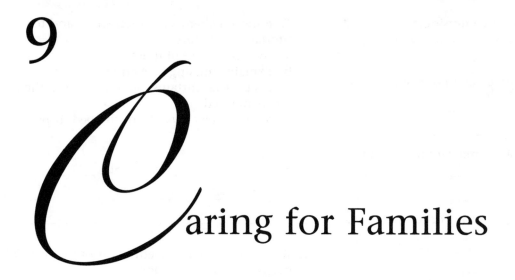

9

*C*aring for Families

*P*reliminary Reading

Chapter 9, pp. 139-154

*C*omprehensive Understanding

The Family

- Define the three important attributes that characterize contemporary families.

    a. *Durability:* _____

    b. *Resiliency:* _____

    c. *Diversity:* _____

Concept of Family

- A family is a: _____

    _____

Definition: What Is a Family?

- The family can be defined as _____, _____, or as a _____.

- To effectively provide care, nurses must understand that individual attitudes about family are deeply ingrained and deserve respect.

- To provide individualized care, the nurse must understand that families take many forms and have diverse cultural and ethnic orientations.

Current Trends and New Family Forms

- Summarize the various family forms.

  a. Nuclear family: _____

  _____

  _____

  b. Extended family: _____

  _____

  _____

  c. Single-parent family: _____

  _____

  _____

  d. Blended family: _____

  _____

  _____

  e. Alternative: _____

  _____

  _____

- Identify at least four current trends that challenge the family.

  a. _____

  b. _____

  c. _____

  d. _____

- Explain the following threats and concerns facing the family.

  a. Changing economic status: _____

  _____

  _____

  b. Homelessness: _____

  _____

  _____

  c. Family violence: _____

  _____

  _____

  d. Human immunodeficiency virus (HIV):

  _____

  _____

Theoretical Approaches: An Overview

- Summarize the following general perspectives when working with or studying families.

  a. Family health system: _____

  _____

  _____

  b. Developmental stages: _____

  _____

  _____

Attributes of Families

Structure
- Structure and function are closely related and continually interact with one another.

- Structure is based on ongoing membership of the family and the pattern of relationships.

- Structure may enhance or detract from the family's ability to respond to stressors. Briefly explain each of the following.

  a. Rigid structure: _____

  _____

  _____

  b. Open structure: _____

  _____

  _____

Function
- Family functioning focuses on the processes used by the family to achieve its goals. Identify these processes. _____

  _____

  _____

  _____

The Family and Health

- The health of the family is influenced by its relative position in society.

- Identify the variables that affect the structure, function, and health of a family. _____

  _____

  _____

  _____

- The family strongly influences the health behaviors of its members. In turn, the health status of each individual influences how the family unit functions and its ability to achieve goals.

- Family environment is crucial because health behavior reinforced in early life has a strong influence on later health practices.

Attributes of Healthy Families

- The crisis-proof or effective family is able to integrate the need for stability with the need for growth and change. Explain. _____

  _____

  _____

- Define *family hardiness*. _____

  _____

Family Nursing

- The goal of family nursing is to: _____

  _____

  _____

- Identify the three levels and focuses proposed for family nursing practice. Briefly explain each.

  a. Family as context: _____

     _____

     _____

  b. Family as client: _____

     _____

     _____

  c. Family as system: _____

     _____

     _____

Nursing Process for the Family

- Three factors underlie the family approach to the nursing process. Name them.

  a. _____

  b. _____

  c. _____

Assessing the Needs of the Family

- Identify areas to include in the family assessment. _____

  _____

  _____

  _____

  _____

Family-Focused Care

- Collaboration with family members is an essential component of family-focused care, whether the family is the client or the context of care. Briefly explain each.

  a. Family as client: _____

     _____

     _____

  b. Family as context: _____

     _____

     _____

- Explain the purpose of a culturalgram. _____

  _____

  _____

- The goals the nurse sets in caring for the family must be _____,

  _____, and _____.

Challenges for Family Nursing

- Summarize the challenges for family nursing in relation to each of the following.

  a. Discharge planning: _____

     _____

     _____

b. Cultural diversity: _____

Implementing Family-Centered Care
- Nursing interventions aim to: _____

_____

_____

Health Promotion
- Health promotion interventions are needed to:

_____

_____

- Family strengths include: _____

_____

_____

Acute Care

- Summarize the challenges of family nursing in the acute care setting: _____

_____

_____

_____

Restorative Care

- In restorative care settings, the challenge in family nursing is to _____. Give some examples: _____

_____

- Whenever an individual becomes dependent on another family member for care and assistance, there is significant stress affecting both the caregiver and the recipient. Explain.

_____

_____

- Caregiving occurs within the context of the family.

- Explain the concept of reciprocity. _____

_____

_____

- Identify available family and community resources. _____

_____

_____

_____

Review Questions

The student should select the appropriate answer and cite the rationale for choosing that particular answer.

1. Family functioning can best be described as:
   a. The processes that a family uses to meet its goal
   b. The way the family members communicate with each other
   c. Interrelated with family structure
   d. Adaptive behaviors that foster health

Answer: _____ Rationale: _____

_____

_____

2. Family structure can best be described as:
   a. A basic pattern of predictable stages
   b. Flexible patterns that contribute to adequate functioning
   c. The pattern of relationships and ongoing membership
   d. A complex set of relationships

Answer: _____ Rationale: _____

_____

_____

3. The majority of families today:
   a. Consist of a mother, father, and one or more children
   b. Include stepchildren
   c. Include a woman who works outside the home
   d. Are very similar to families of the past

Answer: _____ Rationale: _____

_____

_____

4. When planning care for a client and using the concept of family as client, the nurse:
   a. Understands that the client's family will always be a help to the client's health goals.
   b. Considers the developmental stage of the client and not the family.
   c. Realizes that cultural background is an important variable when assessing the family.
   d. Includes only the client and his or her significant other.

Answer: _____ Rationale: _____

_____

_____

5. Interventions used by the nurse when providing care to a rigidly structured family include:
   a. Exploring with them the benefits of moving toward more flexible modes of action
   b. Attempting to change the family structure
   c. Providing solutions for problems as they arise
   d. Administering nursing care in a manner that provides minimal opportunity for change

Answer: _____ Rationale: _____

_____

_____

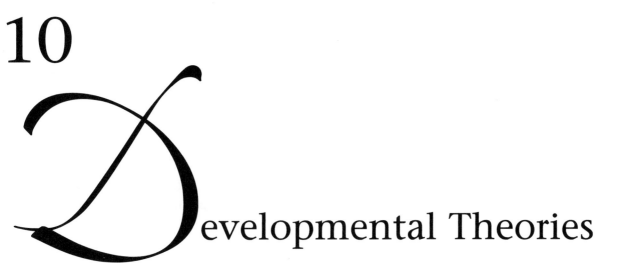

10

Developmental Theories

Preliminary Reading

Chapter 10, pp. 155-170

Comprehensive Understanding

Growth and Development

- Define *growth*. _____

- Define *development*. _____

Major Factors Influencing Growth and Development
- Identify the processes of growth and development.

  a. Physical growth: _____

  _____

  b. Development: _____

  _____

  c. Maturation: _____

  _____

  d. Differentiation: _____

  _____

Developmental Theories

- Explain briefly the four areas of theory development.

    a. Biophysical development: _____

    _____

    b. Psychoanalytic/psychosocial development:

    _____

    _____

    c. Cognitive development: _____

    _____

    d. Moral development: _____

    _____

Biophysical Developmental Theories

- Briefly summarize Gesell's theory. _____

    _____

    _____

Psychoanalytic/Psychosocial Theory

- Briefly describe. _____

    _____

    _____

- Briefly explain Sigmund Freud's theory regarding personality development. _____

    _____

    _____

    _____

- Explain the five psychosexual developmental stages of Freud's theory.

    a. Stage 1: Oral: _____

    _____

    _____

    b. Stage 2: Anal: _____

    _____

    _____

    c. Stage 3: Phallic: _____

    _____

    _____

    d. Stage 4: Latency: _____

    _____

    _____

    e. Stage 5: Genital: _____

    _____

    _____

Erik Erickson

- Erickson extended Freud's model by placing psychoanalytic theory within a social/cultural perspective.

- Erickson defined eight stages of life. Each stage builds on a successful resolution of the previous development. Explain each.

    a. Trust versus mistrust: _____

    _____

    _____

    b. Autonomy versus shame and doubt: _____

    _____

    _____

    c. Initiative versus guilt: _____

    _____

    _____

    d. Industry versus inferiority: _____

    _____

    _____

    e. Identity versus role confusion: _____

    _____

    _____

    f. Intimacy versus isolation: _____

    _____

    _____

    g. Generativity versus stagnation: _____

    _____

    _____

    h. Integrity versus despair: _____

    _____

    _____

Robert Havighurst's Development Tasks

- Havighurst defined a series of essential tasks that arise from predictable and external pressures. These pressures include _____, _____, and _____.

- Identify a limitation to this theory. _____
  _____
  _____

Roger Gould's Themes of Adult Development

- Gould's research supports stage theory in adult development with a set of themes. Briefly explain the five themes identified.

  a. _____
  _____

  b. _____
  _____

  c. _____
  _____

  d. _____
  _____

  e. _____
  _____

Stella Chess and Alexander Thomas's Temperament Factor

- Temperament is: _____
  _____

- Three personality types were identified as _____, _____, and _____. One of the factors in the development of problems for these children was the inability of the parent and the environment to be flexible and understand the needs of the child given the personality structure.

Cognitive Development Theory

Jean Piaget's Theory of Cognitive Development

- Jean Piaget created a cognitive development theory that includes four periods and recognizes that children move through these specific periods at different rates but in the same sequence. Explain each of these periods.

  a. Sensorimotor: _____
  _____
  _____

  b. Preoperational: _____
  _____
  _____

  c. Concrete operations: _____
  _____
  _____

  d. Formal operations: _____
  _____
  _____

Moral Developmental Theory

- Moral development theories try to explain:
  _____
  _____

Jean Piaget's Moral Developmental Theory

- Explain the three stages of Piaget's moral development theory.

  a. Premoral stage: _____
  _____
  _____

  b. Conventional stage: _____
  _____
  _____

  c. Autonomous stage: _____
  _____
  _____

Lawrence Kohlberg's Moral Developmental Theory

- Kohlberg identified six stages of moral development under three levels. Briefly explain each.

  a. Level I: Preconventional level: _____
  _____

Stage 1: _____

_____

Stage 2: _____

_____

b. Level II: Conventional level: _____

_____

Stage 3: _____

_____

Stage 4: _____

_____

c. Level III: Postconventional level: _____

_____

Stage 5: _____

_____

Stage 6: _____

_____

- Identify the limitations to Kohlberg's research.

_____

_____

- Briefly explain Gilligan's argument with Kohlberg's theory. _____

_____

_____

$\mathcal{R}$eview Questions

The student should select the appropriate answer and cite the rationale for choosing that particular answer.

1. According to Piaget, the school-age child is in the third stage of cognitive development, which is characterized by:
   a. Conventional thought
   b. Concrete operations
   c. Identity versus role diffusion
   d. Postconventional thought

   Answer: _____ Rationale: _____

   _____

   _____

2. According to Erickson, the developmental task of adolescence is:
   a. Autonomy versus shame and doubt
   b. Self-identity versus role confusion
   c. Industry versus inferiority
   d. Role acceptance versus role confusion

   Answer: _____ Rationale: _____

   _____

   _____

3. According to Erickson's developmental theory, the primary developmental task of the middle years is to:
   a. Achieve generativity
   b. Achieve intimacy
   c. Establish a set of personal values
   d. Establish a sense of personal identity

   Answer: _____ Rationale: _____

   _____

   _____

4. Which of the following behaviors is most characteristic of the concrete operations stage of cognitive development?
   a. Progression from reflex activity to imitative behavior
   b. Inability to put oneself in another's place
   c. Thought processes become increasingly logical and coherent
   d. Ability to think in abstract terms and draw logical conclusions

   Answer: _____ Rationale: _____

   _____

   _____

5. According to Kohlberg, children develop moral reasoning as they mature. Which of the following is most characteristic of a preschooler's stage of moral development?
   a. Obeying the rules of correct behavior.
   b. Showing respect for authority is important behavior.
   c. Behavior that pleases others is considered good.
   d. Actions are determined as good or bad in terms of their consequences.

   Answer: _____ Rationale: _____

   _____

   _____

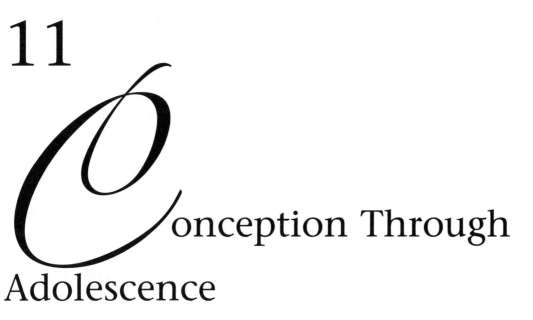

11

Conception Through Adolescence

$\mathcal{P}$reliminary Reading

Chapter 11, pp. 171-215

$\mathcal{C}$omprehensive Understanding

Growth and Development

- Human growth and development are continuous and intricate, complex processes that are often divided into stages organized by age groups.

Selecting a Developmental Framework for Nursing

- Providing nursing care that is developmentally appropriate is easier when planning on a theoretical framework.

- A developmental approach encourages organized care directed at the child's current level of functioning to motivate self-direction and health promotion.

Conception

Intrauterine Life

- Define the following terms/events.

  a. *Nagele's rule:* _____

  _____

  b. *Fertilization:* _____

  _____

c. *Zygote:* _____

_____

d. *Morula:* _____

_____

e. *Blastocyst:* _____

_____

f. *Embryo:* _____

_____

g. *Placenta:* _____

_____

h. *Implantation:* _____

_____

- Explain the development process and health concerns for the following trimesters.

  a. *First trimester*

  Physical changes: _____

  Health promotion: _____

  _____

  Teratogens: _____

  _____

  b. *Second trimester*

  Physical changes: _____

  _____

  Health promotion: _____

  _____

  c. *Third trimester*

  Physical changes: _____

  _____

  Health promotion: _____

  _____

  Cognitive changes: _____

  _____

  Psychosocial changes: _____

  _____

Transition from Intrauterine to Extrauterine Life

- _____, _____, and _____ influence adjustment to the external environment.

Physical Changes

- An immediate assessment of the neonate's condition is performed because the first concern is the _____

  _____

  _____

- List the five physiological parameters evaluated through the Apgar assessment.

  a. _____

  b. _____

  c. _____

  d. _____

  e. _____

Psychosocial Changes

- Which two factors are most important in promoting closeness of the parents and neonate?

  _____

  _____

  _____

- Define *bonding*. _____

  _____

  _____

Health Risks

- Briefly explain the three most important physical needs of the newborn.

  a. Airway: _____

  _____

  b. Temperature: _____

  _____

  c. Prevention of infection: _____

  _____

The Newborn

- The *neonatal period* is defined as: _____

_____

_____

Physical Changes
- Identify the normal characteristics of the newborn.

  a. Height: _____

  b. Weight: _____

  c. Head circumference: _____

  d. Vital signs: _____

  _____

  e. Physical characteristics: _____

  _____

  _____

  f. Neurological function: _____

  _____

  _____

  g. Behavioral characteristics: _____

  _____

  _____

Cognitive Changes
Early cognitive development begins with innate behavior, reflexes, and sensory functions.

Identify the sensory functions that contribute to cognitive development in the newborn.

_____

_____

_____

Psychosocial Changes
- Explain the interactions that foster deep attachment between the infant and parents.

_____

_____

_____

_____

Health Risks
- Define *hyperbilirubinemia*. _____

_____

Health Concerns
- Screening for inborn errors of metabolism applies to: _____

_____

- Circumcision is a common and controversial procedure. Identify the risks and benefits of this procedure.

  a. Risks: _____

  b. Benefits: _____

The Infant

- Infancy is the period from _____ to _____.

_____

Physical Changes
- Summarize the normal characteristics of the infant.

  a. Physical growth: _____

  _____

  b. Vital signs: _____

  _____

  c. Gross motor skills: _____

  _____

  _____

  d. Fine motor skills: _____

  _____

  _____

Cognitive Changes
- Summarize the cognitive development of an infant. _____

_____

_____

Psychosocial Changes
- During the first year, infants begin to differentiate themselves from others as separate beings capable of acting on their own.

- Erickson describes the psychosocial developmental crisis for the infant as trust versus mistrust.

- Define *play*. _____
  _____

- Identify activities appropriate at this stage of development. _____
  _____

Health Risks
- Identify the common types of injury and possible prevention strategies. _____
  _____
  _____

- Child maltreatment includes: _____
  _____

Health Concerns
- The foundation for children's perceptions of their health status is laid early in life.

- Internal body sensations and experiences with the outside world affect self-perceptions.

- The quality of nutrition influences the infant's growth and development.

- Identify the feeding alternatives for an infant.
  _____
  _____
  _____

- Identify some supplementation needs of an infant. _____
  _____
  _____

- Briefly explain health concerns related to the following.
  a. Dentition: _____
     _____
  b. Immunizations: _____
     _____

c. Sleep: _____
   _____

d. Overfeeding: _____
   _____

The Toddler

- Toddlerhood ranges from _____ to _____
  _____
  _____

Physical Changes
- Summarize the normal characteristics of the toddler.
  a. Self-care activities: _____
  b. Motor skills: _____
  c. Vital signs: _____
  d. Head circumference: _____
  e. Weight: _____
  f. Height: _____
  g. Physiological anorexia: _____

Cognitive Changes
- Summarize Piaget's preoperational thought stage. _____
  _____

- Describe language ability at this stage. _____
  _____
  _____

Psychosocial Changes
- Identify Erickson's psychosocial development stage. _____
  _____

- Explain the parental implications of the following developmental states.
  a. Independence: _____
     _____
  b. Social interactions: _____
     _____
  c. Play: _____
     _____

Health Risks

- Describe some developmental abilities for this age period. _____
  _____
  _____

- Identify injury prevention strategies. _____
  _____
  _____

Health Concerns

- Children increasingly recognize internal body sensations but have difficulty pinpointing their location.

- Children who deviate radically from their usual patterns of eating, sleeping, or playing require assessment to determine whether these alterations result from illness.

- Children begin to internalize the labels that parents or health care professionals give to the somatic stages.

- Briefly explain the nutrition requirements for this age group. _____
  _____

The Preschooler

- The preschool period refers to _____
  _____
  _____

Physical Changes

- Summarize the normal characteristics of the preschooler.
  a. Vital signs: _____
  b. Weight: _____
  c. Height: _____
  d. Coordination: _____

Cognitive Changes

- Preschoolers continue to master the preoperational stage of cognition.

- The first phase of this period, _____
  (2 to 4 years), is characterized by _____.

- Define *artificialism*. _____
  _____

- Define *animism*. _____
  _____

- Summarize the intuitive phase of preconceptional thought (4 years). _____
  _____

- The greatest fear of this age-group is: _____
  _____

- Summarize this group's moral development.
  _____
  _____
  _____

- Describe the language ability for this age group. _____
  _____

Psychosocial Changes

- The preschooler's world expands beyond the family into the neighborhood where they meet other children and adults.

- Identify some dependent behaviors that preschoolers may revert to during stress or illness. _____
  _____

- Summarize the pattern of play for the preschooler. _____
  _____
  _____
  _____

Health Risks

- Guidelines for injury prevention in the toddler also apply to the preschooler. _____ and _____ are the top priorities for this age group.

Health Concerns

- Parental beliefs about health, children's bodily sensations, and the ability to perform daily activities help children develop attitudes about their health.

- Explain health concerns related to the following for this group.

    a. Nutrition: _____

    b. Sleep: _____

    c. Vision: _____

The School-Age Child

- The school-age years range from _____ to _____.

- _____ signals the end of middle childhood.

- The school and home influence growth and development, and adjustments by the parents and child are required.

- Parents must learn to allow their child to make decisions, accept responsibility, and learn from life's experiences.

Physical Changes

- Summarize the normal characteristics of the school-age child.

    a. Weight: _____

    b. Height: _____

    c. Cardiovascular functioning: _____

    d. Neuromuscular functioning: _____

    e. Skeletal growth: _____

Cognitive Changes

- Cognitive changes provide the school-age child with the ability to think in a logical manner about the here and now. They are not yet capable of abstract thinking.

- Define the cognitive skills that are developing in this group. _____

- Describe the language development during middle childhood. _____

Psychosocial Changes

- The developmental task for school-age children is _____ versus _____.

- Summarize psychosocial development in relation to the following.

    a. Moral development: _____

    b. Peer relationships: _____

    c. Sexual identity: _____

Health Risks

- _____ and _____ are the leading causes of death or injury.

- Infections account for the majority of all childhood illnesses; respiratory infections are the most prevalent.

- Identify the specific health concerns of children living in poverty. _____

Health Concerns

Perception of wellness is based on _____

_____.

Identify five critical functions of a school-based health promotion program.

a. _____

b. _____

c. _____

d. _____

e. _____

Accidents are the leading cause of death and injury in the school-age period. Children should be encouraged to take responsibility for their own safety.

Identify at least five health promotion activities that are appropriate for the school-age child.

a. _____

b. _____

c. _____

d. _____

e. _____

Identify the nutritional requirements for the

school-age child. _____

_____

Preadolescent

Preadolescence refers to _____.

Physically, preadolescence begins _____.

The Adolescent

Adolescence is the period of development ____

_____.

Define *puberty*, and explain the changes that

occur at this time. _____

_____

_____

Physical Changes

- List the four major physical changes associated with sexual maturation.

  a. _____

  b. _____

  c. _____

  d. _____

  e. _____

- Summarize the weight and skeletal changes

  that occur during adolescence. _____

  _____

  _____

- The hormones responsible for the development of secondary sex characteristics are

  _____ and _____.

- Explain the effects of physical changes on peer

  interactions. _____

  _____

  _____

Cognitive Changes

- Changes that occur within the mind and the widening social environment of the adolescent

  result in _____,

  the highest level of intellectual development.

- During this period of cognitive development, the adolescent develops the ability to solve problems through logical operations.

- For the first time, the young person can move beyond the physical or concrete properties of a situation and use reasoning powers to understand the abstract.

- Briefly explain the cognitive abilities of this

  group: _____

  _____

  _____

Chapter 11: Conception Through Adolescence   53

- Describe the language skills of the adolescent.

  _____

  _____

  _____

Psychosocial Changes

- The search for _____ is the major task of adolescent psychosocial development.

- Teenagers must establish close peer relationships or remain socially isolated.

- Explain identity versus role confusion (Erickson). _____

  _____

- Behaviors indicating negative resolution are _____ and _____.

- Explain the following components of total identity.

  a. Sexual identity: _____

  _____

  b. Group identity: _____

  _____

  c. Family identity: _____

  _____

  d. Vocational identity: _____

  _____

  e. Health identity: _____

  _____

  f. Moral identity: _____

  _____

Health Risks

- Identify the leading cause of death and its sources among adolescents. _____

  _____

- _____ is the second leading cause of death.

- Suicide is the third leading cause of death among adolescents. List the six warning signs of suicide for this group.

  a. _____

  b. _____

  c. _____

  d. _____

  e. _____

  f. _____

- Substance abuse is a major concern. Adolescents at risk are _____

- In forming healthy habits of daily living, emphasis is on exercise, sleep, nutrition, and stress reduction.

- Define the two eating disorders that follow.

  a. Anorexia nervosa: _____

  _____

  b. Bulimia nervosa: _____

  _____

- _____ and _____ expectations contribute to early heterosexual and homosexual relations.

- Briefly explain the two prominent consequences of adolescent sexual activity.

  a. Sexually transmitted disease (STD): _____

  _____

  _____

  b. Pregnancy: _____

  _____

  _____

- Identify health promotion interventions for the adolescent in regard to the following.

  a. Unintentional injuries: _____

  _____

  b. Substance abuse: _____

  _____

  c. Sexual activity: _____

  _____

d. Firearms: _____

_____

Health Concerns

• Identify the concerns of the following.

a. Rural adolescents: _____

_____

_____

b. Minority adolescents: _____

_____

_____

$\mathcal{R}$eview Questions

The student should select the appropriate answer and cite the rationale for choosing that particular answer.

1. Which statement about human growth and development is accurate?
   a. Growth and development processes are unpredictable.
   b. Growth and development begins with birth and ends after adolescence.
   c. All individuals progress through the same phases of growth and development.
   d. All individuals accomplish developmental tasks at the same pace.

Answer: _____ Rationale: _____

_____

_____

2. The mother of a 2-year-old expresses concern that her son's appetite has diminished and that he seems to prefer milk to other solid foods. Which response by the nurse reflects knowledge of principles of communication and nutrition?
   a. "Oh, I wouldn't be too worried; children tend to eat when they're hungry. I just wouldn't give him dessert unless he eats his meal."
   b. "That is not uncommon in toddlers. You might consider increasing his milk to 2 quarts per day to be sure he gets enough nutrients."
   c. "Have you considered feeding him when he doesn't seem interested in feeding himself?"
   d. "A toddler's rate of growth normally slows down. It's common to see a toddler's appetite diminish in response to decreased calorie needs."

Answer: _____ Rationale: _____

_____

_____

3. Which neonatal assessment finding would be considered abnormal?
   a. Cyanosis of the hands and feet during activity
   b. Palpable anterior and posterior fontanels
   c. Soft, protuberant abdomen

Answer: _____ Rationale: _____

_____

_____

4. To stimulate cognitive and psychosocial development of the toddler, it is important for parents to:
   a. Set firm and consistent limits
   b Foster sharing of toys with playmates and siblings
   c. Provide clarification about what is right and wrong
   d. Limit confusion by restricting exploration of the environment

   Answer: _____ Rationale: _____

   _____

   _____

5. Which of the following is true of the developmental behaviors of school-age children?
   a. Formal and informal peer group membership is the key in forming self-esteem.
   b. Fears center on the loss of self-control.
   c. Positive feedback from parents and teachers is crucial to development.
   d. A full range of defense mechanisms is used including rationalization and intellectualization.

   Answer: _____ Rationale: _____

   _____

   _____

6. Adolescents have mastered age-appropriate sexuality when they feel comfortable with their sexual:
   a. Behaviors
   b. Choices
   c. Relationships
   d. All of the above

   Answer: _____ Rationale: _____

   _____

   _____

12

Young to Middle Adult

Comprehensive Understanding

• Young adulthood is the period from _____ to _____.

• Individuals in young adulthood _____, _____, and _____.

• Middle age occurs from _____ to _____.

• The transition into middle age occurs _____.

• Briefly describe the characteristics of the mature adult. _____

_____

_____

• Briefly describe the intellectual and moral developmental differences between men and women during this time. _____

_____

The Young Adult

Physical Changes

- The young adult has completed physical growth

  by the age of _____.

- Identify the personal lifestyle assessment of a

  young adult. _____

  _____

  _____

  _____

Cognitive Changes

- Briefly explain the cognitive development of
  the period in relation to educational, life, and

  occupational experiences. _____

  _____

  _____

Psychosocial Changes

- The emotional health of the young adult is
  related to the individual's ability to address
  and resolve personal and social tasks. Explain
  the patterns of the following age groups.

  a. 23 to 28 years: _____

  _____

  _____

  b. 29 to 34 years: _____

  _____

  _____

  c. 35 to 43 years: _____

  _____

  _____

- The young adult must make decisions concerning a career, marriage, and parenthood.
  Briefly explain the general principles involved.

  a. Lifestyle: _____

  _____

  _____

  b. Career: _____

  _____

  _____

c. Sexuality: _____

_____

_____

d. Childbearing cycle: _____

_____

_____

e. Lactation: _____

_____

_____

- Describe the following types of families.

  a. Singlehood: _____

  _____

  _____

  b. Marriage: _____

  _____

  _____

- Identify five tasks to be completed prior to
  marriage.

  a. _____

  b. _____

  c. _____

  d. _____

  e. _____

- Identify six tasks in the establishment of a
  household.

  a. _____

  b. _____

  c. _____

  d. _____

  e. _____

  f. _____

- Identify the hallmarks of parenthood and

  alternative family structures. _____

  _____

  _____

Identify the hallmarks of emotional health.

_____

_____

_____

Health Risks

- Briefly explain the risk factors for young adults in regard to the following.

  a. Family history: _____

  _____

  _____

  _____

  b. Personal hygiene habits: _____

  _____

  _____

  _____

  c. Violent death and injury: _____

  _____

  _____

  _____

  d. Substance abuse: _____

  _____

  _____

  _____

  e. Unplanned pregnancies: _____

  _____

  _____

  _____

  f. Sexually transmitted diseases: _____

  _____

  _____

  _____

  g. Environmental and occupational risks:

  _____

  _____

  _____

  _____

Health Concerns

- Briefly explain the following.

  a. Health promotion: _____

  _____

  _____

  b. Exercise: _____

  _____

  _____

  c. Routine health screening: _____

  _____

  _____

  d. Psychosocial health: _____

  _____

  _____

- The psychosocial concerns of the young adult are often related to stress. Briefly explain each of the following sources of stress.

  a. Job stress: _____

  _____

  _____

  b. Family stress: _____

  _____

  _____

- Explain the health practices of a woman anticipating pregnancy. _____

  _____

  _____

  _____

- Explain the physiological changes that occur during pregnancy and childbirth.

  a. Prenatal care: _____

  _____

  _____

  _____

b. Physiologic changes—first, second, and third trimester: _____

_____

_____

_____

c. Puerperium: _____

_____

_____

_____

d. Cognitive changes: _____

_____

_____

_____

e. Sensory perception: _____

_____

_____

_____

f. Needs for education: _____

_____

_____

_____

g. Psychosocial changes: _____

_____

_____

_____

h. Health concerns: _____

_____

_____

_____

- Acute care for young adults is frequently related to: _____

_____

- Causes of chronic illness and disability in the young adult are: _____

_____

The Middle Adult

- Briefly explain the characteristics of the middle adult years. _____

_____

_____

Physical Changes

- Briefly explain the major physiological changes that occur between 30 and 65 years of age.

_____

_____

_____

_____

_____

- Define *menopause.* _____

_____

- Define *climacteric.* _____

_____

Cognitive Changes

- Changes in cognitive function of middle adults are rare except in cases of illness or trauma.

Psychosocial Changes

- Summarize the psychosocial development of the middle adult in the following areas.

a. Career transition: _____

_____

_____

b. Sexuality: _____

_____

_____

c. Singlehood: _____

_____

_____

d. Marital changes: _____

_____

_____

e. Family transitions: _____

_____

_____

f. Care of aging parents: _____

_____

_____

• Define *sandwich generation.* _____

_____

_____

Health Concerns

• The following are physiological concerns for the middle adult. Briefly explain each one.

a. Stress and stress reduction: _____

_____

_____

b. Level of wellness: _____

_____

_____

c. Forming positive health habits: _____

_____

_____

d. Obesity: _____

_____

_____

• Summarize two psychosocial concerns of the middle adult.

a. Anxiety: _____

_____

_____

b. Depression: _____

_____

_____

• Identify some common community health programs for the middle adult. _____

_____

Acute Care

• Identify the acute illnesses and injuries that occur in middle adulthood. _____

_____

_____

_____

Restorative and Continuing Care

• Identify some chronic illnesses and/or issues that occur in middle adulthood. _____

_____

_____

_____

$\mathcal{R}$eview Questions

The student should select the appropriate answer and cite the rationale for choosing that particular answer.

1. The greatest cause of illness and death in the young adult population is:
   a. Sexually transmitted disease
   b. Violence
   c. Cardiovascular disease
   d. Substance abuse

   Answer: _____ Rationale: _____

   _____

   _____

2. Psychosocial changes of pregnancy commonly involve all of the following areas except:
   a. Body image
   b. Anxiety and depression
   c. Role changes
   d. Sexuality

   Answer: _____ Rationale: _____

   _____

   _____

3. Which physiological change would be a normal assessment finding in a middle adult?
   a. Increased breast size
   b. Abdominal tenderness and organomegaly
   c. Increased anteroposterior diameter of thorax
   d. Reduced auditory acuity

Answer: _____ Rationale: _____

_____

_____

4. Which of the following characteristics would the nurse have to consider in planning care for a client in middle adulthood?
   a. Declining sexual interest
   b. Declining motor coordination
   c. Decreasing creativity
   d. Declining thinking ability

Answer: _____ Rationale: _____

_____

_____

5. In planning client education for Mrs. Smith, a 45-year-old woman who had an ovarian cyst removed, which of the following facts is true about the sexuality of the middle-aged adult?
   a. Menstruation ceases after menopause.
   b. Estrogen is produced after menopause.
   c. After reaching climacteric, a male is unable to father a child.
   d. With removal of the ovarian cyst, pregnancy cannot occur.

Answer: _____ Rationale: _____

_____

_____

13

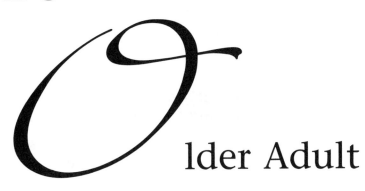

Older Adult

Preliminary Reading

Chapter 13, pp. 234-257

Comprehensive Understanding

• Older adulthood begins usually: _____

_____

Variability Among Older Adults

• Briefly explain the challenges of the older adult.

a. Physiological: _____

_____

b. Cognitive: _____

_____

c. Psychosocial: _____

_____

• Explain the following terminology.

a. Geriatrics: _____

_____

b. Gerontology: _____

_____

c. Gerontological nursing: _____

_____

d. Gerotonic nursing: _____

_____

Myths and Stereotypes

- Identify at least five myths and/or stereotypes regarding the older adult. _____

_____

_____

- Define *ageism.* _____

_____

Nurses' Attitudes Toward Older Adults

- The attitude of the nurse toward older adults comes in part from _____,

_____, _____,

and _____.

Theories of Aging

- Give a brief description of the following biological theories.

  a. Stochastic theories: _____

  _____

  _____

  b. Nonstochastic theories: _____

  _____

  _____

- Describe the three classic psychosocial theories of aging. _____

  _____

  _____

  _____

Developmental Tasks of Older Adults

- List the seven developmental tasks of the older adult.

  a. _____

  b. _____

c. _____

d. _____

e. _____

f. _____

g. _____

Community-Based and Institutional Health Care Services

- Briefly describe the following health services that are used by the older population.

  a. Retirement communities: _____

  _____

  _____

  b. Home care: _____

  _____

  _____

  c. Day care: _____

  _____

  _____

  d. Respite care: _____

  _____

  _____

  e. Long-term care: _____

  _____

  _____

Assessing the Needs of Older Adults

- Nurses need to take into account five key points to ensure an age-specific approach.

  a. _____

  b. _____

  c. _____

  d. _____

  e. _____

List some techniques to use for the older adult with visual impairments.

a. _____

b. _____

c. _____

List some techniques to use with the older adult with hearing impairment.

a. _____

b. _____

c. _____

d. _____

Physiological Changes

- Identify the physiological changes that occur in the older adult with regard to the following:

a. General survey: _____

_____

_____

_____

b. Integumentary system: _____

_____

_____

_____

c. Head and neck: _____

_____

_____

_____

d. Thorax and lungs: _____

_____

_____

_____

e. Heart and vascular system: _____

_____

_____

_____

f. Breasts: _____

_____

_____

_____

g. Gastrointestinal system and abdomen:

_____

_____

_____

_____

h. Reproductive system: _____

_____

_____

_____

i. Urinary system: _____

_____

_____

_____

_____

j. Musculoskeletal system: _____

_____

_____

_____

k. Neurological system: _____

_____

_____

_____

Cognitive Changes

- The structural and physiological changes that occur in the brain during aging do not necessarily affect adaptive and functional abilities.

- Define:

a. *Dementia:* _____

_____

b. *Delirium:* _____

_____

- Identify the characteristic progressive symptoms of Alzheimer's disease.

a. _____

b. _____

c. _____

- Identify the symptoms of Lewy body disease (LBD). _____
  _____
  _____

- Identify the symptoms in frontotemporal dementia. _____
  _____
  _____

- Identify the symptoms in vascular dementia.
  _____
  _____

- Explain depression in the older adult. _____
  _____
  _____

Psychosocial Changes

- Identify at least five areas that should be addressed when counseling an older adult about retirement.
  a. _____
  b. _____
  c. _____
  d. _____
  e. _____

- Briefly explain some of the reasons older adults experience social isolation. _____
  _____
  _____

- Briefly describe the sexual changes that occur in the older adult. _____
  _____
  _____

- List four factors to assess when assisting older adults with housing needs.
  a. _____
  b. _____
  c. _____
  d. _____

- A common misconception is that the death of an older adult is a blessing and the culmination of a full life.

- Many dying older adults still have goals and are not emotionally prepared to die.

Addressing the Health Concerns of Older Adults

- The three most common causes of death in the older adult are _____, _____, and _____.

- *Healthy People 2010* lists seven essential elements of health promotion:
  a. _____
  b. _____
  c. _____
  d. _____
  e. _____
  f. _____
  g. _____

Health Promotion and Maintenance: Physiological Concerns

- Summarize the physiological health concerns related to each of the following.
  a. Heart disease: _____
     _____
     _____
  b. Cancer: _____
     _____
     _____
  c. Stroke: _____
     _____
     _____
  d. Smoking: _____
     _____
     _____
  e. Alcohol abuse: _____
     _____
     _____

f. Nutrition: _____

_____

g. Dental problems: _____

_____

h. Exercise: _____

_____

i. Arthritis: _____

_____

j. Falls: _____

_____

k. Sensory impairments: _____

_____

l. Pain: _____

_____

_____

m. Medication use: _____

_____

_____

• Briefly explain the age-related changes affecting drug therapy in adults over the age of 65.

_____

_____

_____

Health Promotion and Maintenance: Psychosocial Health Concerns

• Briefly describe the interventions used to maintain the psychosocial health of the older adult.

a. Therapeutic communication: _____

_____

_____

b. Touch: _____

_____

c. Reality orientation: _____

_____

d. Validation therapy: _____

_____

e. Reminiscence: _____

_____

f. Body-image interventions: _____

_____

_____

Older Adults and the Acute Care Setting

• Older adults in the acute care setting are at increased risk for adverse events such as:

_____,

_____, _____,

_____, _____,

and _____.

• Explain why the older adult is at risk for each of the following.

a. Delirium: _____

_____

_____

b. Dehydration: _____

_____

_____

c. Malnutrition: _____

_____

_____

d. Nosocomial infections: _____

_____

_____

e. Urinary incontinence: _____

_____

f. Falls: _____

_____

_____

Older Adults and Restorative Care

- Summarize the two types of ongoing care for the older adult and identify the focus of each.

_____

_____

_____

_____

Review Questions

The student should select the appropriate answer and cite the rationale for choosing that particular answer.

1. Which statement about older adults is accurate?
   a. Older adults are institutionalized.
   b. Most older adults live on a fixed income.
   c. Most older adults cannot learn to care for themselves.
   d. Most older adults have no sexual desire.

   Answer: _____ Rationale: _____

   _____

   _____

2. Which statement describing delirium is correct?
   a. Persons with delirium may experience delusions and hallucinations.
   b. The onset of delirium is slow and insidious.
   c. Symptoms of delirium are stable and unchanging.
   d. Symptoms of delirium are irreversible.

   Answer: _____ Rationale: _____

   _____

   _____

3. Nutritional needs of the older adult:
   a. Are exactly the same as those of young and middle adults
   b. Include increased amounts of vitamin C, vitamin A, and calcium
   c. Include increased kilocalories to support metabolism and activity
   d. Include increased proteins and carbohydrates

   Answer: _____ Rationale: _____

   _____

   _____

4. Ms. Dale states that she does not need the TV turned on because she cannot see very well. Normal visual changes in older adults include all of the following except:
   a. Decreased visual acuity
   b. Decreased accommodation to darkness
   c. Double vision
   d. Sensitivity to glare

   Answer: _____ Rationale: _____

   _____

   _____

5. Mr. DeLone states that he is worried about his parents' plans to retire. All of the following would be appropriate responses regarding retirement of the older adult except:
   a. Positive adjustment is often related to how much a person planned for the retirement.
   b. Retirement for most persons represents a sudden shock that is irreversibly damaging to self-image and self-esteem.
   c. Reactions to retirement are influenced by the importance that has been attached to the work role.
   d. Retirement may affect an individual's physical and psychological functioning.

   Answer: _____ Rationale: _____

   _____

   _____

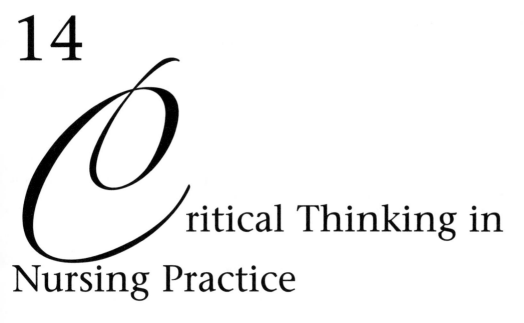

14

Critical Thinking in Nursing Practice

Preliminary Reading

Chapter 14, pp. 260-276

Comprehensive Understanding

Critical Decisions in Nursing Practice

- Critical decision making separates professional nurses from technical or ancillary personnel.

- Describe the process of critical thinking in nursing. _____

  _____

- To think critically, the nurse must be able to:
  a. _____
  b. _____
  c. _____
  d. _____
  e. _____

Critical Thinking Defined

- Define *critical thinking.* _____

- Identify the APA core critical thinking skills that apply to nursing.

    a. _____

    b. _____

    c. _____

    d. _____

    e. _____

- Learning to think critically helps a nurse to care for clients as their advocate and to make better informed choices about their care.

Reflection
- Define *reflection*. _____

_____

- Briefly summarize seven tips to facilitate critical thinking.

    a. _____

    b. _____

    c. _____

    d. _____

    e. _____

    f. _____

    g. _____

- Provide some examples of how a nurse can use

    reflection. _____

    _____

- Identify a common approach to reflection that

    a student nurse may use. _____

    _____

Language
- To become a critical thinker, a nurse must be able to use language precisely and clearly. It is important not only to communicate clearly with clients and families, but to be able to communicate findings clearly to other health professionals.

Intuition
- Define *intuition*. _____

_____

- Cite some examples of how a nurse gains intuitive knowledge. _____

_____

_____

Levels of Critical Thinking in Nursing

- Three levels of critical thinking in nursing have been identified. Briefly describe each.

    a. Basic: _____

    _____

    b. Complex: _____

    _____

    c. Commitment: _____

    _____

Critical Thinking Competencies

- Critical thinking competencies are the cognitive processes a nurse uses to make judgments.

Scientific Method
- Define *scientific method*. _____

_____

- List the steps of the scientific method.

    a. _____

    b. _____

    c. _____

    d. _____

    e. _____

Problem Solving
- Define *problem solving*. _____

_____

- Solving a problem in one situation allows the nurse to apply the knowledge to future client situations.

Decision Making
- Define *decision making*. _____

_____

- Explain the process that an individual needs to go through to make a decision. _____

Diagnostic Reasoning and Inferences

- Explain the process of diagnostic reasoning.

_____

_____

_____

Clinical Decision Making

- The clinical decision making process requires

_____.

- List the criteria for decision making (Strader, 1992).

    a. _____

    b. _____

    c. _____

- After determining a client's priorities, a nurse selects therapies most likely to solve each problem.

- Cite some examples of how nurses make decisions about their clients.

_____

Nursing Process as a Competency

- The nursing process is a systematic and comprehensive approach for nursing care. List the five steps of the nursing process.

    a. _____

    b. _____

    c. _____

    d. _____

    e. _____

Critical Thinking Model

- Summarize the critical thinking model and list its five components. _____

_____

_____

_____

Specific Knowledge Base

- Identify what constitutes a nurse's knowledge base. _____

_____

Experience

- Identify the ways that critical thinking is developed through experience. _____

_____

Attitudes for Critical Thinking

- The following attributes are important for critical thinking. Briefly explain each of them.

    a. Confidence: _____

    _____

    _____

    b. Thinking independently: _____

    _____

    _____

    c. Fairness: _____

    _____

    _____

    d. Responsibility and accountability: _____

    _____

    _____

    e. Risk taking: _____

    _____

    _____

    f. Discipline: _____

    _____

    _____

    g. Perseverance: _____

    _____

    _____

    h. Creativity: _____

    _____

    _____

    i. Curiosity: _____

    _____

    _____

j. Integrity: _____

_____

_____

k. Humility: _____

_____

_____

Standards for Critical Thinking

- The fifth component of critical thinking includes _____ and _____.

- Intellectual standards refer to _____.

- Professional standards refer to _____.

Critical Thinking Synthesis

- *Critical thinking* is defined as: _____

_____

- The nursing process is the traditional critical thinking competency which allows nurses to make clinical judgments and take actions based on reason.

- Briefly explain how the nursing process and the critical thinking model work together.

_____

_____

$\mathcal{R}$eview Questions

The student should select the appropriate answer and cite the rationale for choosing that particular answer.

1. Clinical decision making requires the nurse to:
   a. Improve a client's health
   b. Establish and weigh criteria in deciding the best choice of therapy for a client
   c. Follow the physician's orders for client care
   d. Standardize care for the client

Answer: _____ Rationale: _____

_____

_____

2. Which of the following is *not* one of the five steps of the nursing process?
   a. Planning
   b. Evaluation
   c. Hypothesis testing
   d. Assessment

Answer: _____ Rationale: _____

_____

_____

3. Gathering, verifying, and communicating data about the client to establish a database is an example of which component of the nursing process?
   a. Assessment
   b. Planning
   c. Evaluation
   d. Nursing diagnosis
   e. Implementation

Answer: _____ Rationale: _____

_____

_____

4. Completing nursing actions necessary for accomplishing a care plan is an example of which component of the nursing process?
   a. Assessment
   b. Planning
   c. Evaluation
   d. Nursing diagnosis
   e. Implementation

Answer: _____ Rationale: _____

_____

_____

15

$\mathcal{N}$ursing Assessment

$\mathcal{P}$reliminary Reading

Chapter 15, pp. 277-298

$\mathcal{C}$omprehensive Understanding

Nursing Process Overview

- The nursing process is used to _____, _____, and _____.

- The nursing process is one variation of scientific reasoning that allows nurses to _____, _____, and _____ nursing practice.

A Critical Thinking Approach to Assessment

- Nursing assessment is the systematic process of _____, _____, and _____ data about a client.

- This phase of the nursing process includes two steps. Name them.

  a. _____

  b. _____

- Identify the purpose of the assessment. _____
  _____

- As the nurse initiates the assessment component for a specific client, the nurse is also synthesizing critical knowledge, experience, standards, and attitudes simultaneously.

- A comprehensive database includes: _____

- List Gordon's 11 functional health patterns.

  a. _____

  b. _____

  c. _____

  d. _____

  e. _____

  f. _____

  g. _____

  h. _____

  i. _____

  j. _____

  k. _____

- Briefly explain the problem-focused approach to assessment. _____

  _____

  _____

- Whichever approach is used, the nurse must cluster cues of information and identify emerging patterns and potential problems.

Organization of Data Gathering
- Accurate assessment makes it possible to develop appropriate nursing diagnoses and to devise appropriate goals and strategies.

- It is important for the nurse's assessment to first consider the _____.

- Identify some nonverbal behavior that a nurse may observe during an assessment.

  _____

  _____

  _____

Data Collection
- Assessment does not include inferences or interpretative statements that are unsupported with data.

- Descriptive data originate in:

  a. _____

  b. _____

c. _____

d. _____

- The collection of inaccurate, incomplete, or inappropriate data leads to incorrect identification of the client's health care needs and subsequent inaccurate, incomplete, or inappropriate nursing diagnoses. Data are incomplete

  if the nurse _____,

  _____, or _____.

Types of Data

- Define each of the following:

  a. *Subjective data:* _____

  _____

  _____

  b. *Objective data:* _____

  _____

  _____

Sources of Data

- Each source provides information about the client's level of wellness, anticipated prognosis, risk factors, health practices and goals, and patterns of health and illness.

Client
- Identify the types of information a client can provide.

  a. _____

  b. _____

  c. _____

  d. _____

  e. _____

Family and Significant Others
- Families can be an important secondary source of information about the client's health status. Give an example. _____

  _____

  _____

- Identify the ways that health care team members identify data.

  a. _____

  b. _____

  c. _____

Medical Records

- By reviewing medical records, the nurse can

  _____, _____, and

  _____.

Other Records

- Identify records that may contain pertinent

  health care information. _____

  _____

Literature Review

- Reviewing nursing, medical, and pharmacological literature about an illness helps the nurse complete the database.

Nurse's Experience

- A nurse's ability to make an assessment will

  improve as he or she uses _____,

  applies _____, and focuses _____.

Methods of Data Collection

Interview

- During an interview nurses have the opportunity to:

  a. _____

  b. _____

  c. _____

  d. _____

  e. _____

  f. _____

- Define *nurse-client relationship.* _____

  _____

- Describe the phases of the interview.

  a. _____

  b. _____

  c. _____

- The nurse uses various types of interview techniques. Define the following types.

  a. *Open-ended questions:* _____

  _____

  b. *Back-channeling:* _____

  _____

  c. *Problem-seeking:* _____

  _____

  d. *Closed-ended questions:* _____

  _____

Nursing Health History

- The nursing health history is data collected about:

  a. _____

  b. _____

  c. _____

  d. _____

  e. _____

- Identify the four purposes (objectives) for obtaining a nursing health history.

  a. _____

  b. _____

  c. _____

  d. _____

- Briefly explain each of the following components of a health history.

  a. Biographical information: _____

  _____

  _____

  b. Reason for seeking health care: _____

  _____

  _____

  c. Client expectations: _____

  _____

  _____

  d. Present illness or health concerns: _____

  _____

e. Health history: _____

_____

f. Family history: _____

_____

g. Environmental history: _____

_____

g. Psychosocial history: _____

_____

h. Spiritual health: _____

_____

i. Review of systems (ROS): _____

_____

Physical Examination

- The physical examination and the collection of diagnostic and laboratory data involve the

_____

_____.

Order of Examination

- The exam is carried out in a systematic manner. Explain. _____

_____

- Define the following physical examination techniques.

a. *Inspection:* _____

_____

b. *Palpation:* _____

_____

c. *Percussion:* _____

_____

d. *Auscultation:* _____

_____

- Identify at least two contributions that laboratory data make to the nursing assessment.

a. _____

b. _____

Formulating Nursing Judgments

- Through a process of inferential reasoning and judgment, the nurse decides what information has meaning in relation to the client's health status.

Data Validation and Interpretation

- Define inferential reasoning. _____

_____

Data Clustering

- After collecting and validating subjective and objective data and interpreting the data, the nurse organizes the information into meaningful clusters. This depends on recognizing

_____.

- During data clustering, the nurse organizes data and focuses attention on client functions needing support and assistance for recovery.

Data Documentation

- Identify the two essential reasons for thoroughness in data documentation.

a. _____

b. _____

*R*eview Questions

The student should select the appropriate answer and cite the rationale for choosing that particular answer.

1. In most circumstances, the best source of information for nursing assessment of the adult client is the:
   a. Nursing literature
   b. Physician
   c. Client
   d. Medical record

Answer: _____ Rationale: _____

_____

_____

2. The interview technique that is most effective in strengthening the nurse-client relationship by demonstrating the nurse's willingness to hear the client's thoughts is:
   a. Open-ended question
   b. Direct question
   c. Problem-solving
   d. Problem-seeking

Answer: _____ Rationale: _____
_____
_____

3. While obtaining a health history, the nurse asks Mr. Jones if he has noted any change in his activity tolerance. This is an example of which interview technique?
   a. Direct question
   b. Problem-seeking
   c. Problem-solving
   d. Open-ended question

Answer: _____ Rationale: _____
_____
_____

4. Mr. Davis tells the nurse that he has been experiencing more frequent episodes of indigestion. The nurse asks if the indigestion is associated with meals or a reclining position and about what relieves the indigestion. This is an example of which interview technique?
   a. Problem-seeking
   b. Problem-solving
   c. Direct question
   d. Open-ended question

Answer: _____ Rationale: _____
_____
_____

5. The information obtained in a review of systems (ROS) is:
   a. Objective
   b. Subjective
   c. Based on physical examination findings
   d. Based on the nurse's perspective

Answer: _____ Rationale: _____
_____
_____

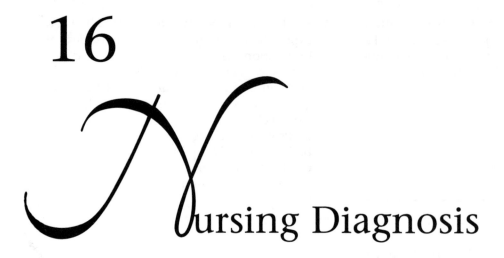

16

$\mathcal{N}$ursing Diagnosis

$\mathcal{P}$reliminary Reading

Chapter 16, pp. 299-316

$\mathcal{C}$omprehensive Understanding

- Define *nursing diagnosis.* _____
- Define *medical diagnosis.* _____

Evolution of Nursing Diagnosis

- Briefly summarize the evolution of nursing diagnosis. _____

_____

- Explain the purpose of NANDA. _____

_____

- Explain the purpose of using nursing diagnoses. _____

_____

Critical Thinking and the Nursing Diagnostic Process

Diagnostic Process

- The diagnostic reasoning process includes: _____

- The diagnostic process is dynamic and requires the nurse to reflect on existing assessment data and health care needs of the client.

Analysis and Interpretation of Data

- Data analysis involves recognizing _____, comparing _____, and drawing _____.

- Defining characteristics are: _____

  _____

- Defining characteristics that are beyond healthy norms form the basis for problem identification.

Formulation of the Nursing Diagnosis

- NANDA has identified three types of nursing diagnoses. Briefly explain each one.

  _____

  _____

  _____

- An actual nursing diagnosis describes: _____

  _____

- An at risk nursing diagnosis describes: _____

  _____

- A wellness nursing diagnosis describes: _____

  _____

Components of a Nursing Diagnosis

- Nursing diagnoses are stated in a two-part format. The _____ followed by a

  _____.

- The diagnostic label of the nursing diagnosis is:

  _____

- The related factors of the nursing diagnosis are

  _____

- The etiology of the nursing diagnosis is: _____

  _____

- NANDA approves a definition for each diagnosis following clinical use and testing.

- Risk factors are: _____

  _____

- Nursing assessment data must support the diagnostic label, and the related factors must support the etiology.

Mind-Mapping Nursing Diagnosis

- Briefly explain the benefits of mind-mapping.

  _____

  _____

Sources of Diagnosis Errors

Errors in Data Collection

- Identify the four practices that are essential during assessment to avoid data collection errors.

  a. _____

  b. _____

  c. _____

  d. _____

Errors in Interpretation and Analysis of Data

- Identify three ways the nurse can determine if data are accurate and complete.

  a. _____

  b. _____

  c. _____

Errors in Data Clustering

- Identify three ways that incorrect data clustering occurs.

  a. _____

  b. _____

  c. _____

Errors in the Diagnostic Statement

- Identify some common guidelines developed to reduce errors in the diagnostic statement.

  a. _____

  b. _____

  c. _____

  d. _____

  e. _____

  f. _____

  g. _____

h. _____

i _____

j. _____

k. _____

l. _____

Nursing Diagnosis and Other Health Care Problems

- Compare the characteristics of medical and nursing diagnoses. _____
_____
_____

- A collaborative problem is: _____
_____
_____

Nursing Diagnosis: Application to Care Planning

- The formulated nursing diagnoses provide direction for the planning process and the selection of nursing interventions to achieve the desired outcomes.

Advantages of Nursing Diagnoses

- Explain the advantages of nursing diagnoses to each of the following.

    a. Communication tool: _____
_____
_____

    b. Documentation: _____
_____
_____

    c. Discharge teaching: _____
_____
_____

    d. Quality assurance and improvement: _____
_____
_____

e. Professionally: _____
_____
_____

Limitations of Nursing Diagnoses

- List two limitations of nursing diagnoses.

    a. _____

    b. _____

$\mathcal{R}$eview Questions

The student should select the appropriate answer and cite the rationale for choosing that particular answer.

1. A nursing diagnosis:
    a. Is a statement of a client response to a health problem that requires nursing intervention
    b. Identifies nursing problems
    c. Is derived from the physician's history and physical examination
    d. Is not changed during the course of a client's hospitalization

Answer: _____ Rationale: _____
_____
_____

2. The first part of the nursing diagnosis statement:
    a. Identifies an actual or potential health problem
    b. Identifies the cause of the client problem
    c. May be stated as a medical diagnosis
    d. Identifies appropriate nursing interventions

Answer: _____ Rationale: _____
_____
_____

3. The second part of the nursing diagnosis statement:
   a. Is connected to the first part of the statement with the phrase "due to"
   b. Identifies the probable cause of the client problem
   c. Identifies the expected outcomes of nursing care
   d. Is usually stated as a medical diagnosis

Answer: _____ Rationale: _____

_____

_____

4. Which of the following is the correctly stated nursing diagnosis?
   a. Needs to be fed related to broken right arm
   b. Abnormal breath sounds caused by weak cough reflex
   c. Impaired physical mobility related to rheumatoid arthritis
   d. Impaired skin integrity related to fecal incontinence

Answer: _____ Rationale: _____

_____

_____

5. Mr. Margauz, a 52-year-old business executive, is admitted to the coronary care unit. During his admission interview he denies chest pain or shortness of breath. His pulse and blood pressure are normal. He appears tense and does not want the nurse to leave his bedside. When questioned, he states that he is very nervous. At this moment, which nursing diagnosis is most appropriate?
   a. Alteration in comfort, chest pain
   b. Alteration in bowel elimination related to restricted mobility
   c. High risk for altered cardiac output related to heart attack
   d. Anxiety related to intensive care unit admission

Answer: _____ Rationale: _____

_____

_____

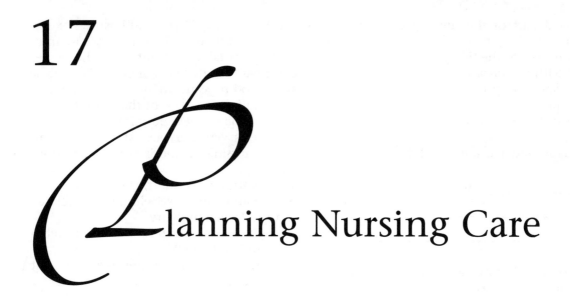

17 Planning Nursing Care

Preliminary Reading

Chapter 17, pp. 317-338

Comprehensive Understanding

Establishing Priorities

- Priority setting involves ranking nursing diagnoses in order of importance.

- Priorities are classified as high, immediate, or low. Give an example of each. _____

  _____

  _____

  _____

Critical Thinking in Establishing Goals and Expected Outcomes

- Establishing goals and expected outcomes requires that the nurse critically evaluate the _____

  _____, the _____, and the _____.

- Goals and expected outcomes are specific statements of client _____ or _____
  that the nurse anticipates from the nursing care.

- Identify the two purposes for writing goals and expected outcomes.

  a. _____

  b. _____

- Each goal and expected outcome statement must have a time frame for evaluation.

Goals of Care
- Define the following.

  a. *Client-centered goal:* _____

  _____

  b. *Short-term goal:* _____

  _____

  c. *Long-term goal:* _____

  _____

Expected Outcomes
- Define *expected outcomes.* _____

  _____

  _____

- Outcomes are desired responses of the client's

  condition in the _____,

  _____, _____,

  _____, or _____ dimensions.

- The expected outcomes should be written in measurable behavioral terms sequentially, with time frames.

- Identify the functions of an expected outcome.

  a. _____

  b. _____

  c. _____

  d. _____

- The rationale for several expected outcomes is:

  _____

  _____

  _____

Guidelines for Writing Goals and Expected Outcomes

There are seven guidelines to follow when writing goals and expected outcomes. Define and give an example of each.

  a. Client-centered factors: _____

  _____

  b. Singular factors: _____

  _____

  c. Observable factors: _____

  _____

  d. Measurable factors: _____

  _____

  e. Time-limited factors: _____

  _____

  f. Mutual factors: _____

  _____

  g. Realistic factors: _____

  _____

Critical Thinking in Designing Nursing Interventions

- Nursing interventions are those actions designed to assist the client in moving from the present level of health to that described in the expected outcome.

Types of Interventions
- There are three categories of interventions, and category selection is based on the client's needs. Define and give an example of each.

  a. Nurse-initiated: _____

  _____

  b. Physician-initiated: _____

  _____

  c. Collaborative: _____

  _____

Selection of Interventions
- Identify the six factors the nurse uses to select nursing interventions for a specific client.

  a. _____

  b. _____

  c. _____

  d. _____

  e. _____

  f. _____

- Define *collaboration.* _____

  _____

  _____

- The advantages of the taxonomy of nursing interventions are:

  a. _____

  b. _____

  c. _____

  d. _____

Planning Nursing Care

- Define *nursing care plan.* _____

  _____

  _____

Purpose of Care Plans
- Briefly explain the purpose of a nursing care plan in relation to the following.

  a. Communication: _____

  _____

  b. Identification and coordination of resources: _____

  _____

  c. Continuity of care: _____

  _____

  d. Change-of-shift reports: _____

  _____

  e. Long-term needs of client: _____

  _____

  f. Expected outcome criteria: _____

  _____

- The complete care plan is the blueprint for nursing action. It provides direction for implementation of the plan and a framework for evaluation of the client's response to nursing actions.

- Briefly explain each of the following.

  a. Institutional care plans:

  _____

  _____

  b. Computerized care plans: _____

  _____

  _____

  c. Student care plans: _____

  _____

  _____

  d. Concept maps: _____

  _____

  _____

  e. Critical pathways: _____

  _____

  _____

Consulting Other Health Care Professionals

- Consultation is a process in which _____

  _____

  _____

- Consultation is based on the problem-solving approach, and the consultant is the stimulus for change.

When to Consult
- The need to consult occurs when the nurse has identified a problem that cannot be solved using personal knowledge, skills, and resources.

How to Consult
- List the six responsibilities of the nurse when seeking consultation.

  a. _____

  b. _____

  c. _____

  d. _____

  e. _____

  f. _____

*R*eview Questions

The student should select the appropriate answer and cite the rationale for choosing that particular answer.

1. Well-formulated, client-centered goals should:
   a. Meet immediate client needs
   b. Include preventive health care
   c. Include rehabilitation needs
   d. All of the above

   Answer: _____ Rationale: _____

   _____

   _____

2. The following statement appears on the nursing care plan for an immunosuppressed client: The client will remain free from infection throughout hospitalization. This statement is an example of a (an):
   a. Nursing diagnosis
   b. Short-term goal
   c. Long-term goal
   d. Expected outcome

   Answer: _____ Rationale: _____

   _____

   _____

3. The following statements appear on a nursing care plan for a client after a mastectomy: Incision site approximated; absence of drainage or prolonged erythema at incision site; and client remains afebrile. These statements are examples of:
   a. Nursing interventions
   b. Short-term goals
   c. Long-term goals
   d. Expected outcomes

   Answer: _____ Rationale: _____

   _____

   _____

4. The planning step of the nursing process includes which of the following activities?
   a. Assessing and diagnosing
   b. Evaluating goal achievement
   c. Performing nursing actions and documenting them
   d. Setting goals and selecting interventions

   Answer: _____ Rationale: _____

   _____

   _____

5. The nursing care plan is:
   a. A written guideline for implementation and evaluation
   b. A documentation of client care
   c. A projection of potential alterations in client behaviors
   d. A tool to set goals and project outcomes

   Answer: _____ Rationale: _____

   _____

   _____

18

$\mathcal{I}$mplementing Nursing Care

$\mathcal{P}$reliminary Reading

Chapter 18, pp. 339-353

$\mathcal{C}$omprehensive Understanding

- Implementation describes: _____
  _____
  _____

- A nursing intervention is: _____
  _____

- Define each.
  a. *Direct care interventions:* _____
     _____

  b. *Indirect care interventions:* _____
     _____

Types of Nursing Interventions

Independent Nursing Interventions
- Describe an independent nursing intervention and a collaborative intervention. _____
  _____
  _____

Protocols and Standing Orders

Nursing interventions can be based on protocols an standings orders. Briefly explain each and provide an example of where they are commonly used.

a. Protocols: _____

_____

b. Standing orders: _____

_____

Critical Thinking in Implementing Nursing Interventions

Identify the factors that should be considered when choosing interventions.

a. _____

b. _____

c. _____

d. _____

e. _____

f. _____

When making decisions about implementing care, the nurse needs to consider the following.

a. _____

b. _____

c. _____

d. _____

Implementation Process

Reassessing the Client

When new data are obtained and a new need is identified, the nurse modifies nursing care.

Reviewing and Revising the Existing Nursing Care Plan

If the client's status has changed and the nursing diagnosis and related nursing interventions are no longer appropriate, the nursing care plan needs to be modified.

• Modification of the existing care plan includes several steps. Identify them.

a. _____

b. _____

c. _____

d. _____

Organizing Resources and Care Delivery

• Before implementing care, the nurse evaluates the plan to determine the need for assistance and the type of assistance required.

• Describe how each of the following contribute to the preparation of care delivered.

a. Equipment: _____

_____

b. Personnel: _____

_____

c. Environment: _____

_____

d. Client: _____

_____

e. Anticipating and preventing complications: _____

_____

f. Identifying areas of assistance: _____

_____

Implementing Skills

• Nursing practice is composed of three skills. Define and give an example of each.

a. *Cognitive:* _____

_____

_____

b. *Interpersonal:* _____

_____

c. *Psychomotor:* _____

_____

_____

Chapter 18: Implementing Nursing Care   87

Direct Care

Activities of Daily Living
- Define *activities of daily living* (ADLs). _____

  _____

  _____

- Conditions that result in the need for assistance with ADLs can be temporary, permanent, or rehabilitative.

Instrumental Activities of Daily Living (IADLs)
- IADLs include: _____

  _____

  _____

- A life-saving measure is: _____

  _____

  _____

Counseling
- *Counseling* is defined as: _____

  _____

  _____

- Identify some areas in which clients or families may need counseling.

  a. _____

  b. _____

  c. _____

Teaching
- Define the following.

  a. *Teaching:* _____

  _____

  b. *Teaching-learning process:* _____

  _____

Controlling for Adverse Reactions
- An adverse reaction is: _____

  _____

  _____

Preventive Measures
- Preventive nursing actions are: _____

  _____

  _____

Indirect Care
Communicating Nursing Interventions
- Nursing interventions are written (via the nursing care plan and medical record) or communicated orally (one nurse to another or to another health care professional).

- Define *interdisciplinary plan.* _____

  _____

  _____

Delegating, Supervising, and Evaluating the Work of Other Staff Members
- Give an example of what tasks you could delegate to each of the following.

  a. Certified nurse assistant: _____

  _____

  _____

  b. LPN: _____

  _____

  _____

Achieving Client Goals
- The client's health care goals can be achieved by:

  a. _____

  b. _____

  c. _____

  d. _____

Review Questions

The student should select the appropriate answer and cite the rationale for choosing that particular answer.

1. Which of the following is not true of standing orders?
   a. Standing orders are approved and signed by the physician in charge of care before implementation.
   b. With standing orders, the nurse relies on the physician's judgment to determine if the intervention is appropriate.
   c. Standing orders are commonly found in critical care and community health settings.
   d. With standing orders, nurses have the legal protection to intervene appropriately in the client's best interest.

Answer: _____ Rationale: _____

_____

_____

2. The nursing care plan calls for the client, a 300 lb. woman, to be turned every 2 hours. The client is unable to assist with turning. The nurse knows that she may hurt her back if she attempts to turn the client by herself. The nurse should:
   a. Rewrite the care plan to eliminate the need for turning
   b. Ignore the intervention related to turning in the care plan
   c. Turn the client by herself
   d. Ask another nurse to help her turn the client

Answer: _____ Rationale: _____

_____

_____

3. Being alert to the possibility of the client becoming nauseated after general anesthesia is an example of which type of nursing skill?
   a. Cognitive
   b. Interpersonal
   c. Technical
   d. Psychosocial

Answer: _____ Rationale: _____

_____

_____

4. Mrs. Kay comes to the family clinic for birth control. The nurse obtains a health history and performs a pelvic examination and Pap smear. The nurse is functioning according to:
   a. Protocol
   b. Standing order
   c. Nursing care plan
   d. Intervention strategy

Answer: _____ Rationale: _____

_____

_____

5. Mary Jones is a newly diagnosed diabetic patient. The nurse shows Mary how to administer an injection. This intervention activity is:
   a. Counseling
   b. Communicating
   c. Teaching
   d. Managing

Answer: _____ Rationale: _____

_____

_____

19

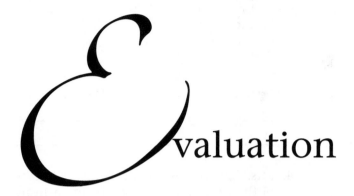

Evaluation

Preliminary Reading

Chapter 19, pp. 354-369

Comprehensive Understanding

Critical Thinking and Evaluation

- Evaluation of care requires the nurse to reflect on the client's responses to nursing interventions and to determine their effectiveness in promoting the client's well-being.

- Evaluation is the step in the nursing process whereby the nurse continually redirects nursing care to meet client needs.

- Explain the two types of evaluations.

  a. Positive: _____

  b. Negative: _____

- A client whose health status changes continuously requires frequent evaluation.

Evaluation Process

- Identify the five elements of the evaluation process.

  a. _____

  b. _____

  c. _____

  d. _____

  e. _____

- A goal specifies: _____

  _____

  _____

- Expected outcomes are: _____

  _____

  _____

- The purposes of the Nursing Outcomes Classification (NOC) are:

  a. _____

  b. _____

  c. _____

Collecting Evaluative Measures
- Identify the two aspects of care that need to be identified.

  a. _____

  b. _____

- The primary source of data for evaluation is:

  _____

  _____

  _____

Interpreting and Summarizing Findings
- To objectively evaluate the success in achieving a goal, the nurse should use the following steps.

  a. _____

  b. _____

  c. _____

  d. _____

  e. _____

- When documenting the client's response to interventions, the nurse always includes the same evaluative measures gathered during assessment.

Care Plan Revision and Critical Thinking
- Accurate evaluation leads to the appropriate revision of ineffective care plans and discontinuation of therapy that has been successful.

Discontinuing a Care Plan
- After determining that expected outcomes and goals have been achieved, the nurse confirms this evaluation with the client and discontinues that care plan.

Modifying a Care Plan
- When goals are not met, the nurse identifies the factors that interfered with goal achievement.

- Lack of goal achievement may also result from an error in nursing judgment or failure to follow each step of the nursing process.

- When there is failure to achieve a goal, the entire _____ sequence is repeated to discover changes that need to be made to _____ or _____ the client's health.

- A complete reassessment of all client factors relating to the nursing diagnosis and etiology is the first step in reevaluating the nursing process. Briefly explain the following.

  a. Reassessment: _____

  _____

  b. Nursing diagnosis: _____

  _____

  c. Goals and expected outcomes: _____

  _____

  d. Interventions: _____

  _____

  e. Evaluation: _____

  _____

Quality Improvement
- The evaluation of health care is a process used to determine the quality of care and service provided to clients.

- JCAHO defines quality improvement (QI) as:

_____

_____

_____

_____

- Explain the following steps in relation to improving the quality of nursing care and taking appropriate action to resolve any problems.

    a. Quality improvement: _____

    _____

    b. Outcomes management: _____

    _____

    c. Professional outcomes: _____

    _____

    d. Client outcomes: _____

    _____

$\mathcal{R}$eview Questions

The student should select the appropriate answer and cite the rationale for choosing that particular answer.

1. Measuring the client's response to nursing interventions and his or her progress toward achieving goals occurs during which phase of the nursing process?
    a. Planning
    b. Nursing diagnosis
    c. Evaluation
    d. Assessment

    Answer: _____ Rationale: _____

    _____

    _____

2. Evaluation is:
    a. Begun immediately before the client's discharge
    b. Only necessary if the physician orders it
    c. An integrated, ongoing nursing care activity
    d. Performed primarily by nurses in the quality assurance department

    Answer: _____ Rationale: _____

    _____

    _____

3. The criteria used to determine the effectiveness of a nursing action are based on the:
    a. Nursing diagnosis
    b. Expected outcomes
    c. Client's satisfaction
    d. Nursing interventions

    Answer: _____ Rationale: _____

    _____

    _____

4. The primary source of data for evaluation is the:
    a. Physician
    b. Client
    c. Nurse
    d. Medical record

    Answer: _____ Rationale: _____

    _____

    _____

5. When a client-centered goal has not been met in the projected time frame, the most appropriate action by the nurse would be to:
    a. Repeat the entire sequence of the nursing process to discover needed changes
    b. Conclude that the goal was inappropriate or unrealistic and eliminate it from the plan
    c. Continue with the same plan until the goal is met
    d. Rewrite the plan using different interventions

    Answer: _____ Rationale: _____

    _____

    _____

20

$\mathcal{M}$anaging Client Care

$\mathcal{P}$reliminary Reading

Chapter 20, pp. 370-385

$\mathcal{C}$omprehensive Understanding

Building a Nursing Team

• Building an empowered nursing team begins with the nurse executive.

• Define *philosophy of care*. _____

_____

_____

Nursing Care Delivery Models

• Care delivery must be effective in helping nurses achieve desirable outcomes for their clients.

• Briefly explain the following delivery systems.

  a. Functional nursing: _____

  _____

  _____

  b. Team nursing: _____

  _____

  _____

c. Total patient care: _____

_____

_____

d. Primary nursing: _____

_____

_____

e. Case management: _____

_____

_____

Decentralized Decision Making

- Briefly explain the following management structures.

  a. Centralized management: _____

  _____

  b. Decentralized management: _____

  _____

  c. Matrix: _____

  _____

- Identify the responsibilities of a nurse manager.

  _____

  _____

  _____

- The following are key elements in empowering staff and establishing decentralized decision making. Briefly explain each one.

  a. Responsibility: _____

  _____

  _____

  b. Authority: _____

  _____

  _____

  c. Accountability: _____

  _____

  _____

- The nurse manager nurtures and supports staff involvement through the following approaches. Briefly explain each.

  a. Shared governance: _____

  _____

  _____

  b. Nurse/physician collaborative practice:

  _____

  _____

  _____

  c. Interdisciplinary collaboration:

  _____

  _____

  d. Staff communication: _____

  _____

  _____

  e. Staff education: _____

  _____

  _____

Leadership Skills for Nursing Students

- Identify the leadership skills a student nurse may develop and summarize each.

  a. Clinical care coordination: _____

  _____

  b. Clinical decisions: _____

  _____

  c. Priority setting: _____

  _____

  d. Organizational skills: _____

  _____

  e. Use of resources: _____

  _____

  f. Time management: _____

  _____

  g. Evaluation: _____

  _____

- Summarize the following principles of time management.

  a. Goal setting: _____

  _____

  b. Time analysis: _____

  _____

  c. Set priorities: _____

  _____

  d. Interruption control: _____

  _____

  e. Evaluation: _____

  _____

- Give an example of team communication.

  _____

  _____

  _____

- *Delegation* is defined as: _____

  _____

  _____

- Identify the five rights of delegation.

  a. _____

  b. _____

  c. _____

  d. _____

  e. _____

- Identify the purposes of delegation. _____

  _____

  _____

- Summarize the requirements for appropriate delegation.

  a. _____

  b. _____

  c. _____

  d. _____

  e. _____

- List some ways that professional nurses build on their current knowledge base. _____

  _____

  _____

  _____

Quality Management

- List the principles of total quality improvement (TQI).

  a. _____

  b. _____

  c. _____

  d. _____

  e. _____

  f. _____

Quality in Nursing Practice

- *Quality improvement* is defined as: _____

  _____

  _____

- The quality of nursing practice is defined by each of the following.

  a. Professional standards: _____

  _____

  _____

  b. Care guidelines: _____

  _____

  _____

  c. Outcomes: _____

  _____

  _____

- Differentiate between the two types of outcomes.

  a. Professional outcomes: _____

  _____

  b. Client outcomes: _____

  _____

- Differentiate between the two different types of quality improvement teams.

    a. Organization-wide: _____

    _____

    b. Unit-based: _____

    _____

- Identify JCAHO's 10 steps to quality improvement.

    a. _____

    b. _____

    c. _____

    d. _____

    e. _____

    f. _____

    g. _____

    h. _____

    i _____

    j. _____

- Identify who is responsible for the QI program.

    _____

    _____

- A unit's scope of service includes: _____

    _____

    _____

- Some key aspects of service include: _____

    _____

    _____

- A *quality indicator* is defined as: _____

    _____

    _____

- Explain the following three types of quality indicators.

    a. Structure: _____

    _____

    _____

    b. Process: _____

    _____

    _____

    c. Outcome: _____

    _____

    _____

- List some processes and related outcomes that may be in need of improvement. _____

    _____

    _____

- *Threshold* is defined as: _____

    _____

    _____

- When QI is an ongoing process, staff continuously work to improve outcomes or performance by raising thresholds.

- Explain the purpose of data collection and analysis. _____

    _____

    _____

    _____

- Explain the model FOCUS-PDCA. _____

    _____

    _____

- After evaluating quality problems, the staff needs to do the following. Explain each.

    a. Resolve problems: _____

    _____

    _____

    b. Evaluate improvement: _____

    _____

    _____

    c. Communicate results: _____

    _____

    _____

Review Questions

The student should select the appropriate answer and cite the rationale for choosing that particular answer.

1. One difference between a leader and a manager is that a manager:
   a. Is responsible for day-to-day operations and stability
   b. Has a vision or a goal for the group
   c. Influences others to follow his or her direction
   d. Focuses on innovation and change

   Answer: _____ Rationale: _____

   _____

   _____

2. A student nurse practicing primary leadership skills would demonstrate all of the following *except*:
   a. Being sensitive to the group's feelings
   b. Recognizing others for their contribution
   c. Assuming primary responsibility for planning, implementation, follow-up, and evaluation
   d. Developing listening skills and being aware of personal motivation

   Answer: _____ Rationale: _____

   _____

   _____

3. Mr. Jones is the team leader on a busy surgical floor. The team members are upset with the evening client assignments. Mr. Jones tells the team members to work things out for themselves and that whatever they decide will be satisfactory. Mr. Jones' leadership style could best be described as:
   a. Authoritarian
   b. Democratic
   c. Laissez-faire
   d. Situational

   Answer: _____ Rationale: _____

   _____

   _____

4. The effective nurse manager is able to use different styles and leadership skills depending on the specific situation and the maturity of the employees. This is an example of which leadership style?
   a. Authoritarian
   b. Democratic
   c. Laissez-faire
   d. Situational

   Answer: _____ Rationale: _____

   _____

   _____

5. During a cardiac arrest, which leadership style would be most effective?
   a. Authoritarian
   b. Democratic
   c. Laissez-faire
   d. Situational

   Answer: _____ Rationale: _____

   _____

   _____

21

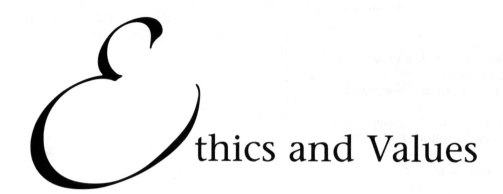

Ethics and Values

Preliminary Reading

Chapter 21, pp. 386-404

Comprehensive Understanding

- Define a *code of ethics*. _____

  _____

  _____

- Explain the field of bioethics. _____

  _____

  _____

Ethics

- Define *ethics*. _____

  _____

  _____

- Define the following basic terms within the context of ethics.

  a. *Autonomy:* _____

  _____

  b. *Beneficence:* _____

  _____

c. *Nonmaleficence:* _____

_____

d. *Justice:* _____

_____

e. *Fidelity:* _____

_____

Professional Nursing

- A code of ethics is a set of _____,

which serve to _____.

_____

_____

- Accountability refers to: _____

_____

_____

- Responsibility refers to: _____

_____

_____

- Describe the concept of confidentiality. _____

_____

_____

- Veracity means: _____

_____

_____

Values

- A *value* is defined as: _____

_____

_____

- Briefly explain the modes of values formation.

_____

_____

_____

_____

- The process of value clarification is: _____

_____

_____

_____

- Identify and explain the three steps of values clarification.

a. _____

b. _____

c. _____

- Define the following terms.

a. *Cultural values:* _____

_____

b. *Ethnocentrism:* _____

_____

Bioethics

- The notion of autonomy was developed to explain and define a society's growing desire to protect clients from scientific endeavors. The notion of client autonomy reflects a change in society's definitions of power and knowledge.

Philosophical Constructs

- Briefly explain the following philosophical constructs in relation to ethical systems.

a. Deontology: _____

_____

_____

b. Utilitarianism/consequentialism: _____

_____

_____

c. Feminist ethics: _____

_____

_____

d. Ethics of care: _____

_____

_____

Consensus in Bioethics

- Consensus bioethics proposes: _____

_____

_____

Nursing Point of View

- Briefly summarize the nurse's point of view in relation to addressing an ethical dilemma.

_____

_____

_____

_____

How to Process an Ethical Dilemma

- Processing an ethical dilemma differs from the nursing process as _____

_____

_____

- To distinguish an ethical problem from questions of procedure, legality, or medical diagnosis, the nurse must decide whether the problem has one or more of the following characteristics.

   a. _____

   b. _____

   c. _____

- The nurse uses the following guidelines for ethical processing and decision making. Briefly describe each one.

   a. Is this an ethical dilemma? _____

   _____

   _____

   b. Gather the relevant information. _____

   _____

   _____

   c. Examine and determine one's own values.

   _____

   _____

   _____

   d. Verbalize the problem. _____

   _____

   _____

   e. Propose alternative courses of action. _____

   _____

   _____

   f. Negotiate the outcome. _____

   _____

   _____

   g. Evaluate the action. _____

   _____

   _____

Institutional Resources

- Identify the functions of ethics committees.

_____

_____

_____

Issues in Bioethics

- Briefly describe the following issues that are common in health care settings.

   a. Quality of life: _____

   _____

   _____

   b. Genetic screening: _____

   _____

   _____

   c. Futile care: _____

   _____

   _____

   d. Allocation of scarce resources: medical technologies: _____

   _____

   _____

   e. Allocation of scarce resources: the nursing shortage: _____

   _____

   _____

Review Questions

The student should select the appropriate answer and cite the rationale for choosing that particular answer.

1. A health care issue often becomes an ethical dilemma because:
   a. A client's legal rights coexist with a health professional's obligations.
   b. Decisions must be made quickly, often under stressful conditions.
   c. Decisions must be made based on value systems.
   d. The choices involved do not appear to be clearly right or wrong.

   Answer: _____ Rationale: _____

   _____

   _____

2. A document that lists the medical treatment a person chooses to refuse if unable to make decisions is the:
   a. Durable power of attorney
   b. Informed consent
   c. Living will
   d. Advance directives

   Answer: _____ Rationale: _____

   _____

   _____

3. Which statement about an institutional ethics committee is correct?
   a. The ethics committee is an additional resource for clients and health care professionals.
   b. The ethics committee relieves health care professionals from dealing with ethical issues.
   c. The ethics committee would be the first option in addressing an ethical dilemma.
   d. The ethics committee replaces decision making by the client and health care providers.

   Answer: _____ Rationale: _____

   _____

   _____

4. The nurse is working with parents of a seriously ill newborn. Surgery has been proposed for the infant, but the chances of success are unclear. In helping the parents resolve this ethical conflict, the nurse knows that the first step is:
   a. Exploring reasonable courses of action
   b. Collecting all available information about the situation
   c. Clarifying values related to the cause of the dilemma
   d. Identifying people who can solve the difficulty

   Answer: _____ Rationale: _____

   _____

   _____

5. Mrs. G., an 88-year-old woman, believes that life should not be prolonged when hope is gone. She has decided that she does not want extraordinary measures taken when her life is at its end. Because she feels this way, she has talked with her daughter about her desires, completed a living will, and left directions with her physician. This is an example of:
   a. Affirming a value
   b. Choosing a value
   c. Prizing a value
   d. Reflecting a value

   Answer: _____ Rationale: _____

   _____

   _____

22

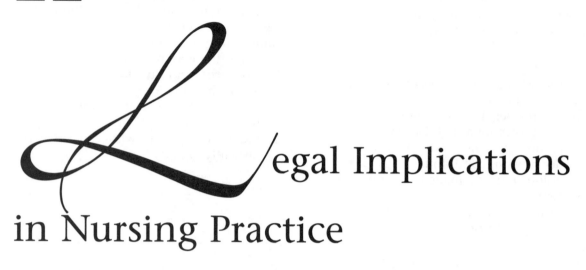

*L*egal Implications in Nursing Practice

*P*reliminary Reading

Chapter 22, pp. 405-422

*C*omprehensive Understanding

Legal Limits of Nursing

- Professional nurses must understand the legal limits influencing their daily practice.

Sources of Law

- The legal guidelines that nurses must follow are derived from the following. Briefly explain each one.

  a. Statutory law: _____

  _____

  b. Nurse Practice Acts: _____

  _____

  c. Regulatory law: _____

  _____

  d. Common law: _____

  _____

- Define the following statutory laws.

  a. *Criminal law:* _____

  _____

  _____

  _____

b. *Crime:* _____

_____

_____

c. *Felony:* _____

_____

_____

_____

d. *Misdemeanor:* _____

_____

_____

e. *Civil law:* _____

_____

_____

_____

Standards of Care

- Standards of care are the legal guidelines for nursing practice and are defined by the: _____

_____

_____

- The Nurse Practice Acts establish: _____

_____

_____

- In a malpractice lawsuit, these standards are used to determine: _____

_____

_____

- All nurses should know the standards of care they are expected to meet within their specialty and work setting. Ignorance of the law or of standards of care is not a defense to malpractice.

- Briefly summarize the case of Darling v. Charleston Community Memorial Hospital and the Illinois Supreme Court's decision.

_____

_____

_____

Federal Statutory Issues in Nursing Practice
- Briefly explain the following.

a. Americans with Disabilities Act: _____

_____

b. EMTALA: _____

_____

c. Mental Health Parity Act: _____

_____

_____

d. Advance directives: _____

_____

_____

e. Living wills: _____

_____

_____

f. Doctrine of autonomy: _____

_____

_____

g. DNR: _____

_____

_____

h. Uniform Anatomical Gift Act: _____

_____

_____

i. HIPAA _____

_____

_____

Chapter 22: Legal Implications in Nursing Practice   103

- State the most frequent indications for the use of restraints:

  a. _____

  b. _____

  c. _____

State Statutory Issues in Nursing Practice

Licensure
- All states use the National Council Licensure Examinations (NCLEX) for registered nurse and licensed nurse examinations.

Good Samaritan Laws
- Briefly explain the nurse's legal coverage under this law. _____

  _____

  _____

Public Health Laws
- Explain the purpose of these laws. _____

  _____

  _____

The Uniform Determination of Death Act
- Explain the legal definition of *death*. _____

  _____

  _____

Physician-Assisted Suicide
- Briefly explain this statute: _____

  _____

  _____

Civil and Common Law Issues in Nursing Practice

- Define the following.

  a. *Tort:* _____

  _____

  b. *Malpractice:* _____

  _____

  c. *Assault:* _____

  _____

d. *Battery:* _____

  _____

Consent
- A signed consent form is required for all routine treatment, hazardous procedures, some treatment programs such as chemotherapy, and research involving clients.

- Informed consent is a person's agreement to:

  _____

  _____

- The following factors must be verified for a consent to be valid.

  a. _____

  b. _____

  c. _____

  d. _____

  e. _____

  f. _____

- The nurse assumes the responsibility for witnessing the client's signature on the consent form but does not legally assume the duty of obtaining consent.

- The nurse's signature witnessing the consent means: _____

  _____

  _____

- Only a person who can understand the explanations provided and who can truly understand the decision they are making can provide informed consent.

- A client who refuses surgery or any other medical treatment must be informed of any harmful consequences.

Abortion Issues
- Summarize the legal rights of women relative to abortion.

  a. Roe v. Wade: _____

  _____

b. Webster v. Reproductive Health Services:

_____

_____

c. Planned Parenthood of Southeastern Pennsylvania v. Casey: _____

_____

Invasion of Privacy

- Briefly explain the four types of invasion of privacy torts.

  a. Intrusion on seclusion: _____

  _____

  b. Appropriation of name: _____

  _____

  c. Publication of private facts: _____

  _____

  d. Publicity in a false light: _____

  _____

Defamation of Character

- Define the following.

  a. *Malice:* _____

  _____

  b. *Slander:* _____

  _____

  c. *Libel:* _____

  _____

Unintentional Torts

- Define the following.

  a. *Negligence:* _____

  _____

  b. *Malpractice:* _____

  _____

- Briefly explain how a nurse can avoid being liable for negligence. _____

  _____

  _____

Student Nurses

- If a client is harmed as a direct result of a nursing student's actions or lack of action, the liability for the incorrect action is generally shared by the student, instructor, hospital or health care facility, and university or educational institution.

- When students are employed as nursing assistants or nurse's aides when not attending classes, they should not perform tasks that do not appear in a job description for a nurses' aide or assistant.

- Briefly explain what malpractice insurance provides for. _____

  _____

  _____

Legal Relationships in Nursing Practice

Short Staffing

- The JCAHO requires institutions to establish guidelines for determining the number of nurses required to give care to a specific number of clients (staffing ratios).

- Nursing supervisors should be informed when a nurse is assigned to care for more clients than is reasonable, and a written protest should be filed to document such an assignment.

- When staffing is inadequate, nurses should not walk out because charges of abandonment can be made.

Floating

- Nurses who float should inform the supervisor of any lack of experience they may have caring for the type of clients on the nursing unit.

- A supervisor can be held liable if a staff nurse is given an assignment he or she cannot safely handle.

Physicians' Orders

- The physician is responsible for directing the medical treatment.

- Nurses are obligated to follow the physician's orders unless: _____

  _____

  _____

- A nurse should not perform a physician's order if it is foreseeable that harm will come to the client.

- If a verbal order is necessary, it should be written out and signed by the physician within 24 hours.

Risk Management
- Risk management is: _____

  _____

  _____

- The steps involved in risk management include:

  a. _____

  b. _____

  c. _____

  d. _____

- A tool used by risk managers is the: _____

  _____

  _____

- Risk management includes documentation. It

  should be: _____

  _____

  _____

Professional Involvement
- Nurses must be involved in their professional organizations and on committees that define the standards of care for nursing practice.

- Nurses become more powerful and more effective as a profession when they are organized and cohesive.

Review Questions

The student should select the appropriate answer and cite the rationale for choosing that particular answer.

1. The scope of nursing practice is legally defined by:
   a. State Nurse Practice Acts
   b. Professional nursing organizations
   c. Hospital policy and procedure manuals
   d. Physicians in the employing institutions

   Answer: _____ Rationale: _____

   _____

   _____

2. A student nurse who is employed as a nursing assistant may perform any functions that:
   a. Have been learned in school
   b. Are expected of a nurse at that level
   c. Are identified in the position's job description
   d. Require technical rather than professional skill

   Answer: _____ Rationale: _____

   _____

   _____

3. A confused client who fell out of bed because side rails were not used is an example of which type of liability?
   a. Felony
   b. Assault
   c. Battery
   d. Negligence

   Answer: _____ Rationale: _____

   _____

   _____

4. The nurse puts a restraint jacket on a client without the client's permission and without a physician's order. The nurse may be guilty of:
   a. Assault
   b. Battery
   c. Invasion of privacy
   d. Neglect

Answer: _____ Rationale: _____

_____

_____

5. In a situation in which there is insufficient staff to implement competent care, a nurse should:
   a. Organize a strike
   b. Inform the clients of the situation
   c. Refuse the assignment
   d. Accept the assignment but make a protest in writing to the administration

Answer: _____ Rationale: _____

_____

_____

23

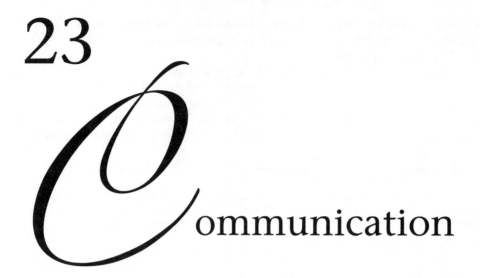

ommunication

Preliminary Reading

Chapter 23, pp. 423-447

Comprehensive Understanding

Communication and Nursing Practice

- Communication is a lifelong process. This process allows: _____
  _____
  _____

- Competency in communication helps the nurse maintain effective relationships with the entire sphere of professional practice and helps meet legal, ethical, and clinical standards of care.

Communication and Interpersonal Relationships
- Communication is the means to establishing helping-healing relationships.

- Communication is essential to the nurse-client relationship because:

  a. _____

  b. _____

- Nurses with expertise in communication can express caring by: _____
  _____
  _____

- The nurse's ability to relate to others is:

_____

_____

Developing Communication Skills
- Briefly explain the qualities of critical thinking in relation to the communication process.

_____

_____

_____

- Critical thinking can help the nurse overcome perceptual biases _____

_____

_____

- Nurses use communication skills to gather, analyze, and transmit information and to accomplish the work of each phase.

Levels of Communication

- Summarize the following communication interactions.

  a. Intrapersonal: _____

  _____

  _____

  b. Interpersonal: _____

  _____

  _____

  c. Transpersonal: _____

  _____

  _____

  d. Small-group: _____

  _____

  _____

  e. Public: _____

  _____

  _____

Basic Elements of the Communication Process

- Briefly summarize the following elements of communication.

  a. Referent: _____

  _____

  _____

  b. Sender: _____

  _____

  _____

  c. Receiver: _____

  _____

  _____

  d. Message: _____

  _____

  _____

  e. Channels: _____

  _____

  _____

  f. Feedback: _____

  _____

  _____

  g. Interpersonal variables: _____

  _____

  _____

  h. Environment: _____

  _____

Forms of Communication

- Messages are conveyed verbally and nonverbally, concretely and symbolically.

Verbal Communication
- Verbal communication involves spoken or written words. Verbal language is a code that conveys specific meaning as words are combined.

- Briefly explain the important aspects of verbal communication listed below.

  a. Vocabulary: _____

  _____

  _____

  b. Denotative and connotative meaning:

  _____

  _____

  _____

  c. Pacing: _____

  _____

  _____

  d. Intonation: _____

  _____

  _____

  e. Clarity: _____

  _____

  _____

  f. Brevity: _____

  _____

  _____

  g. Timing and relevance: _____

  _____

  _____

Nonverbal Communication
- Nonverbal communication includes: _____

  _____

  _____

- Nonverbal communication is much more powerful than verbal communication.

- Becoming an astute observer of nonverbal behavior takes practice, concentration, and sensitivity to others. Briefly explain the following nonverbal behaviors.

  a. Personal appearance: _____

  _____

  _____

  b. Posture and gait: _____

  _____

  _____

  c. Facial expression: _____

  _____

  _____

  d. Eye contact: _____

  _____

  _____

  e. Gestures: _____

  _____

  _____

  f. Sounds: _____

  _____

  _____

  g. Territoriality and personal space: _____

  _____

  _____

- Identify the zones of personal space. _____

  _____

  _____

  _____

  _____

- Identify the zones of touch. _____

  _____

  _____

  _____

Symbolic Communication
- Summarize symbolic communication. _____

  _____

  _____

Metacommunication
- Define *metacommunication*. _____

  _____

  _____

Professional Nursing Relationships

- Professional relationships are created through

  _____, _____,

  and _____.

Nurse-Client Helping Relationships

- The relationship is therapeutic, promoting a psychological climate that facilitates positive change and growth.

- Acceptance conveys a: _____

  _____

  _____

- The nurse-client relationship is characterized by four goal-directed phases. Explain the phases.

  a. Preinteraction phase: _____

     _____

     _____

  b. Orientation phase: _____

     _____

     _____

  c. Working phase: _____

     _____

     _____

  d. Termination phase: _____

     _____

     _____

- Nurses often encourage clients to share personal

  stories. This is called _____

  _____.

Nurse-Family Relationships

- Summarize the principles related to nurse-

  family relationships. _____

  _____

Nurse-Health Team Relationships

- Communication in nurse-health team relationships is geared by: _____

  _____

  _____

Nurse-Community Relationships

- Communication within the community occurs through channels such as: _____

  _____

  _____

Elements of Professional Communication

- Briefly explain the following elements of professional communication.

  a. Courtesy: _____

     _____

     _____

  b. Use of names: _____

     _____

     _____

  c. Privacy and confidentiality: _____

     _____

     _____

  d. Trustworthiness: _____

     _____

     _____

  e. Autonomy and responsibility: _____

     _____

     _____

  f. Assertiveness: _____

     _____

     _____

Communication Within the Nursing Process

ℳ Assessment

- Assessment of a client's ability to communicate includes gathering data about the many contextual factors that influence communication.

- List the contextual factors that influence communication.

  a. _____

  b. _____

  c. _____

  d. _____

  e. _____

- Identify the psychophysiological factors that influence communication. _____

  _____

  _____

- Physical barriers cause _____,

  _____, or _____.

- Explain how developmental factors influence communication. _____

  _____

  _____

- Summarize how sociocultural factors influence communication. _____

  _____

  _____

- Gender influences communication. Explain how communication differs in regard to gender.

  a. Male: _____

  b. Female: _____

ℳ Nursing Diagnosis

- List three nursing diagnoses appropriate for a client with alterations in communication.

  a. _____

  b. _____

  c. _____

ℳ Planning

- List three goals for effective interpersonal communication.

  a. _____

  b. _____

  c. _____

ℳ Implementation

- Therapeutic communication techniques are specific responses that encourage the expression of feelings and ideas and convey the nurse's acceptance and respect. Briefly explain the following techniques.

  a. Active listening: _____

  _____

  _____

  b. Sharing observations: _____

  _____

  _____

  c. Sharing empathy: _____

  _____

  _____

  d. Sharing hope: _____

  _____

  _____

  e. Sharing humor: _____

  _____

  _____

  f. Sharing feelings: _____

  _____

  _____

g. Using touch: _____

_____

h. Using silence: _____

_____

i. Providing information: _____

_____

j. Clarifying: _____

_____

k. Focusing: _____

_____

l. Paraphrasing: _____

_____

m. Asking relevant questions: _____

_____

n. Summarizing: _____

_____

_____

o. Self-disclosing: _____

_____

_____

p. Confronting: _____

_____

_____

• Certain communication techniques can hin-
der or damage professional relationships.
These techniques are referred to as *nonthera-
peutic*. Briefly explain the following nonthera-
peutic techniques.

a. Asking personal questions. _____

_____

_____

b. Giving personal opinions: _____

_____

c. Changing the subject: _____

_____

d. Automatic responses: _____

_____

e. False reassurance: _____

_____

_____

f. Sympathy: _____

_____

g. Asking for explanations: _____

_____

h. Approval or disapproval: _____

_____

_____

i. Defensive responses: _____

_____

_____

j. Passive or aggressive responses: _____

_____

_____

k. Arguing: _____

_____

_____

• Briefly identify the communication techniques
to use with the client with special needs.

a. Clients who cannot speak clearly: _____

_____

_____

b. Clients who are cognitively impaired: _____

_____

_____

c. Clients who are unresponsive: _____

_____

_____

d. Clients who do not speak English: _____

_____

_____

Evaluation

- List four expected outcomes for the client with impaired communication.

a. _____

b. _____

c. _____

d. _____

Review Questions

The student should select the appropriate answer and cite the rationale for choosing that particular answer.

1. In demonstrating the method for deep-breathing exercises, the nurse places his or her hands on the client's abdomen to explain diaphragmatic movement. This technique involves the use of which communication element?
   a. Feedback
   b. Tactile channel
   c. Referent
   d. Message

Answer: _____ Rationale: _____

_____

_____

2. Which statement about nonverbal communication is correct?
   a. It is easy for a nurse to judge the meaning of a client's facial expression.
   b. The nurse's verbal messages should be reinforced by nonverbal cues.

c. The physical appearance of the nurse rarely influences nurse-client interaction.
   d. Words convey meanings that are usually more significant than nonverbal communication.

Answer: _____ Rationale: _____

_____

_____

3. The term referring to the sender's attitude toward the self, the message, and the listener is:
   a. Nonverbal communication
   b. Metacommunication
   c. Connotative meaning
   d. Denotative meaning

Answer: _____ Rationale: _____

_____

_____

4. The referent in the communication process is:
   a. That which motivates the communication
   b. The means of conveying messages
   c. Information shared by the sender
   d. The person who initiates the communication

Answer: _____ Rationale: _____

_____

_____

5. The nurse is conducting an admission interview with the client. To maintain the client's territoriality and maximize communication, the nurse should sit:
   a. 0 to 18 inches from the client
   b. 18 inches to 4 feet from the client
   c. 4 to 12 feet from the client
   d. 12 feet or more from the client

Answer: _____ Rationale: _____

_____

_____

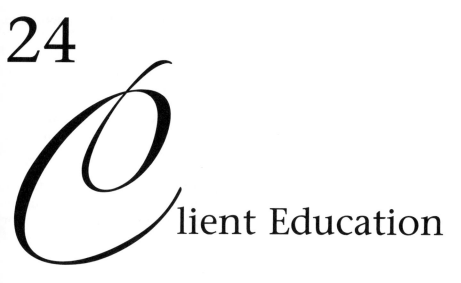

24

Client Education

Preliminary Reading

Chapter 24, pp. 448-475

Comprehensive Understanding

Standards for Client Education

- Briefly summarize the standards for client and family education (JCAHO, 1998).

    a. Standard 1: _____

    _____

    b. Standard 2: _____

    _____

    c. Standard 3: _____

    _____

    d. Standard 4: _____

    _____

- Evidence of successful client education must be noted in the client's medical record.

Purposes of Client Education

- Comprehensive client education includes three important purposes, each involving a separate phase of health care.

Maintenance and Promotion of Health and Illness Prevention

- The nurse is a visible, competent resource for clients intent on improving their physical and psychological well-being. In the school, home, clinic, or workplace, the nurse provides information and skills that will allow clients to practice healthier behaviors.

- Promoting healthy behaviors through education increases self-esteem by allowing clients to assume more responsibility for their health.

- Greater knowledge can result in better health maintenance habits.

Restoration of Health

- Injured or ill clients need information and skills that will help them regain or maintain their levels of health.

- The family is a vital part of a client's return to health, and family members may need as much information as the client.

- The nurse should not assume that the family should be involved and must first assess the client-family relationship.

Coping with Impaired Functioning

- In the case of a serious disability, the client's family role may change, making understanding and acceptance by family members necessary.

- The family's ability to provide support can result from education, which begins as soon as the client's needs are identified and the family displays a willingness to help.

Teaching and Learning

- Define the following.

  a. *Teaching:* _____

  _____

  b. *Learning:* _____

  _____

- Teaching is most effective when it responds to a learner's needs.

- Interpersonal communication is essential for successful teaching.

Role of the Nurse in Teaching and Learning

- The nurse has an ethical responsibility to teach his or her clients.

- The nurse clarifies information provided by physicians and may become the primary source of information for adjusting to health problems.

Teaching as Communication

- The teaching process closely parallels the communication process.

- A learning objective is: _____

  _____

  _____

- Define the following terms in relation to the teaching-learning process.

  a. *Referent:* _____

  _____

  b. *Sender:* _____

  _____

  c. *Message:* _____

  _____

  d. *Channels:* _____

  _____

  e. *Receiver:* _____

  _____

  f. *Feedback:* _____

  _____

Domains of Learning

- Learning occurs in (understandings), (attitudes), and (motor skills) domains.

- The characteristics of learning within each domain affect the teaching and evaluation methods used.

Cognitive Learning

- Bloom (1956) classifies cognitive behaviors in an ordered hierarchy. Summarize each one.

  a. Knowledge: _____

  _____

  b. Comprehension: _____

  _____

  c. Application: _____

  _____

  d. Analysis: _____

  _____

  e. Synthesis: _____

  _____

  f. Evaluation: _____

  _____

Affective Learning

- Affective learning deals with the expression of feelings and the acceptance of attitudes, opinions, and values.

- Summarize the following hierarchy behaviors.

  a. Receiving: _____

  _____

  _____

  b. Responding: _____

  _____

  _____

  c. Valuing: _____

  _____

  _____

  d. Organizing: _____

  _____

  _____

  e. Characterizing: _____

  _____

  _____

Psychomotor Learning

Psychomotor learning involves acquiring skills that require the integration of mental and muscular activity.

- Summarize the following hierarchy behaviors.

  a. Perception: _____

  _____

  _____

  b. Set: _____

  _____

  _____

  c. Guided response: _____

  _____

  _____

  d. Mechanism: _____

  _____

  _____

  e. Complex overt response: _____

  _____

  _____

  f. Adaptation: _____

  _____

  _____

  g. Origination: _____

  _____

  _____

Basic Learning Principles

- Learning depends on the motivation to learn, the ability to learn, and the learning environment.

- The ability to learn depends on _____,

  _____, _____, and

  _____.

Motivation to Learn

- An attentional set is: _____

  _____

  _____

- Briefly explain how the following distractions influence the ability to learn.

  a. Physical discomfort: _____

  b. Anxiety: _____

  c. Environment: _____

- Motivation is: _____

  _____

  _____

- Briefly explain how the following can affect motivation.

  a. Social mastery: _____

  _____

  b. Task mastery: _____

  _____

  c. Physical mastery: _____

  _____

- Compliance is: _____

  _____

  _____

- Self-efficacy is: _____

  _____

  _____

- The process of grieving gives clients time to adapt psychologically to the emotional and physical implications of illness.

- Readiness to learn is significantly related to the stage of grieving.

- When the client enters the stage of acceptance, which is compatible with learning, the nurse introduces a teaching plan.

- Teaching continues as long as the client remains in a stage conducive to learning.

- The client is not seen as a passive recipient or consumer of health care and education but as an active partner in the provision of care.

Ability to Learn
- Summarize how each of the following influence the ability to learn.

  a. Developmental capability: _____

  _____

  _____

  b. Learning in children: _____

  _____

  _____

  c. Adult learning: _____

  _____

  _____

  d. Physical capability: _____

  _____

  _____

Learning Environment
- Factors in the physical environment where teaching takes place can make learning pleasant or difficult. List five factors to consider when selecting the learning setting.

  a. _____

  b. _____

  c. _____

  d. _____

  e. _____

Integrating the Nursing and Teaching Processes

- The nurse sets specific learning objectives and implements the teaching plan using teaching and learning principles to ensure: _____

  _____

  _____

- The nursing and teaching processes are not the same. The nursing process requires: _____

  _____

  _____

- The teaching process focuses on: _____

  _____

  _____

𝒩𝒫 Assessment

- The client requires the nurse to assess the following factors. Summarize each one.

Learning Needs

a. _____

b. _____

c. _____

d. _____

Motivation to Learn

a. _____

b. _____

c. _____

d. _____

e. _____

f. _____

g. _____

h. _____

i. _____

Ability to Learn

a. _____

b. _____

c. _____

d. _____

Teaching Environment

a. _____

b. _____

c. _____

Resources for Learning

a. _____

b. _____

c. _____

d. _____

e. _____

Nursing Diagnosis

- Classifying diagnoses by the three learning domains helps the nurse focus specifically on subject matter and teaching methods.

Planning

- After determining the nursing diagnoses that identify a client's learning needs, the nurse develops a teaching plan, determines goals and expected outcomes, and involves the client in selecting learning experiences. Expected outcomes guide the: _____

_____

_____

- A learning objective identifies the _____ of a planned learning experience and helps _____ for learning.

- A learning objective includes the same criteria as goals or outcomes in a nursing care plan. These are:

  a. _____

  b. _____

  c. _____

  d. _____

- The principles of teaching are techniques that incorporate the principles of learning. Explain the following principles.

  a. Setting priorities: _____

  _____

  b. Timing: _____

  _____

  _____

  c. Organizing teaching material: _____

  _____

  _____

d. Maintaining learning attention and participation: _____

_____

_____

e. Building on existing knowledge: _____

_____

_____

f. Selection of teaching methods: _____

_____

_____

g. Availability of teaching resources: _____

_____

_____

h. Writing teaching plans: _____

_____

_____

Implementation

- Briefly explain the following teaching approaches.

  a. Telling: _____

  _____

  b. Selling: _____

  _____

  c. Participating: _____

  _____

  d. Entrusting: _____

  _____

  e. Reinforcing: _____

  _____

- Summarize the following instructional methods.

  a. One-to-one discussion: _____

  _____

  b. Group instruction: _____

  _____

c. Preparatory instruction: _____

_____

d. Demonstrations: _____

_____

e. Analogies: _____

_____

f. Role playing: _____

_____

g. Discovery: _____

_____

- Identify some teaching tools to be used with the following.

  a. Functional disability: _____

  _____

  b. Illiteracy: _____

  _____

  c. Cultural diversity: _____

  _____

  d. Children's needs: _____

  _____

  e. Older adults: _____

  _____

Evaluation

- Evaluation reinforces correct behavior by the learner, helps learners realize how they should change incorrect behavior, and helps the teacher determine the adequacy of teaching.

- Identify some evaluation measures. _____

_____

_____

- List the three areas to be included when documenting client teaching.

  a. _____

  b. _____

  c. _____

Review Questions

The student should select the appropriate answer and cite the rationale for choosing that particular answer.

1. An internal impulse that causes a person to take action is:
   a. Anxiety
   b. Motivation
   c. Compliance
   d. Adaptation

   Answer: _____ Rationale: _____

   _____

   _____

2. Demonstration of the principles of body mechanics used when transferring clients from bed to chair would be classified under which domain of learning?
   a. Cognitive
   b. Social
   c. Psychomotor
   d. Affective

   Answer: _____ Rationale: _____

   _____

   _____

3. Which of the following clients is most ready to begin a patient-teaching session?
   a. Ms. Hernandez, who is unwilling to accept that her back injury may result in permanent paralysis
   b. Mr. Frank, a newly diagnosed diabetic, who is complaining that he was awake all night because of his noisy roommate
   c. Mrs. Brown, a client with irritable bowel syndrome, who has just returned from a morning of testing in the GI lab
   d. Mr. Jones, a client who had a heart attack 4 days ago and now seems somewhat anxious about how this will affect his future

   Answer: _____ Rationale: _____

   _____

   _____

4. The nurse works with pediatric clients who have diabetes. Which is the youngest age group to which the nurse can effectively teach psychomotor skills such as insulin administration?
   a. Toddler
   b. Adolescent
   c. School-age
   d. Preschool

   Answer: _____ Rationale: _____

   _____

   _____

5. Which of the following is an appropriately stated learning objective for Mr. Ryan, a newly diagnosed diabetic?
   a. Mr. Ryan will be taught self-administration of insulin by 5/2.
   b. Mr. Ryan will perform blood glucose monitoring with the EZ-Check Monitor by the time of discharge.
   c. Mr. Ryan will know the signs and symptoms of low blood sugar by 5/5.
   d. Mr. Ryan will understand diabetes.

   Answer: _____ Rationale: _____

   _____

   _____

Chapter 24: Client Education 121

25

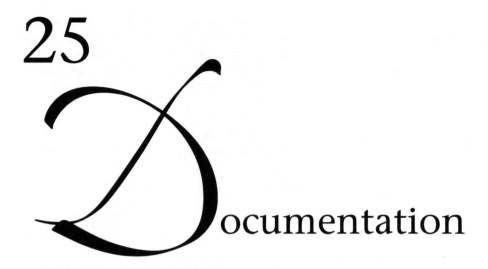

$\mathcal{D}$ocumentation

$\mathcal{P}$reliminary Reading

Chapter 25, pp. 476-497

$\mathcal{C}$omprehensive Understanding

- Define the following terms.

    a. *Documentation:* _____

    b. *Accreditation:* _____

    c. *Diagnosis-related group (DRG):* _____

Confidentiality

- Explain the new rights for patients related to HIPAA.

    a. _____

    b. _____

    c. _____

    d. _____

Standards

Multidisciplinary Communication Within the Health Care Team

- Caregivers use a variety of ways to exchange information about clients. Briefly explain the following.

    a. Client record: _____

    _____

    b. Reports: _____

    _____

Purposes of Records

- Briefly explain the following purposes of a record.

  a. Communication: _____

  b. Legal documentation: _____

  c. Financial billing: _____

  d. Education: _____

  e. Nursing process: _____

  f. Research: _____

  g. Auditing: _____

Guidelines for Quality Documentation and Reporting

- Five important guidelines must be followed to ensure quality documentation and reporting. Explain each one.

  a. Factual: _____
  _____

  b. Accurate: _____
  _____

  c. Complete: _____
  _____

  d. Current: _____
  _____

  e. Organized: _____
  _____

Methods of Recording

- Narrative documentation is a storylike format that documents information specific to client conditions and nursing care. The disadvantages of this style are:

  a. _____

  b. _____

  c. _____

- Problem-oriented medical records (POMR) place emphasis on the client's problems. The method corresponds to the nursing process and facilitates communication of client needs. Explain the following major sections of the POMR.

  a. Database: _____
  _____

  b. Problem list: _____
  _____

  c. Care plan: _____
  _____

  d. Progress notes: _____
  _____

- Focus charting or DAR includes: _____
  _____
  _____

- Briefly explain the POMR forms of documentation.

  a. SOAP notes: _____
  _____

  b. PIE format: _____
  _____

  c. DAR: _____

- Briefly explain these forms of documentation.

  a. Source records: _____
  _____

  b. Charting by exception: _____
  _____

  c. Case management and critical pathways:
  _____
  _____

Common Record-Keeping Forms

- Briefly explain the following formats used for record keeping.

  a. Admission nursing history forms: _____
  _____
  _____

  b. Flow sheets and graphic records: _____
  _____
  _____

c. Nursing Kardex: _____

_____

_____

d. Acuity recording systems: _____

_____

_____

e. Standardized care plans: _____

_____

_____

f. Discharge summary forms: _____

_____

_____

- The JCAHO has established the following standards for client education.

a. _____

b. _____

c. _____

d. _____

e. _____

f. _____

g. _____

Home Health Care Documentation
- Documentation in the home health care system has different implications than it does in other areas of nursing. The primary difference is: _____

_____

_____

- Documentation is both quality control and justification for reimbursement from Medicare, Medicaid, or private insurance companies.

- The nurse is the pivotal person in the documentation of home health care delivery.

Long-Term Health Care Documentation
- Long-term care documentation supports a multidisciplinary approach in the _____ and _____ process.

Computerized Documentation
- Explain the many benefits of computerized documentation. _____

_____

_____

Reporting

- Nurses communicate information about clients so that all members of the health care team can make informed decisions about the client and his or her care.

Change-of-Shift Reports
- Identify the eight major areas to include in a change-of-shift report.

a. _____

b. _____

c. _____

d. _____

e. _____

f. _____

g. _____

h. _____

Telephone Reports
- It is important that information in a telephone report be clear, accurate, and concise.

Telephone or Verbal Orders
- List the guidelines the nurse should follow when receiving telephone orders from physicians.

a. _____

b. _____

c. _____

d. _____

e. _____

f. _____

Transfer Reports

- List the nine major information areas in a transfer report.

a. _____

b. _____

c. _____

d. _____

e. _____

f. _____

g. _____

h. _____

i. _____

Incident Reports

- Define the purpose of an incident report.

_____

_____

$\mathcal{R}$eview Questions

The student should select the appropriate answer and cite the rationale for choosing that particular answer.

1. The primary purpose of a client's medical record is to:
   a. Satisfy requirements of accreditation agencies
   b. Communicate accurate, timely information about the client
   c. Provide validation for hospital charges
   d. Provide the nurse with a defense against malpractice

Answer: _____ Rationale: _____

_____

_____

2. Which of the following is correctly charted according to the six guidelines for quality recording?
   a. "Respirations rapid; lung sounds clear."
   b. "Was depressed today."
   c. "Crying. States she doesn't want visitors to see her like this."
   d. "Had a good day. Up and about in room."

Answer: _____ Rationale: _____

_____

_____

3. During a change-of-shift report:
   a. Two or more nurses always visit all clients to review their plan of care.
   b. Nurses should exchange judgments they have made about client attitudes.
   c. The nurse should identify nursing diagnoses and clarify client priorities.
   d. Client information is communicated from a nurse on a sending unit to a nurse on a receiving unit.

Answer: _____ Rationale: _____

_____

_____

4. An incident report is:
   a. A legal claim against a nurse for negligent nursing care
   b. A summary report of all falls occurring on a nursing unit
   c. A report of an event inconsistent with the routine care of a client
   d. A report of a nurse's behavior submitted to the hospital administration

Answer: _____ Rationale: _____

_____

_____

5. If an error is made while recording, the nurse should:
   a. Erase it or scratch it out
   b. Obtain a new nurse's note and rewrite the entries
   c. Leave a blank space in the note
   d. Draw a single line through the error and initial it

Answer: _____ Rationale: _____

_____

_____

26

*S*elf-Concept

*P*reliminary Reading

Chapter 26, pp. 500-521

*C*omprehensive Understanding

Self-Concept

- Each stage of development has specific activities that assist the client in developing a positive self-concept. Identify some activities for each stage.

a. 0 to 1 year: _____
_____
_____

b. 1 to 3 years: _____
_____
_____

c. 3 to 6 years: _____
_____
_____

d. 6 to 12 years: _____
_____
_____

e. 12 to 20 years: _____
_____
_____

f. Mid-20s to mid-40s: _____

_____

_____

g. Mid-40s to mid-60s: _____

_____

_____

h. Late 60s on: _____

_____

_____

Nursing Knowledge Base

Development of Self-Concept

- The four components of self-concept are

_____, _____,

_____, and _____.

- Self-concept is a dynamic perception that is based on the following.

a. _____

b. _____

c. _____

d. _____

e. _____

f. _____

g. _____

h. _____

i. _____

- A healthy self-concept has a high degree of stability and generates positive or negative feelings toward the self.

- Briefly explain the four significant components of self-concept.

a. Identity: _____

_____

_____

_____

b. Body image: _____

_____

_____

_____

c. Self-esteem: _____

_____

_____

_____

d. Role performance: _____

_____

_____

_____

- List the processes through which a child learns appropriate behaviors.

a. _____

b. _____

c. _____

d. _____

e. _____

Stressors Affecting Self-Concept

- Stressors challenge a person's adaptive capacities.

- A self-concept stressor is any: _____

_____

_____

- Being able to adapt to stressors is likely to lead to a positive sense of self, whereas failure to adapt often leads to a negative sense of self.

- Any change in health can be a stressor that affects self-concept.

- A physical change in the body leads to an altered body image. Identity and self-esteem can also be affected.

- A crisis occurs when a person cannot overcome obstacles with the usual methods of problem solving and adapting.

- *Identity* is defined as: _____

_____

_____

- Stressors throughout life affect identity. Give an example of a stressor for each developmental stage.

  a. Adolescence: _____

  _____

  b. Adulthood: _____

  _____

  c. Retirement: _____

  _____

- Changes in the appearance, structure, or function of a body part will require change in body image. Identify at least five stressors that affect body image.

  a. _____
  b. _____
  c. _____
  d. _____
  e. _____

- Transitions within one's roles may lead to the following. Explain.

  a. Role conflict: _____

  _____

  b. Role ambiguity: _____

  _____

  c. Role strain: _____

  _____

  d. Role overload: _____

  _____

  e. Self-esteem stressors: _____

  _____

  f. High self-esteem: _____

  _____

  g. Low self-esteem: _____

  _____

Family Effect on Self-Concept Development

- The family plays a key role in creating and maintaining its members' self-concepts.

- Children learn from their parents and siblings a basic sense of who they are and how they are expected to live.

The Nurse's Effect on the Client's Self-Concept

- A nurse's acceptance of a client with an altered self-concept helps stimulate positive rehabilitation.

- List five areas the nurse must clarify and assess about him-or herself in order to promote a positive self-concept in clients.

  a. _____
  b. _____
  c. _____
  d. _____
  e. _____

Self-Concept and the Nursing Process

Assessment

- In assessing self-concept, the nurse should focus on each component of self-concept (_____, _____, _____, and _____); behaviors suggestive of an altered self-concept; actual and potential self-concept stressors; and _____ patterns.

- Much of the data regarding self-concept are most effectively gathered through observation of a client's nonverbal behavior and by paying attention to the content of the client's conversation rather than through direct questioning.

- The nursing assessment should include consideration of previous coping behaviors: the _____, _____, and _____ of the stressors; and the client's _____ and _____ resources.

- As the nurse identifies previous coping patterns it is useful to consider if these patterns have contributed to healthy functioning or created more problems.

- Exploring resources and strengths, such as helpful significant others or prior use of community resources, can be important in formulating a realistic and effective plan.

- Asking the client how he or she believes interventions will make a difference in the problem can provide useful information regarding the client's expectations and provide an opportunity to discuss the client's goals. Give an example. _____

_____

_____

Nursing Diagnosis

- Accurate development of a nursing diagnosis requires discussing the problem with the client and the family.

- Before involving the family, the nurse needs to consider the _____ and

_____.

Planning

- The nurse, client, and family need to plan care directed at helping the client regain or maintain a healthy self-concept.

- Interventions focus on helping the client and on coping methods.

- The nurse looks for strengths in both the individual and the family and provides resources and education to turn limitations into strengths.

Implementation

Promoting a Healthy Self-Concept

Health Promotion

- List some healthy lifestyle measures that contribute to a healthy self-concept. _____

_____

_____

Acute Care

- In acute care, the nurse is likely to encounter clients who are experiencing _____ to their self-concept due to the nature of the treatment and diagnostic procedure.

- Identify ways a nurse can assist a client in the adjustment to a change in physical appearance.

_____

_____

_____

Restorative Care

- Identify goals to help a client attain a more positive self-concept.

   a. _____

   b. _____

   c. _____

   d. _____

   e. _____

- Identify seven nursing interventions for the client to engage in self-exploration.

   a. _____

   b. _____

   c. _____

   d. _____

   e. _____

   f. _____

   g. _____

Evaluation

- Client care evaluates the actual care delivered by the health team based on expected outcomes. Briefly explain the expected outcomes for a self-concept disturbance. _____

_____

_____

_____

- Client expectations evaluate care from the client's perspective. Give an example. _____

_____

_____

_____

Review Questions

The student should select the appropriate answer and cite the rationale for choosing that particular answer.

1. Which developmental stage is particularly crucial for identity development?
   a. Infancy
   b. Preschool age
   c. Adolescence
   d. Young adult

Answer: _____ Rationale: _____

_____

_____

2. Which of the following statements about body image is correct?
   a. Physical changes are quickly incorporated into a person's body image.
   b. Body image refers only to the external appearance of a person's body.
   c. Body image is a combination of a person's actual and perceived (ideal) body.
   d. Perceptions by other persons have no influence on a person's body image.

Answer: _____ Rationale: _____

_____

_____

3. Robert, who is 2 years old, is praised for using his potty instead of wetting his pants. This is an example of learning a behavior by:
   a. Identification
   b. Imitation
   c. Substitution
   d. Reinforcement-extinction

Answer: _____ Rationale: _____

_____

_____

4. Mrs. Watson has just undergone a radical mastectomy. The nurse is aware that Mrs. Watson will probably have considerable anxiety over:
   a. Role performance
   b. Self-identity
   c. Body image
   d. Self-esteem

Answer: _____ Rationale: _____

_____

_____

5. Which of the following statements demonstrates that the nurse's self-concept is positively affecting the client?
   a. "You've got to take a more active part in caring for your ostomy."
   b. "I know your ostomy is difficult to look at, but you will get used to it in time."
   c. (While grimacing) "Ostomy care isn't so bad."
   d. "Let me show you how to place the bag on your stoma."

Answer: _____ Rationale: _____

_____

_____

Critical Thinking Model for Nursing Care Plan Alterations in Self-Concept

Imagine that you are the student nurse, Jan, in the Care Plan on page 515 of your text. Complete the *Assessment phase* of the critical thinking model by writing in the appropriate boxes of the model on p. 132. Think about the following.

- In developing Mr. Johnson's plan of care, what knowledge did Jan apply?

- In what way might Jan's previous experience apply in this case?

- What intellectual or professional standards were applied to Mr. Johnson?

- What critical thinking attitudes did you use in assessing Mr. Johnson?

- As you review your assessment, what key areas did you cover?

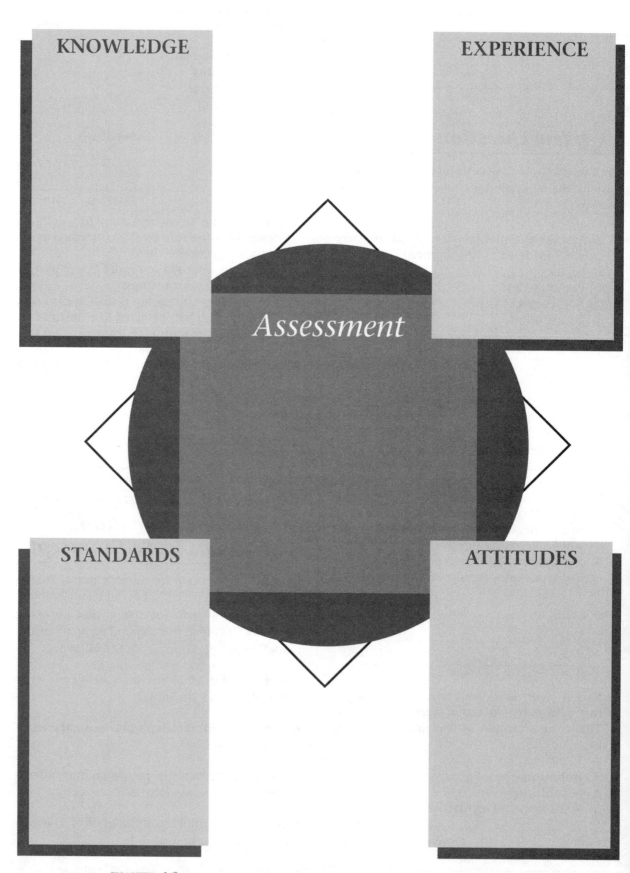

KNOWLEDGE

EXPERIENCE

Assessment

STANDARDS

ATTITUDES

CHAPTER 26 Critical Thinking Model for Nursing Care Plan for *Alterations in Self-Concept*

See answers on page 534.

27

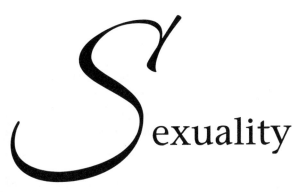

Sexuality

Preliminary Reading

Chapter 27, pp. 522-542

Comprehensive Understanding

Scientific Knowledge Base

Sexual Development

- Each stage of development brings changes in sexual functioning and the role of sexuality in relationships. Explain each stage.

  a. Infancy and early childhood: _____

  _____

  b. School-age: _____

  _____

  c. Puberty/adolescence: _____

  _____

  d. Young adulthood: _____

  _____

  e. Middle adulthood: _____

  _____

  f. Older adulthood: _____

  _____

Sexual Response Cycle
- The three phases of the sexual response cycle

  are _____, _____,

  and_____.

- These phases are the result of vasocongestion and myotonia. Explain each of these physiological responses.

  a. Female: _____

  _____

  b. Male: _____

  _____

Sexual Orientation
- *Sexual orientation* is defined as: _____

  _____

  _____

- Human sexual orientation is a continuum

  between _____ and

  _____ orientations.

Contraception
- There are numerous contraceptive options available. Briefly list the options available under the following categories.

  a. Nonprescriptive methods: _____

  _____

  _____

  b. Methods requiring a health care provider:

  _____

  _____

  _____

Sexually Transmitted Diseases
- The highest prevalence is among

  _____ and _____.

- List the prevalent STDs.

  a. _____

  b. _____

  c. _____

  d. _____

  e. _____

- Identify the primary routes of HIV transmission. _____

  _____

  _____

- Those primarily vulnerable to HIV infec-

  tions are _____, _____,

  _____, and _____.

Nursing Knowledge Base

Sociocultural Dimensions of Sexuality
- Global cultural diversity creates considerable variability in sexual norms and represents a wide spectrum of beliefs and values.

- Common areas of diversity include the following.

  a. _____

  b. _____

  c. _____

  d. _____

  e. _____

  f. _____

- Briefly summarize the impact of pregnancy

  and menstruation on sexuality. _____

  _____

  _____

- Identify the issues regarding the difficulty the nurse has in discussing sexuality with clients.

  a. _____

  b. _____

  c. _____

  d. _____

Decisional Issues
- Briefly discuss the following decisional issues.

  a. Contraception: _____

  _____

  _____

  b. Abortion: _____

  _____

  _____

  c. STD prevention: _____

  _____

  _____

Alterations in Sexual Health
- Explain the following issues.

  a. Infertility: _____

  _____

  _____

  b. Sexual abuse: _____

  _____

  _____

  c. Personal and emotional conflicts: _____

  _____

  _____

  d. Sexual dysfunction: _____

  _____

  _____

Sexuality and the Nursing Process

- A person's sexuality has physical, psychological, social, and cultural elements.

Assessment
- Briefly explain the following factors that affect sexuality.

  a. Physical: _____

  _____

  _____

  _____

  b. Self-concept: _____

  _____

  _____

  _____

  c. Relationship: _____

  _____

  _____

  _____

  d. Self-esteem: _____

  _____

  _____

  _____

- List the questions a nurse may use to elicit a brief sexual history from an adult.

  a. _____

  b. _____

  c. _____

  d. _____

- Explain how the nurse is able to anticipate when a client is at risk for sexual dysfunction.

  _____

  _____

  _____

- Briefly explain the physical assessment in evaluating the cause of sexual concerns or problems.

    a. Female: _____

    _____

    b. Male: _____

    _____

Nursing Diagnosis

- Identify clues that may signal risk for or an actual nursing diagnosis related to sexuality.

    a. _____

    b. _____

    c. _____

    d. _____

    e. _____

Planning

- The PLISSIT model developed by Annon (1976) guides the planning phases. Explain each of the following.

    a. P: _____

    b. LI: _____

    c. SS: _____

    d. IT: _____

Implementation

Health Promotion

- Topics of education vary, depending on the defining characteristics and related factors. Describe some situations. _____

    _____

    _____

    _____

    _____

    _____

Acute Care

- Nursing interventions that address alterations in sexuality are aimed at _____,

    _____, and/or

    _____.

- The client should be encouraged to investigate and acknowledge social and ethical values and analyze the role of sexuality in his or her self-concept.

- Identify situational and developmental crises that prompt education. _____

    _____

    _____

    _____

    _____

    _____

Restorative Care

- In the home it is important to assist individuals in creating an environment comfortable for sexual activity.

- In the long-term care setting, facilities should make proper arrangements for privacy during resident's sexual experiences.

Evaluation

- Client care evaluates the actual care delivered by the health care team based on the expected outcomes.

- Client or spouse verbalizations determine if goals and outcomes have been achieved.

- Sexuality is felt more than observed, and sexual expression requires an intimacy not amenable to observation.

- All people involved may need to be reminded of the individual nature of sexual expression and the multiple factors that affect perceptions and responses.

- Client expectations evaluate care from the client's perspective. Briefly explain the client's perspective. _____

_____

_____

_____

_____

$\mathcal{R}$eview Questions

The student should select the appropriate answer and cite the rationale for choosing that particular answer.

1. At what developmental stage is it particularly important for children reared in single-parent families to be exposed to same-sex adults?
   a. Infancy
   b. Toddlerhood and preschool years
   c. School-age
   d. Adolescence

Answer: _____ Rationale: _____

_____

_____

2. In the school-age child, learning and reinforcement of gender-appropriate behaviors are most commonly derived from:
   a. Parents
   b. Teachers
   c. Siblings
   d. Peers

Answer: _____ Rationale: _____

_____

_____

3. Which statement about sexual response in the older adult is correct?
   a. The resolution phase is slower.
   b. The orgasm phase is prolonged.
   c. The plateau phase is prolonged.
   d. The refractory phase is more rapid.

Answer: _____ Rationale: _____

_____

_____

4. The least effective means of preventing pregnancy is:
   a. Coitus interruptus
   b. Calendar (rhythm) method
   c. Body temperature method
   d. Mucus method

Answer: _____ Rationale: _____

_____

_____

5. The only 100% effective method to avoid contracting a disease through sex is:
   a. Using condoms
   b. Avoiding sex with partners at risk
   c. Knowing the sexual partner's health history
   d. Abstinence

Answer: _____ Rationale: _____

_____

_____

Critical Thinking Model for Nursing Care Plan for Sexual Dysfunction

Imagine that you are Jack, the nurse in the Care Plan on page 536 of your text. Complete the *Assessment phase* of the critical thinking model by writing your answers in the appropriate boxes of the model shown. Think about the following.

- In developing Mr. Clement's plan of care, what knowledge did Jack apply?

- In what way might Jack's previous experience assist in this case?

- What intellectual or professional standards were applied to Mr. Clement?

- What critical thinking attitudes did you utilize in assessing Mr. Clement?

- As you review your assessment, what key areas did you cover?

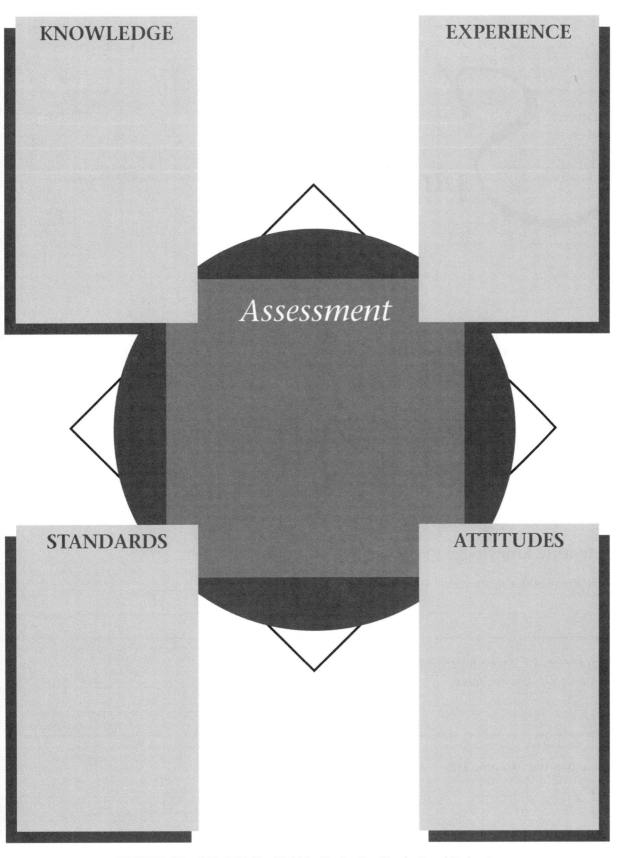

KNOWLEDGE

EXPERIENCE

Assessment

STANDARDS

ATTITUDES

CHAPTER 27 Critical Thinking Model for Nursing Care Plan for *Sexual Dysfunction*

See answers on page 535.

28

Spiritual Health

Preliminary Reading

Chapter 28, pp. 543-566

Comprehensive Understanding

- Spirituality is: _____
  _____
  _____

Scientific Knowledge Base

- Summarize the relationship of spirituality and healing. _____
  _____
  _____

Framework of Systemic Organization
- Briefly explain this model. _____
  _____
  _____

- Identify the two processes to achieve control.

  a. _____

  b. _____

- Define the system processes that an individual uses to strive for spirituality.

  a. Coherence: _____

  b. Individuation: _____

Traditional Concepts in Spiritual Health

- The concepts of _____, _____, _____, and _____ give direction in understanding the views each individual has of life and its value.

- Individuals' definitions of spirituality are influenced by their own _____, _____, _____, and _____.

- Identify the two important characteristics of spirituality.

  a. _____

  b. _____

- Explain how the following view spirituality.

  a. Atheists: _____

  b. Agnostics: _____

- Explain the concept of faith. _____

_____

_____

- The belief that comes with faith involves _____, or an awareness of that which one cannot see or know in ordinary ways.

- Define *religion*. _____

_____

_____

- Religion serves different purposes in people's lives.

- Explain the differences between the terms spirituality and religion. _____

_____

_____

- Summarize the concept of hope. _____

_____

_____

Spiritual Problems

- Spiritual distress is: _____

_____

_____

- Briefly explain each of the following causes of spiritual distress.

  a. Acute illness: _____

  _____

  _____

  b. Chronic illness: _____

  _____

  _____

  c. Terminal illness: _____

  _____

  _____

  d. Near-death experience: _____

  _____

  _____

Nursing Process

- An element of quality health care is to exhibit caring for the client so that a relationship of trust forms. Trust is strengthened when the caregiver _____ and _____.

- Briefly explain shared community and compassion. _____

_____

_____

- It is important for nurses to sort out value judgments about other people's belief systems.

- The nurse must be willing to share and discover another person's meaning and purpose in life, sickness, and health.

𝒩𝒫 Assessment

- The assessment should focus on aspects of spirituality most likely to be influenced by life experiences, events, and questions in the case of illness and hospitalization.

- The JAREL spirituality well-being scale provides nurses and other health care professionals with a tool for assessing client's spiritual well-being. Briefly summarize the three dimensions.

  a. Faith/belief dimension: _____

  _____

  _____

  b. Life/self-responsibility: _____

  _____

  _____

  c. Life-satisfaction/self-actualization: _____

  _____

  _____

- Explain how the following can affect a client's spiritual health.

  a. Fellowship and community: _____

  _____

  _____

  b. Ritual and practice: _____

  _____

  _____

  c. Vocation: _____

  _____

  _____

𝒩𝒫 Nursing Diagnosis

- When reviewing a spiritual assessment and integrating the information into an appropriate nursing diagnosis, the nurse should consider the client's current health status from a holistic perspective, with spirituality as the unifying principle.

- State the defining characteristics for the following two diagnoses.

  a. Spiritual well-being: _____

  _____

  _____

  b. Spiritual distress: _____

  _____

  _____

𝒩𝒫 Planning

- In order to develop an individualized plan of care, the nurse integrates knowledge gathered from the assessment and relating to resources and therapies available for spiritual care.

- Identify the three goals for spiritual caregiving.

  a. _____

  b. _____

  c. _____

𝒩𝒫 Implementation

Health Promotion

- Spiritual care should be a central theme in promoting an individual's overall well-being.

- Briefly explain the following interventions and how they are helpful in maintaining or promoting a client's spiritual health.

  a. Establishing presence: _____

  _____

  _____

  b. Supporting a healing relationship: _____

  _____

  _____

Acute Care

- Within acute care settings, clients experience multiple stressors that threaten to overwhelm their coping resources.

- Explain how the following interventions are helpful in the client's therapeutic plan.

  a. Support systems: _____
  _____
  _____

  b. Diet therapies: _____
  _____
  _____

  c. Supporting rituals: _____
  _____
  _____

  d. Prayer: _____
  _____
  _____

  e. Meditation: _____
  _____
  _____

  f. Supporting grief work: _____
  _____
  _____

Evaluation

Client Care

- Client care evaluates the actual care delivered by the health team based on the expected outcomes. Give some examples.
  _____
  _____
  _____
  _____

Client Expectations

- A client's expectation evaluates care from the client perspective. Give some examples.
  _____
  _____
  _____
  _____

Review Questions

The student should select the appropriate answer and cite the rationale for choosing that particular answer.

1. When planning care to include spiritual needs for a client of the Moslem faith, the religious practices the nurse should understand include all of the following *except:*
   a. A priest must be present to conduct rituals.
   b. Strength is gained through group prayer.
   c. Family members are a source of comfort.
   d. Faith healing provides psychological support.

   Answer: _____ Rationale: _____
   _____
   _____

2. When consulting with the dietary department regarding meals for a client of the Hindu religion, which of the following dietary items would not be included on the meal trays?
   a. Meats
   b. Dairy products
   c. Vegetable entrees
   d. Fruits

   Answer: _____ Rationale: _____
   _____
   _____

3. If an Islamic client dies, the nurse should be aware of what religious practice?
   a. Only relatives and friends may touch the body.
   b. Members of a ritual burial society cleanse the body.
   c. Last rites are mandatory.
   d. The body is always cremated.

   Answer: _____ Rationale: _____
   _____
   _____

Chapter 28: Spiritual Health   143

4. If a nurse were to use a nursing diagnosis to relate concerns about spiritual health, which of the following would be used?
   a. Spiritual distress
   b. Inability to adjust
   c. Lack of faith
   d. Religious dilemma

Answer: _____ Rationale: _____

_____

_____

5. Mr. Phillips was recently diagnosed with a malignant tumor. The staff had observed him crying on several occasions, and now he cries as he reads from his Bible. Interventions to help Mr. Phillips cope with his illness would include:
   a. Asking the hospital chaplain to visit him daily
   b. Engaging Mr. Phillips in diversional activities to reduce feelings of hopelessness
   c. Supporting his use of inner resources by providing time for meditation
   d. Praying with Mr. Phillips as often as possible

Answer: _____ Rationale: _____

_____

_____

Critical Thinking Model for Nursing Care Plan for Spiritual Well-Being

Imagine that you are Leah, the nurse in the Care Plan on page 558 of your text. Complete the *Planning phase* of the critical thinking model by writing your answers in the appropriate boxes of the model shown. Think about the following.

- In developing James' plan of care, what knowledge did Leah apply?

- In what way might Leah's previous experience assist in developing a plan of care for James?

- When developing a plan of care, what intellectual and professional standards were applied?

- What critical thinking attitudes might have been applied developing James' plan?

- How will Leah accomplish the goals?

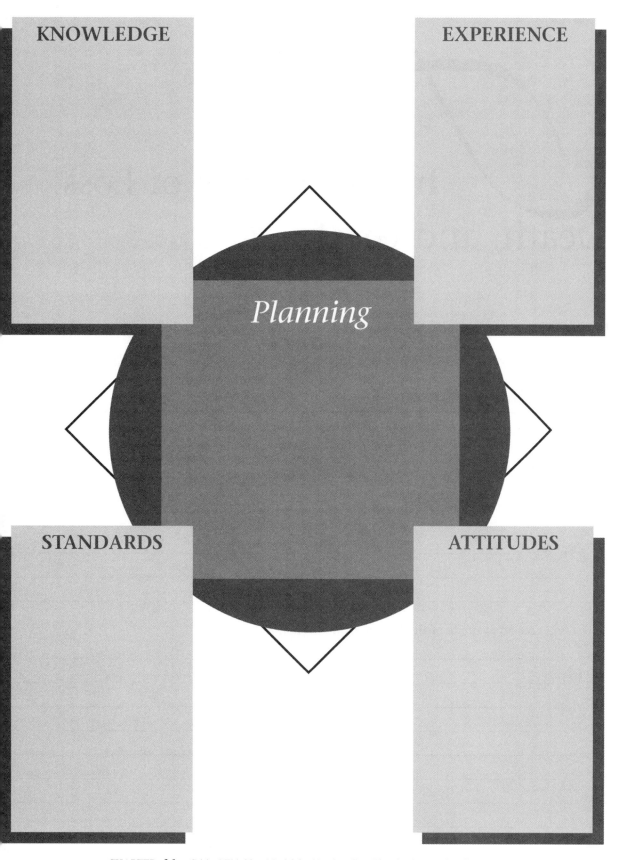

KNOWLEDGE

EXPERIENCE

Planning

STANDARDS

ATTITUDES

CHAPTER 28   Critical Thinking Model for Nursing Care Plan for *Spiritual Well-Being*

See answers on page 536.

29

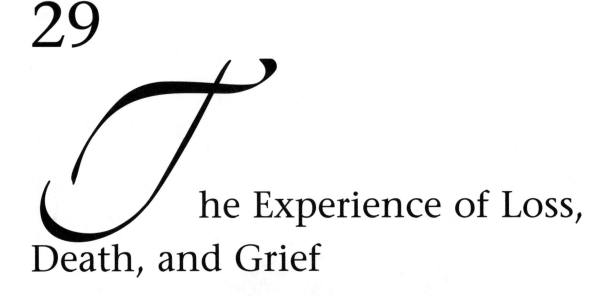

The Experience of Loss, Death, and Grief

Preliminary Reading

Chapter 29, pp. 567-594

Comprehensive Understanding

Scientific Knowledge Base

Loss

- Define *loss*. _____

  _____

  _____

- List and give an example of the five categories of loss.

  a. _____

  _____

  b. _____

  _____

  c. _____

  _____

  d. _____

  _____

  e. _____

  _____

Grief

• Describe the following terms.

a. Grief: _____

b. Mourning: _____

c. Bereavement: _____

Theories of the Grieving Process

• List the phases of the grieving process proposed by each of the theorists listed below.

Kübler-Ross's Stages of Dying

a. _____

b. _____

c. _____

d. _____

e. _____

Bowler's Phases of Mourning

a. _____

b. _____

c. _____

d. _____

e. _____

Worden's Four Tasks of Mourning

a. _____

b. _____

c. _____

d. _____

e. _____

• Briefly describe the following types of grief.

a. Normal grief: _____
_____

b. Anticipatory grief: _____
_____

c. Complicated grief: _____
_____

d. Disenfranchised grief: _____
_____

Nursing Knowledge Base

• Briefly explain the factors that influence loss and grief.

a. Human development: _____
_____

b. Psychosocial perspectives: _____
_____

c. Socioeconomic status: _____
_____

d. Personal relationships: _____
_____

e. Nature of the loss: _____
_____

f. Culture and ethnicity: _____
_____

• Explain how the mechanism of hope is used to cope with grief and loss.
_____
_____
_____

The Nursing Process and Grief Assessment

• The nurse should avoid assuming that a particular behavior indicates grief and allow persons to share what is happening in their own ways.

• It is important for the nurse to assess type and stage of grief the client is in.

• Identify some symptoms of normal grief. _____
_____
_____

• Briefly explain end-of-life decisions. _____
_____
_____

- Assess your own experience with grief. _____

  _____

  _____

Nursing Diagnosis

- List four nursing diagnoses for the following groups.

  a. The individual: _____

  _____

  _____

  _____

  b. The family: _____

  _____

  _____

  _____

  c. The community: _____

  _____

  _____

  _____

Planning

- Grieving has a therapeutic value that enables people to work through their losses, recollect their thoughts and feelings, and resume life with new insights and direction.

- List three goals appropriate for a client dealing with loss.

  a. _____

  b. _____

  c. _____

- List the three most crucial needs of the dying client.

  a. _____

  b. _____

  c. _____

Implementation

- To deliver the client's plan of care appropriately, the nurse must consider all levels of health. Briefly explain each of the following.

  a. Health promotion: _____

  _____

  _____

  b. Acute care: _____

  _____

  _____

- The nurse must schedule adequate private time with the client and family to promote open communication, accomplishing the following goals.

  a. _____

  b. _____

  c. _____

- Give an example of a nursing strategy for each dimension of hope.

  a. Affective dimension: _____

  _____

  b. Cognitive dimension: _____

  _____

  c. Behavioral dimension: _____

  _____

  d. Affiliative dimension: _____

  _____

  e. Temporal dimension: _____

  _____

  f. Contextual dimension: _____

  _____

Identify the nursing strategies to facilitate mourning for the client.

a. _____

b. _____

c. _____

d. _____

e. _____

f. _____

g. _____

Acute Care

- When health care providers deliver palliative care they do:

a. _____

b. _____

c. _____

d. _____

e. _____

f. _____

g. _____

- Give examples of how the following contribute to comfort for the dying patient.

a. Symptom control: _____

_____

b. Maintaining dignity and self-esteem: _____

_____

c. Preventing abandonment and isolation: ___

_____

d. Providing a comfortable and peaceful environment: _____

_____

Hospice Care

- Identify the components of hospice care.

_____

_____

Care After Death

- Care after death includes caring for the body with dignity and sensitivity. Identify the physiological changes that take place after death and the appropriate nursing interventions.

_____

_____

_____

_____

_____

Evaluation

Client Care

- Grieving is an individual process, and resolution of loss does not follow a set schedule.

- The care of the dying client requires the nurse to evaluate the client's level of comfort with illness and the client's quality of life.

Client Expectations

- Client expectations evaluate care from the client perspective. The client expects individualization of care, including comfort, dignity, and cooperation, to maximize the client's quality of life.

Review Questions

The student should select the appropriate answer and cite the rationale for choosing that particular answer.

1. Which statement about loss is accurate?
   a. Loss is only experienced when there is an actual absence of something valued.
   b. The more an individual has invested in what is lost, the less the feeling of loss.
   c. Loss may be maturational, situational, or both.
   d. The degree of stress experienced is unrelated to the type of loss.

   Answer: _____ Rationale: _____

   _____

   _____

2. The developmental stage at which the child is first able to understand logical explanations about death is:
   a. Toddlerhood
   b. Preschool age
   c. School-age
   d. Adolescence

   Answer: _____ Rationale: _____

   _____

   _____

3. A hospice program emphasizes:
   a. Curative treatment and alleviation of symptoms
   b. Palliative treatment and control of symptoms
   c. Hospital-based care
   d. Prolongation of life

   Answer: _____ Rationale: _____

   _____

   _____

4. Trying questionable and experimental forms of therapy is a behavior that is characteristic of which stage of dying?
   a. Anger
   b. Depression
   c. Bargaining
   d. Acceptance

   Answer: _____ Rationale: _____

   _____

   _____

5. All of the following are crucial needs of the dying client except:
   a. Control of pain
   b. Preservation of dignity and self-worth
   c. Love and belonging
   d. Freedom from decision making

   Answer: _____ Rationale: _____

   _____

   _____

Critical Thinking Model for Nursing Care Plan for Grief and Loss

Imagine that you are the student nurse in the Care Plan on page 582 of your text. Complete the *Evaluation phase* of the critical thinking model by writing your answers in the appropriate boxes of the model shown. Think about the following.

- In evaluating Mr. Miller's plan of care, what knowledge did you apply?

- In what way might your previous experience influence your evaluation of Mr. Miller's care?

- During evaluation, what intellectual and professional standards were applied to Mr. Miller's care?

- In what way do critical thinking attitudes play a role in how you approach evaluation of Mr. Miller's care?

- How might you adjust Mr. Miller's care?

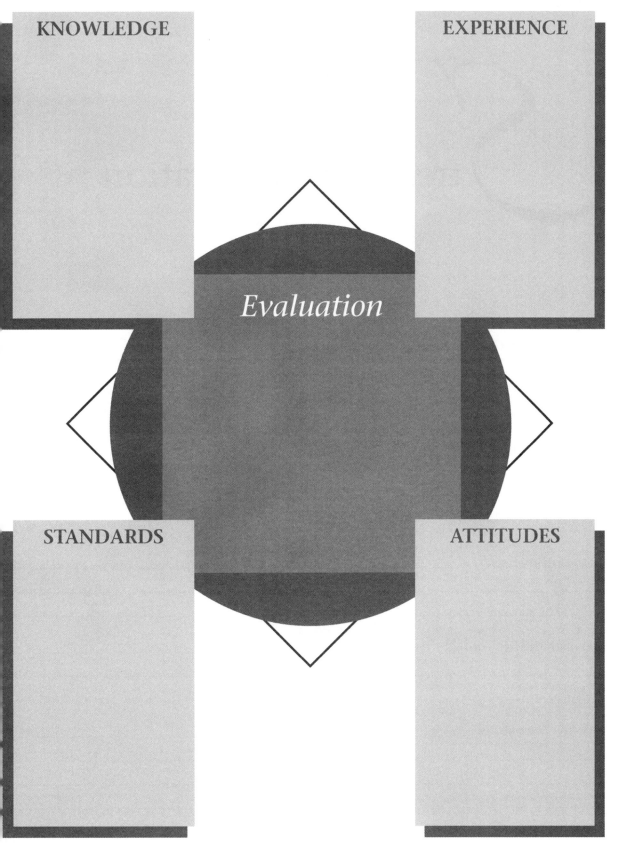

KNOWLEDGE

EXPERIENCE

Evaluation

STANDARDS

ATTITUDES

CHAPTER *29*   Critical Thinking Model for Nursing Care Plan for *Grief and Loss*

See answers on page 537.

30

_S_tress and Adaptation

_P_reliminary Reading

Chapter 30, pp. 595-614

_C_omprehensive Understanding

Scientific Knowledge Base

- Stress is: _____

_____

_____

- Stressors represent an: _____

_____

_____

- Explain the fight-or-flight response to stress. _____

_____

_____

- Define _homeostasis._ _____

_____

_____

_____

152   Chapter 30: Stress and Adaptation

- Explain the three major mechanisms of response to a stressor.

  a. Medulla oblongata: _____

  _____

  _____

  b. Reticular formation: _____

  _____

  _____

  c. Pituitary gland: _____

  _____

  _____

General Adaptation Syndrome

- List (in sequence) and briefly describe the three stages of the general adaptation syndrome (GAS).

  a. _____

  b. _____

  c. _____

Reaction to Psychological Stress

- Explain the following terms.

  a. Primary appraisal: _____

  _____

  b. Secondary appraisal: _____

  _____

  c. Coping: _____

  _____

  d. Ego-defense mechanisms: _____

  _____

- Distinguish between the two different types of stress.

  a. Distress: _____

  _____

  b. Eustress: _____

  _____

- Explain posttraumatic stress disorder.

  _____

  _____

- Explain the two types of crisis.

  a. Developmental crisis: _____

  _____

  b. Situational crisis: _____

  _____

Nursing Knowledge Base

- Summarize the following models related to stress and coping.

  a. Neuman's systems model: _____

  _____

  b. Pender's health promotion model: _____

  _____

- The following factors can potentially be stressors. Explain.

  a. Situational factors: _____

  _____

  _____

  b. Maturational factors: _____

  _____

  _____

  c. Sociocultural factors: _____

  _____

  _____

Nursing Process

Assessment

- Some individuals experience stress and difficulty coping while others are also experiencing the stress in their own ways.

- Give an example of each of the following factors to assess.

  a. Perception of stressor: _____

  _____

  b. Coping resources: _____

  _____

  c. Maladaptive coping resources: _____

  _____

Chapter 30: Stress and Adaptation   153

d. Adherence to healthy practices: _____

_____

- Identify six physical indicators of stress.

    a. _____

    b. _____

    c. _____

    d. _____

    e. _____

    f. _____

Nursing Diagnosis

- Stress can result in multiple diagnostic statements.

Planning

- Desirable outcomes for persons experiencing stress are:

    a. _____

    b. _____

    c. _____

    d. _____

- Nursing interventions are designed within the framework of primary, secondary, and tertiary prevention.

Implementation

Health Promotion

- Identify the primary modes of intervention for stress.

    a. _____

    b. _____

    c. _____

- Explain how the following methods reduce stressors.

    a. Time management: _____

    _____

    b. Regular exercise: _____

    _____

c. Guided imagery and visualization: _____

_____

d. Support systems: _____

_____

e. Progressive muscle relaxation: _____

_____

f. Assertiveness training: _____

_____

g. Journal writing: _____

_____

h. Stress management in the workplace: _____

_____

Acute Care

- Crisis intervention is: _____

_____

_____

- Crises occur: _____

_____

_____

Restorative Care

- Briefly explain when recovery from stress occurs. _____

_____

_____

Evaluation

- Briefly explain the client's care in relation to:

    a. Client's perceptions of stress: _____

    _____

    b. Client's expectations: _____

    _____

Review Questions

The student should select the appropriate answer and cite the rationale for choosing that particular answer.

1. Which definition does *not* characterize stress?
   a. Any situation in which a nonspecific demand requires an individual to respond or take action
   b. A phenomenon affecting social, psychological, developmental, spiritual, and physiological dimensions
   c. A condition eliciting an intellectual, behavioral, or metabolic response
   d. Efforts to maintain relative constancy within the internal environment

   Answer: _____ Rationale: _____

   _____

   _____

2. Which statement about homeostasis is inaccurate?
   a. Homeostatic mechanisms provide long-term and short-term control over the body's equilibrium.
   b. Homeostatic mechanisms are self-regulatory.
   c. Homeostatic mechanisms function through negative feedback.
   d. Illness may inhibit normal homeostatic mechanisms.

   Answer: _____ Rationale: _____

   _____

   _____

3. Major homeostatic mechanisms are controlled by all of the following except:
   a. Thymus gland
   b. Medulla oblongata
   c. Reticular formation
   d. Pituitary gland

   Answer: _____ Rationale: _____

   _____

   _____

4. Which of the following is an example of the local adaptation syndrome?
   a. Alarm reaction
   b. Fight-or-flight response
   c. Ego-defense mechanisms
   d. Inflammatory response

   Answer: _____ Rationale: _____

   _____

   _____

5. The general adaptation syndrome consists of three stages. During which stage does the body stabilize and hormone levels return to normal?
   a. Exhaustion
   b. Regeneration
   c. Resistance
   d. Compensation

   Answer: _____ Rationale: _____

   _____

   _____

6. Crisis intervention is a specific measure used for helping a client resolve a particular, immediate stress problem. This approach is based on:
   a. The ability of the nurse to solve the client's problems
   b. An in-depth analysis of a client's situation
   c. Teaching the client how to use ego-defense mechanisms
   d. Effective communication between the nurse and client

   Answer: _____ Rationale: _____

   _____

   _____

Chapter 30: Stress and Adaptation   155

Critical Thinking Model for Nursing Care Plan for Caregiver Role Strain

Imagine that you are Janet, the nurse in the Care Plan on page 609 of your text. Complete the *Evaluation phase* of the critical thinking model by writing your answers in the appropriate boxes of the model shown. Think about the following.

- In evaluating the care of Carl and Evelyn, what knowledge did Janet apply?

- In what way might Janet's previous experience influence the evaluation of Carl's care?

- During evaluation, what intellectual and professional standards were applied to Carl's care?

- In what way do critical thinking attitudes play a role in how Janet approaches the evaluation of Carl's care?

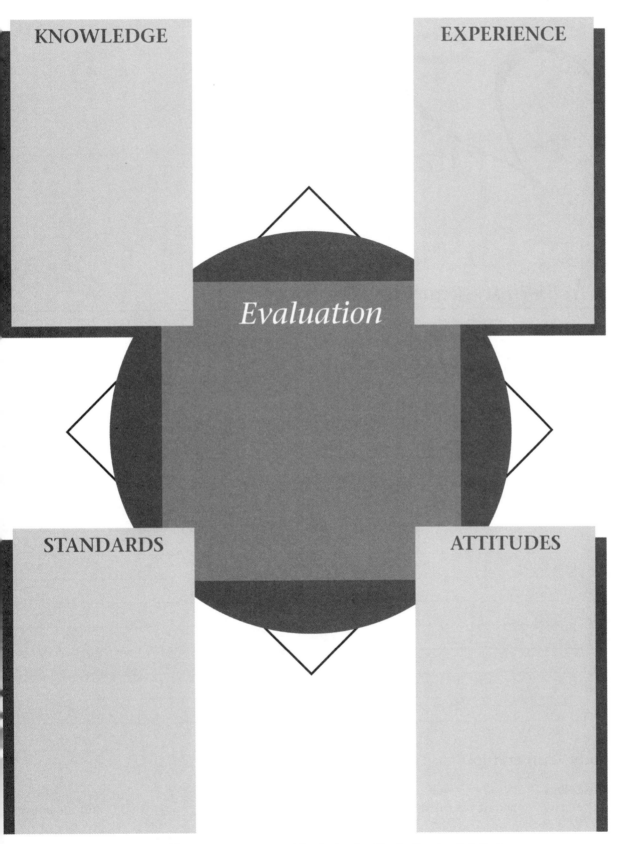

KNOWLEDGE

EXPERIENCE

Evaluation

STANDARDS

ATTITUDES

CHAPTER *30*   Critical Thinking Model for Nursing Care Plan for *Caregiver Role Strain*

See answers on page 538.

31

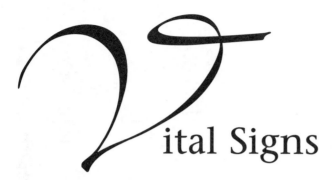

Vital Signs

Preliminary Reading

Chapter 31, pp. 617-670

Comprehensive Understanding

Guidelines for Taking Vital Signs

- Identify the guidelines that assist the nurse to incorporate vital sign measurement into practice.

    a. _____

    b. _____

    c. _____

    d. _____

    e. _____

    f. _____

    g. _____

    h. _____

    i. _____

    j. _____

    k. _____

    l. _____

Body Temperature

Physiology
- The body temperature is the difference between the _____ and the amount

    _____.

- Define *core temperature*. _____

_____

- Define *thermoregulation*. _____

_____

_____

- Briefly summarize how neural and vascular mechanisms control body temperature. _____

_____

_____

- List four sources, or mechanisms, for heat production.

   a. _____

   b. _____

   c. _____

   d. _____

- Explain the following mechanisms of body heat loss, and give an example of each.

   a. Radiation: _____

   _____

   b. Conduction: _____

   _____

   c. Convection: _____

   _____

   d. Evaporation: _____

   _____

   e. Diaphoresis: _____

   _____

Skin in Temperature Regulation

- Briefly explain the skin's role in temperature regulation.

   a. Insulation of the body: _____

   _____

   _____

   b. Vasoconstriction: _____

   _____

   _____

   c. Temperature sensation: _____

   _____

   _____

Behavioral Control

- Identify four factors that must be present for a person to control body temperature.

   a. _____

   b. _____

   c. _____

   d. _____

Factors Affecting Body Temperature

- Changes in body temperature within the normal range occur when the relationship between heat production and heat loss is altered by physiological or behavioral variables. Summarize the following variables.

   a. Age: _____

   _____

   b. Exercise: _____

   _____

   _____

   c. Circadian rhythm: _____

   _____

   _____

   d. Stress: _____

   _____

   _____

   e. Environment: _____

   _____

   _____

- Temperature alterations can be related to

_____, _____,

_____, or any combination of

these alterations.

- Pyrexia, or fever, occurs because _____
  _____
  _____

- Explain how a fever works as an important defense mechanism. _____
  _____
  _____

- Explain how a fever serves a diagnostic purpose. _____
  _____
  _____

- Explain how a fever affects metabolism._____
  _____
  _____

- Define the following terms.
  a. *Hyperthermia:* _____
     _____

  b. *Malignant hyperthermia:* _____
     _____

- Define and explain the causes of *heat stroke.*
  _____
  _____

- Define and explain the causes of *heat exhaustion.* _____
  _____
  _____

- Define and explain the causes of *hypothermia.*
  _____
  _____
  _____

- Frostbite occurs when: _____
  _____
  _____

Nursing Process and Thermoregulation
- Independent measures can be implemented to increase or minimize heat loss, to promote heat conservation, and to increase comfort.

Assessment

- List the assessment sites for temperature measurement.
  a. _____
  b. _____
  c. _____
  d. _____

- State the formulas for the following conversions.
  a. Fahrenheit to centigrade: _____
  b. Centigrade to Fahrenheit: _____

- Identify the advantages and disadvantages of the types of thermometers.
  a. _____
  b. _____
  c. _____

Nursing Diagnosis

- Identify three nursing diagnoses related to thermoregulation.
  a. _____
  b. _____
  c. _____

Planning

- The plan of care depends on the nurse's assessment of the client's perception and acceptance of the body temperature alteration.

- Care also depends on the extent to which the client's internal compensatory mechanisms and behaviors have adjusted to the temperature alteration.

⁄ℕℙ Implementation

Health Promotion

- Health promotion for clients at risk of altered temperature is directed to: _____

  _____

  _____

- Identify the risk factors. _____

  _____

  _____

Acute Care

- The procedures used to intervene and treat an elevated temperature depend on the fever's cause; its adverse effects; and its strength, intensity, and duration.

- Explain the differences related to febrile states in each of the following.

  a. Children: _____

  _____

  b. Hypersensitivities to drugs: _____

  _____

- Give three examples of each type of fever therapy.

  a. Pharmacological:

  1. _____

  2. _____

  3. _____

  b. Nonpharmacological:

  1. _____

  2. _____

  3. _____

- Identify an independent and a dependent nursing intervention to control shivering.

  _____

  _____

  _____

- First aid treatment for heatstroke is:

  _____

  _____

- Summarize the treatment for hypothermia.

  _____

  _____

  _____

Restorative Care

- Summarize the client teaching in regard to the treatment of a fever.

  _____

  _____

⁄ℕℙ Evaluation

- After any intervention, the nurse measures the client's temperature to evaluate it for any change.

- Other evaluative measures are _____

  and _____.

Pulse

- Define *pulse*. _____

  _____

Physiology and Regulation

- Define the following terms.

  a. *Stroke volume:* _____

  _____

  b. *Cardiac output:* _____

  _____

- _____, _____, and _____ factors regulate the strength of the heart's contractions and its stroke volume.

Assessment of Pulse

- Identify the two most common peripheral pulse sites to assess.

  a. _____

  b. _____

Use of a Stethoscope

- Identify the five major parts of the stethoscope.

  a. _____

  b. _____

  c. _____

  d. _____

  e. _____

Character of the Pulse

- List four characteristics to identify during peripheral pulse assessment. By using an asterisk, specify the two characteristics to identify when assessing an apical pulse.

  a. _____

  b. _____

  c. _____

  d. _____

- Define the following.

  a. *Tachycardia:* _____

  _____

  b. *Bradycardia:* _____

  _____

  c. *Dysrhythmia:* _____

  _____

  d. *Pulse deficit:* _____

  _____

Nursing Process and Pulse Determination

- Pulse assessment determines the general state of cardiovascular health and the response to other system imbalances.

- The nurse evaluates client outcomes by assessing the pulse _____, _____, _____, and _____ following each intervention.

Respiration

- Define the following.

  a. *Ventilation:* _____

  _____

  b. *Diffusion:* _____

  _____

  c. *Perfusion:* _____

  _____

Physiological Control

- Breathing is a passive process. The respiratory center in the brainstem regulates the control of respirations.

- Ventilation is controlled by levels of _____, _____, and _____ in the arterial blood.

- The most important factor in the control of ventilation is the level of _____.

- *Hypoxemia* is: _____

  _____

  _____

Mechanics of Breathing

- Briefly summarize the process of inspiration.

  _____

  _____

  _____

- Define the following terms.

  a. *Tidal volume:* _____

  _____

  b. *Eupnea:* _____

  _____

Assessment of Ventilations

- Accurate measurement requires _____ and _____ of the chest wall movement.

- List three objective measurements used in respiratory status assessment.

  a. _____

  b. _____

  c. _____

- Define the following alterations in breathing patterns.

  a. *Bradypnea:* _____

  _____

  b. *Tachypnea:* _____

  _____

  c. *Hyperpnea:* _____

  _____

  d. *Apnea:* _____

  _____

  e. *Hypoventilation/hyperventilation:* _____

  _____

  f. *Cheyne-Stokes':* _____

  _____

  g. *Kussmaul's:* _____

  _____

  h. *Biot's:* _____

  _____

Assessment of Diffusion and Perfusion

- The respiratory processes of diffusion and perfusion can be evaluated by measuring the oxygen saturation of the blood.

- The saturation of arterial blood is _____,

  and venous blood is _____.

- Explain the purpose of a pulse oximeter.

  _____

  _____

Nursing Process and Respiratory Vital Signs

- Vital sign measurement of respiratory rate, pattern, and depth, along with SvO_2, allows the nurse to assess ventilation, diffusion, and perfusion.

- The nurse evaluates client outcomes by assessing the _____, _____, _____, and _____ following each intervention.

Blood Pressure

- Define the following terms:

  a. *Blood pressure:* _____

  _____

  b. *Systolic:* _____

  _____

  c. *Diastolic:* _____

  _____

- The difference between the systolic and diastolic pressure is the _____

  _____

  _____.

Physiology of Arterial Blood Pressure

- Blood pressure is reflected by the following. Briefly explain each.

  a. Cardiac output: _____

  _____

  _____

  b. Peripheral resistance: _____

  _____

  _____

  c. Blood volume: _____

  _____

  _____

  d. Viscosity:

  _____

  _____

  e. Elasticity: _____

  _____

  _____

Factors Influencing Blood Pressure

- List six factors that influence blood pressure.

    a. _____

    b. _____

    c. _____

    d. _____

    e. _____

    f. _____

Hypertension

- Identify the criteria for the diagnosis of hypertension in an adult. _____

    _____

    _____

- Briefly summarize the physiology of hypertension. _____

    _____

    _____

    _____

- List five risk factors that are linked to hypertension.

    a. _____

    b. _____

    c. _____

    d. _____

    e. _____

Hypotension

- Identify the criteria for the diagnosis of hypotension in an adult. _____

    _____

    _____

    _____

- Explain the physiology of hypotension and its causes. _____

    _____

    _____

    _____

    _____

- Orthostatic hypotension occurs when: _____

    _____

    _____

- Explain how you would assess a client for orthostatic hypotension.

    _____

    _____

    _____

Assessment of Blood Pressure

- Identify two methods for measuring blood pressure.

    a. _____

    b. _____

- Identify the two types of sphygmomanometers, and list their advantages and disadvantages.

    a. _____

    b. _____

- The sounds heard over an artery distal to the blood pressure cuff are Korotkoff sounds.

    a. First: _____

    b. Second: _____

    c. Third: _____

    d. Fourth: _____

    e. Fifth: _____

- During the initial assessment the nurse should obtain and record the blood pressure in

    _____

    arms.

- Pressure differences between the arms greater than _____ indicate vascular problems.

- Identify five common mistakes in measurement.

    a. _____

    b. _____

    c. _____

    d. _____

e. _____

- Identify the four reasons why the measurement of blood pressure in infants and children is difficult.

  a. _____

  b. _____

  c. _____

  d. _____

- Explain the rationale for the use of an ultrasonic stethoscope. _____

  _____

  _____

- Identify the method the nurse may use to assess blood pressure when Korotkoff sounds are not audible with the standard stethoscope.

  _____

  _____

- Define *auscultatory gap*. _____

  _____

  _____

- Give an example of when you would assess a client's blood pressure using his lower extremities. _____

  _____

- Identify the advantage and disadvantage of using automatic blood pressure devices. _____

  _____

  _____

  _____

- List the benefits of blood pressure self-measurement.

  a. _____

  b. _____

  c. _____

  d. _____

Nursing Process and Blood Pressure Determination

- The assessment of blood pressure along with pulse assessment is used to evaluate the general state of cardiovascular health and responses to other system imbalances.

- The nurse evaluates client outcomes by assessing the blood pressure following each intervention.

Health Promotion and Vital Signs

- When teaching clients and their families the importance of vital sign measurements, the client's age is an important factor.

- Identify some of the common variations in the older adult.

  a. Temperature: _____

  _____

  b. Pulse rate: _____

  _____

  c. Blood pressure: _____

  _____

  d. Respirations: _____

  _____

Recording Vital Signs

- In addition to the actual vital sign values, the nurse records in the nurses' notes any accompanying or precipitating symptoms.

- The nurse needs to document any intervention initiated as a result of a vital sign measurement.

Review Questions

The student should select the appropriate answer and cite the rationale for choosing that particular answer.

1. The skin plays a role in temperature regulation by:
   a. Insulating the body
   b. Constricting blood vessels
   c. Sensing external temperature variations
   d. All of the above

   Answer: _____ Rationale: _____

   _____

   _____

2. The nurse bathes the client who has a fever with cool water. The nurse does this to increase heat loss by means of:
   a. Radiation
   b. Convection
   c. Condensation
   d. Conduction

   Answer: _____ Rationale: _____

   _____

   _____

3. The nurse is assessing a client who she suspects has the nursing diagnosis *hyperthermia related to vigorous exercise in hot weather.* In reviewing the data the nurse knows that the most important sign of heatstroke is:
   a. Confusion
   b. Hot, dry skin
   c. Excess thirst
   d. Muscle cramps

   Answer: _____ Rationale: _____

   _____

   _____

4. When the nurse takes the client's radial pulse, he notes a dysrhythmia. His most appropriate action is to:
   a. Inform the physician immediately
   b. Wait 5 minutes and retake the radial pulse
   c. Take the pulse apically for 1 full minute
   d. Check the client's record for the presence of a previous dysrhythmia

   Answer: _____ Rationale: _____

   _____

   _____

5. The nurse is auscultating Mrs. McKinnon's blood pressure. The nurse inflates the cuff to 180 mm Hg. At 156 mm Hg, the nurse hears the onset of a tapping sound. At 130 mm Hg the sound changes to a murmur or swishing. At 100 mm Hg the sound momentarily becomes sharper, and at 92 mm Hg it becomes muffled. At 88 mm Hg the sound disappears. Mr. McKinnon's blood pressure is:
   a. 180/92
   b. 180/130
   c. 156/88
   d. 130/88

   Answer: _____ Rationale: _____

   _____

   _____

32

*H*ealth Assessment and Physical Examination

*P*reliminary Reading

Chapter 32, pp. 671-771

*C*omprehensive Understanding

Purposes of Physical Examination

- List the five nursing purposes for performing a physical assessment.

    a. _____

    b. _____

    c. _____

    d. _____

    e. _____

Gathering a Health History

- The main objective of the nurse/client interaction is for the nurse to find out what is central to the client's concerns and to help the client find solutions.

Developing Nursing Diagnoses and a Care Plan

- After collecting a history, the nurse conducts a physical examination to _____, _____, or _____ the existing database.

- A complete assessment is needed to form a definitive diagnosis.

- The nurse learns to group significant findings into patterns of data that reveal actual or high-risk nursing diagnoses.

- The baseline is: _____

_____

_____.

Managing Client Problems

- The nurse's success in providing care depends on his or her ability to recognize a change in the client's status and to modify therapies so that the client gains the most desirable outcome.

- Physical assessment skills allow the nurse to

_____ and _____.

Evaluating Nursing Care

- Physical assessment skills enhance the evaluation of nursing measures through monitoring

_____ and _____ outcomes of care.

Cultural Sensitivity

- A client's culture will influence his or her willingness to assume responsibility for health. Culture also influences a client's tendency to seek professional health care.

Integration of Physical Assessment with Nursing Care

- Whether a complete or partial physical assessment is performed, an examination should be integrated into routine care.

Skills of Physical Assessment

Inspection
- Define *inspection*. _____

_____

_____

- List six principles to facilitate accurate inspection of body parts.

a. _____

b. _____

c. _____

d. _____

e. _____

f. _____

Palpation
- Define *palpation*. _____

_____

_____

- Identify the parts of the hand used to assess each of the following.

a. Temperature: _____

b. Pulsations: _____

c. Vibrations: _____

d. Turgor: _____

- Briefly explain the following:

a. Light palpation: _____

_____

b. Deep palpation: _____

_____

c. Percussion: _____

_____

- Identify the information obtained through percussion.

_____

_____

_____

- Explain the two types of percussion.

a. Direct: _____

_____

b. Indirect: _____

_____

- Percussion produces five types of sounds. Identify them.

a. _____

b. _____

c. _____

d. _____

e. _____

Auscultation

- Define *auscultation*. _____

_____

_____

- Briefly explain the following characteristics of sound.

a. Frequency: _____

_____

b. Loudness: _____

_____

c. Quality: _____

_____

d. Duration: _____

_____

Olfaction

- Olfaction helps the nurse detect abnormalities that cannot be recognized by any other means.

Preparation for Examination

Infection Control

- Examination techniques cause the nurse to contact body fluids and discharge. Standard precautions should be used throughout the examination.

Environment

- List at least three environmental factors that the nurse should attempt to control before performing a physical examination.

a. _____

b. _____

c. _____

Equipment

- Hand washing is done before equipment preparation and before the examination.

- All equipment should be checked to see that it functions properly.

Physical Preparation of the Client

- Briefly explain the following preparations before an examination.

a. Physical: _____

_____

_____

_____

b. Positioning: _____

_____

_____

_____

c. Psychological: _____

_____

_____

_____

Assessment of Age Groups

- List at least six variations in the nurse's individual style that are appropriate when examining children.

a. _____

b. _____

c. _____

d. _____

e. _____

f. _____

- List at least five variations in the nurse's individual style that are appropriate when examining older adults.

a. _____

b. _____

c. _____

d. _____

e. _____

Organization of the Examination

- List eight principles to follow for a well-organized examination.

a. _____

b. _____

c. _____

d. _____

e. _____

f. _____

g. _____

h. _____

General Survey
- List three assessment components of the general survey.

  a. _____

  b. _____

  c. _____

General Appearance and Behavior
- Summarize the 14 specific observations of the client's general appearance and behavior.

  a. _____

  b. _____

  c. _____

  d. _____

  e. _____

  f. _____

  g. _____

  h. _____

  i _____

  j. _____

  k. _____

  l. _____

  m. _____

  n. _____

Vital Signs
- Assessment of vital signs is the first part of the physical assessment.

Height, Weight, and Circumference
- A person's general level of health can be reflected in the ratio of height and weight.

- List three actions that should be taken to ensure accurate weight measurement of a hospitalized client.

  a. _____

  b. _____

  c. _____

- In the infant a chest circumference can be compared with the head circumference to rule out problems in head or chest size.

Skin, Hair, and Nails

- The skin provides the body's _____ and _____ and acts as a sensory organ for _____, _____, _____, and _____.

- The physical assessment skills of _____ and _____ are used to assess the integument's function and integrity.

Skin
- Assessment of the skin can reveal a variety of conditions including changes in _____, _____, _____, and _____.

- List at least four risks for skin lesions in the hospitalized client.

  a. _____

  b. _____

  c. _____

  d. _____

- Define the following terms:

  a. *Melanoma:* _____

  _____

  b. *Basal cell carcinoma:* _____

  _____

- For each skin color variation, identify the mechanism that produces color change, common causes of the variation, and the optimal sites for assessment. (See the table at the top of next page.)

Skin Color	Mechanisms	Causes	Assessment Sites
Cyanosis			
Pallor			
Jaundice			
Erythema			

- Define *hyperpigmentation* and *hypopigmentation*. _____ _____

- Define *moisture*. _____ _____ _____

- Excessive dryness can worsen skin conditions such as _____ and _____.

- The temperature of the skin depends on the amount of _____ circulating through the dermis.

- The character of the skin's surface and the feel of deeper portions are its _____.

- Define *skin turgor* and describe normal findings. _____ _____

- Petechiae are: _____ _____ _____

- Identify the two causes of edema.
  a. _____
  b. _____

- Explain the following terms related to lesions.
  a. Senile keratosis: _____ _____
  b. Cherry angiomas: _____ _____

- When a lesion is detected, it is inspected for _____, _____, _____, _____, _____, _____, and _____.

- Briefly describe the following primary skin lesions.
  a. Macule: _____
  b. Papule: _____
  c. Nodule: _____
  d. Tumor: _____
  e. Wheal: _____
  f. Vesicle: _____
  g. Pustule: _____
  h. Ulcer: _____
  i. Atrophy: _____

Hair and Scalp
- When inspecting the hair, the nurse notes the _____, _____, _____, _____, and _____.

- Define.

  a. *Alopecia:* _____

  b. *Hirsutism:* _____

- Name the three types of lice.

  a. _____

  b. _____

  c. _____

Nails
- When inspecting the nail bed, the nurse notes

  the _____, _____, _____,

  _____, _____, and _____.

- The nurse palpates the nail base to determine:

  _____

  _____

- Briefly describe the following abnormalities of the nail bed.

  a. Clubbing: _____

  b. Beau's lines: _____

  c. Koilonychia: _____

  d. Splinter hemorrhages: _____

  e. Paronychia: _____

Head and Neck

Head

Inspection	Palpation	Percussion	Auscultation

- Define the following head abnormalities:

  a. *Hydrocephalus:* _____

  b. *Acromegaly:* _____

Eyes

Inspection	Palpation	Percussion	Auscultation
Visual Acuity			
Visual Fields			
Extraocular			
Movements			

External Eye Structures

Inspection	Palpation	Percussion	Auscultation
Eyebrows			
Eyelids			
Lacrimal Apparatus			
Conjunctivae and Sclerae			
Corneas, Pupils, and Irises			

- Define the following common eye and visual abnormalities.

    a. Exophthalmos: _____

    _____

    b. Strabismus: _____

    _____

    c. Hyperopia: _____

    _____

    d. Myopia: _____

    _____

    e. Presbyopia: _____

    _____

    f. Astigmatism: _____

    _____

    g. Nystagmus: _____

- Identify the six structures you would assess in the internal eye.

    a. _____

    b. _____

    c. _____

    d. _____

    e. _____

    f. _____

Ears

Inspection	Palpation	Percussion	Auscultation
External Ear			
Middle Ear			
Inner Ear			

- Identify the mechanisms for sound transmission.

  a. _____

  b. _____

  c. _____

  d. _____

  e. _____

- Identify the types of problems that affect the ear.

  a. _____

  b. _____

  c. _____

  d. _____

- The three types of hearing loss are _____

  _____, _____,

  and _____.

- Define *ototoxicity*. _____

  _____

  _____

- Briefly explain how a tuning fork works.

  _____

  _____

- Define *Weber's test*. _____

  _____

  _____

- Define *Rinne test*. _____

  _____

  _____

Nose and Sinuses

Inspection	Palpation	Percussion	Auscultation
Nose			
Sinuses			

Mouth and Pharynx

Inspection	Palpation	Percussion	Auscultation
Lips			
Buccal Mucosa, Gums, and Teeth			
Tongue and Floor of Mouth			
Palate			
Pharynx			

- Define the following conditions of the mouth:

  a. *Caries:* _____

  b. *Leukoplakia:* _____

  c. *Varicosities:* _____

  d. *Exostosis:* _____

Neck

Inspection	Palpation	Percussion	Auscultation
Neck Muscles			
Lymph Nodes			
Thyroid Gland			
Carotid Artery and Jugular Vein			
Trachea			

Thorax and Lungs

Inspection	Palpation	Percussion	Auscultation
Posterior Thorax			
Lateral Thorax			
Anterior Thorax			

- Accurate physical assessment of the thorax and lungs requires review of the ventilatory and respiratory functions of the lung.

- Define *vocal* or *tactile fremitus*. _____
  _____
  _____

- Identify the normal breath sounds and where they are located. _____
  _____
  _____

- Complete the following table of adventitious breath sounds.

Sound	Auscultation Site	Cause	Character
Crackles			
Rhonchi			
Wheezes			
Pleural Friction Rub			

Heart

- Assessment of heart function involves a review of signs and symptoms from the nursing history, pulse assessment, and direct examination of the heart.

- Answer the following questions regarding the PMI.

  a. What is the PMI? _____

  b. Where is the PMI normally located in the infant and young child? _____
     _____

  c. Where is the PMI located in the older child and adult? _____
     _____

  d. What techniques may be used to locate the PMI? _____
     _____

- Define what occurs during the two phases of the cardiac cycle.

  a. Systole: _____
     _____

  b. Diastole: _____
     _____

- Define the following heart sounds:

  S_1: _____

  S_2: _____

  S_3: _____

  S_4: _____

- Define *dysrhythmia*. _____
  _____
  _____

- Define *murmur.* _____

   _____

   _____

- List the six factors to assess when a murmur is detected.

   a. _____

   b. _____

   c. _____

   d. _____

   e. _____

   f. _____

Mouth and Pharynx

- Define *thrill.* _____

   _____

   _____

Vascular System

- Examination of the vascular system includes measurement of the blood pressure and a thorough assessment of the integrity of the peripheral vascular system.

Inspection	Palpation	Percussion	Auscultation
Carotid Arteries			
Jugular Veins			
Peripheral Arteries			
Peripheral Veins			
Lymphatic System			

Explain the following conditions that are related to the vascular system.

a. Syncope: _____

b. Occlusion: _____

c. Stenosis: _____

d. Atherosclerosis: _____

e. Bruit: _____

Explain the steps the nurse would use to assess venous pressure.

a. _____

b. _____

c. _____

d. _____

e. _____

The Allen's test is used to: _____

_____

_____

The 3 Ps that characterize an occlusion are

_____, _____, and

_____.

Phlebitis is: _____

_____

_____

Breasts

It is important to examine the breasts of female and male clients.

- The American Cancer Society (1998) recommends the following guidelines for early detection of breast cancer.

a. _____

b. _____

c. _____

d. _____

e. _____

- Briefly explain the proper technique for palpating breast tissue. _____

_____

_____

- List seven characteristics that should be included when describing an abnormal breast mass.

a. _____

b. _____

c. _____

d. _____

e. _____

f. _____

g. _____

- Define the following terms.

a. *Metastasize:* _____

_____

b. *Fibrocystic breast disease:* _____

_____

Inspection	Palpation	Percussion	Auscultation
Breasts			

Abdomen

- The abdominal examination includes an assessment of the lower GI tract in addition to the liver, stomach, uterus, ovaries, kidneys, and bladder.

- Describe four techniques used to help the client relax during assessment of the abdomen.

  a. _____

  b. _____

  c. _____

  d. _____

Inspection	Palpation	Percussion	Auscultation
Abdomen			
Liver			

- Define the following.

  a. *Hernias:* _____

  _____

  b. *Distention:* _____

  _____

  c. *Peristalsis:* _____

  _____

  d. *Paralytic ileus:* _____

  _____

  e. *Borborygmi:* _____

  _____

  f. *Rebound tenderness:* _____

  _____

  g. *Aneurysm:* _____

  _____

Female Genitalia and Reproductive Tract

- Briefly explain the preparation of a client for a complete examination of the genitalia and reproductive tract. _____

  _____

  _____

Inspection	Palpation	Percussion	Auscultation
External Genitalia			
Cervix			
Vagina			

Define the following terms.

a. *Chancres:* _____

_____

b. *Cystocele:* _____

_____

c. *Rectocele:* _____

_____

• Speculum examination of the internal genitalia includes: _____

_____

_____

Male Genitalia

• An examination of the male genitalia includes assessment of the external genitalia and the inguinal ring and canal.

Inspection	Palpation	Percussion	Auscultation
Penis			
Scrotum			
Inguinal Ring and Canal			
Rectum and Anus			

Summarize how the nurse would assess sexual maturity. _____

_____

Rectum and Anus

The purpose of digital palpation is: _____

_____

Musculoskeletal System

• The assessment of musculoskeletal function focuses on determining the range of joint motion, muscle strength and tone, and joint and muscle condition.

Inspection	Palpation	Percussion	Auscultation
Joint Motion			

Chapter 32: Health Assessment and Physical Examination   181

- Define.

    a. *Hypertonicity:* _____

    _____

    b. *Hypotonicity:* _____

    _____

    c. *Kyphosis:* _____

    _____

    d. *Osteoporosis:* _____

    _____

    e. *Goniometer:* _____

    _____

Neurological System

- The neurological system is responsible for many functions including _____

    _____

    _____.

Mental and Emotional Status

- There are five areas that Folstein's Mini-Mental State tool assesses. Name them.

    a. _____

    b. _____

    c. _____

    d. _____

    e. _____

- An alteration in mental or emotional status may reflect a disturbance in cerebral functioning.

- List three factors that may change cerebral function.

    a. _____

    b. _____

    c. _____

- Define *delirium* and list the clinical criteria for it. _____

    _____

    _____

- The level of consciousness exists along a continuum, from full awakening, alertness, and cooperation to unresponsiveness to any form of external stimuli.

- Identify the tool and the three factors to assess consciousness. _____

    _____

    _____

- Behavior, moods, hygiene, grooming, and choice of dress reveal pertinent information about mental status.

- Explain the function of the cerebral cortex in language. _____

    _____

    _____

- Intellectual function includes the following. Briefly explain how each is assessed.

    a. Abstract thinking: _____

    _____

    b. Judgment: _____

    _____

    c. Memory: _____

    _____

    d. Knowledge: _____

    _____

- There are two types of aphasia. Describe each one.

    a. _____

    b. _____

Cranial Nerve Function

- Identify the 12 cranial nerves:

    a. _____

    b. _____

    c. _____

    d. _____

    e. _____

    f. _____

g. _____

h. _____

i. _____

j. _____

k. _____

l. _____

Sensory Function

- The sensory pathways of the central nervous system conduct sensations of _____, _____, _____, _____, and _____.

- Summarize how a nurse would assess the client's sensory function. _____
_____
_____

Motor Function

- Identify the functions of the cerebellum. _____
_____
_____

- Describe the maneuvers used to assess balance and gross motor function.

  a. _____

  b. _____

  c. _____

Reflexes

- Eliciting reflex reactions allows the nurse to assess the integrity of sensory and motor pathways of the reflex arc and specific spinal cord segments.

- Briefly explain the two categories of normal reflexes. _____
_____
_____

Review Questions

The student should select the appropriate answer and cite the rationale for choosing that particular answer.

1. The component that should receive the highest priority before a physical examination is:
   a. Preparation of the environment
   b. Preparation of the equipment
   c. Physical preparation of the client
   d. Psychological preparation of the client

   Answer: _____ Rationale: _____
   _____
   _____

2. The nurse assesses the skin turgor of the client by:
   a. Grasping a fold of skin on the back of the forearm and releasing
   b. Palpating the skin with the dorsum of the hand
   c. Pressing the skin for 5 seconds, releasing, and noting each centimeter of depth
   d. Inspecting the buccal mucosa with a penlight

   Answer: _____ Rationale: _____
   _____
   _____

3. While examining Mr. Parker, the nurse notes a circumscribed elevation of skin filled with serous fluid on his upper lip. The lesion is 0.4 cm in diameter. This type of lesion is called a:
   a. Macule
   b. Nodule
   c. Vesicle
   d. Pustule

   Answer: _____ Rationale: _____
   _____
   _____

Chapter 32: Health Assessment and Physical Examination   183

4. When assessing the client's thorax, the nurse should:
   a. Complete the left side and then the right side
   b. Change the position of the stethoscope between inspiration and expiration
   c. Compare symmetrical areas from side to side
   d. Begin with the posterior lobes on the right side

   Answer: _____ Rationale: _____

   _____

   _____

5. In a client with pneumonia, the nurse hears high-pitched, continuous musical sounds over the bronchi on expiration. These sounds are called:
   a. Crackles
   b. Rhonchi
   c. Wheezes
   d. Friction rubs

   Answer: _____ Rationale: _____

   _____

   _____

6. The second heart sound (S2) occurs when:
   a. The mitral and tricuspid valves close
   b. There is rapid ventricular filling
   c. Systole begins
   d. The aortic and pulmonic valves close

   Answer: _____ Rationale: _____

   _____

   _____

33

$\mathcal{I}$nfection Control

$\mathcal{P}$reliminary Reading

Chapter 33, pp. 772-820

$\mathcal{C}$omprehensive Understanding

Nature of Infection

- An infection is an: _____

  _____

  _____

- Define *communicable*. _____

  _____

  _____

Chain of Infection

- Development of an infection occurs in a cycle that depends on the following elements:

  a. _____

  b. _____

  c. _____

  d. _____

  e. _____

  f. _____

- Microorganisms include _____, _____ and

  _____.

- Define.

  a. *Virulence:* _____

  _____

  _____

  b. *Immunocompromised:* _____

  _____

  _____

- The potential for microorganisms or parasites to cause disease depends on four factors. Name them.

  a. _____

  b. _____

  c. _____

  d. _____

- Define *reservoir.* _____

  _____

  _____

- Define *carriers.* _____

  _____

  _____

- To thrive, organisms require the following. Briefly explain each one.

  a. Food: _____

  _____

  b. Oxygen: _____

  _____

  c. Water: _____

  _____

  d. Temperature: _____

  _____

  e. pH: _____

  _____

  f. Light: _____

  _____

- Microorganisms can exit through a variety of sites. Briefly explain each one.

  a. Skin and mucous membranes: _____

  _____

  _____

  b. Respiratory tract: _____

  _____

  _____

  c. Urinary tract: _____

  _____

  _____

  d. Gastrointestinal tract: _____

  _____

  _____

  e. Reproductive tract: _____

  _____

  _____

  f. Blood: _____

  _____

  _____

- List the six routes through which microorganisms are transmitted from the reservoir to the host.

  a. _____

  b. _____

  c. _____

  d. _____

  e. _____

  f. _____

The Infection Process

- The severity of the client's illness depends on the _____ , the _____ , and _____ .

- Describe the two types of infections.
    a. Localized: _____
    _____

    b. Systemic: _____
    _____

Defenses Against Infection

- The inflammatory response is: _____
    _____
    _____

- Explain the normal body defenses against infection.
    a. Normal flora: _____
    _____
    _____

b. Body system defenses: _____
    _____
    _____

c. Inflammation: _____
    _____
    _____

- For each body system or organ in the grid below, identify at least one defense mechanism and the primary action to prevent infection.

System/Organ	Defense Mechanism	Action
Skin		
Mouth		
Respiratory Tract		
Urinary Tract		
Gastrointestinal Tract		

- The inflammatory response includes the following. Explain each briefly.

  a. Vascular and cellular responses: _____

  _____

  _____

  b. Inflammatory exudate: _____

  _____

  _____

  c. Tissue repair: _____

  _____

  _____

- Define *immune response.* _____

  _____

  _____

- Briefly explain the following vascular and cellular responses:

  a. Edema: _____

  _____

  _____

  b. Phagocytosis: _____

  _____

  _____

  c. Inflammatory exudates: _____

  _____

  _____

  d. Tissue repair: _____

  _____

  _____

Nosocomial Infections

- Define *nosocomial infections.* _____

  _____

  _____

- Define the following types of nosocomial infections.

  a. *Iatrogenic:* _____

  _____

  b. *Exogenous:* _____

  _____

  c. *Endogenous:* _____

  _____

- Identify at least three factors that increase a hospitalized client's risk of acquiring a nosocomial infection.

  a. _____

  b. _____

  c. _____

- Identify the major sites for nosocomial infection. _____

  _____

  _____

  _____

The Nursing Process in Infection Control

NP Assessment

- The nurse assesses the client's _____

  _____, and _____.

- Knowing the factors that increase the client's susceptibility or risk for infection, the nurse is better able to plan preventive therapy that includes aseptic technique.

- Any reduction in the body's primary or secondary defenses against infection places a client at risk. List at least four risk factors of each.

  a. Inadequate primary defenses: _____

  _____

  _____

  b. Inadequate secondary sources: _____

  _____

  _____

- The following factors influence client susceptibility. Explain each one.

  a. Age: _____

  _____

  _____

  b. Nutritional status: _____

  _____

  _____

  c. Stress: _____

  _____

  _____

  d. Disease process: _____

  _____

  _____

  e. Medical therapy: _____

  _____

  _____

Clinical Appearance

- Describe the clinical appearance of each type of infection.

  a. Local: _____

  _____

  b. Systemic: _____

  _____

- Describe how an infection is manifested in an older adult. _____

  _____

  _____

Laboratory Data

- List at least five laboratory values that may indicate infection:

  a. _____

  b. _____

  c. _____

  d. _____

  e. _____

Clients with Infection

- The ways in which infection can affect the client's and family's needs may be _____,

  _____, _____,

  _____, or _____.

Nursing Diagnosis

- The nurse may diagnose a risk for infection or make diagnoses that result from the effects of infection on health status.

Planning

- List four common goals for the client with an actual or potential risk for infection.

  a. _____

  b. _____

  c. _____

  d. _____

Implementation

Health Promotion

- List five ways a nurse may prevent an infection from developing or spreading.

  a. _____

  b. _____

  c. _____

  d. _____

  e. _____

- List preventive interventions to protect a client from invasion by pathogens: _____

  _____

  _____

  _____

Acute Care Measures

- The nurse follows certain principles and procedures to prevent infection and to control its spread. Briefly explain each one.

  a. Concept of asepsis: _____

  _____

  b. Medical asepsis: _____

  _____

- Explain the following methods of controlling or eliminating infectious agents.

  a. Proper cleansing: _____

  _____

  b. Disinfection: _____

  _____

  c. Sterilization of objects: _____

  _____

  d. Control or elimination of reservoirs: _____

  _____

  e. Control of portals of exit: _____

  _____

  f. Control of transmission (hand washing):

  _____

  _____

- Nurses should wash their hands in the following situations.

  a. _____

  b. _____

  c. _____

  d. _____

  e. _____

- Many measures that control the exit of microorganisms also control the entrance of pathogens. Give at least five examples.

  a. _____

  b. _____

  c. _____

  d. _____

  e. _____

- A client's resistance to infection improves as the nurse protects the body's normal defenses against infection. Explain. _____

  _____

  _____

- Isolation or barrier precautions include the appropriate use of _____,

  _____, _____

  and _____.

- Barrier protection is indicated for use with clients. Explain. _____

  _____

  _____

- The CDC's new isolation guidelines (1996) contain a two-tiered approach. Explain.

  a. Standard Precautions (Tier 1): _____

  _____

  _____

  _____

  b. Transmission Categories (Tier 2): _____

  _____

  _____

  _____

- Regardless of the type of isolation system, the nurse must follow the following basic principles. _____
  _____
  _____

- Briefly summarize the psychological implications of isolation: _____
  _____
  _____
  _____

- In the grid below, place an X under the barriers required to maintain protective asepsis for each category-specific isolation technique.

Type of Isolation	Room	Gown	Gloves	Mask
Strict				
Content				
Respiratory				
Enteric Precautions				
Tuberculosis Isolation				
Drainage and Secretion Precautions				
Universal Blood and Body Fluid Precautions				
Care of the Severely Compromised Client				

- Explain the techniques for collecting specimens from the client with a suspected infection.

  a. Wound: _____

  _____

  b. Blood: _____

  _____

  c. Stool: _____

  _____

  d. Urine: _____

  _____

- Explain the CDC recommendations for bagging trash or linen. _____

  _____

  _____

- Describe how you would transport a client with an infection. _____

  _____

  _____

Role of the Infection-Control Professional

- List eight responsibilities of the infection-control professional.

  a. _____

  b. _____

  c. _____

  d. _____

  e. _____

  f. _____

  g. _____

  h. _____

Infection Prevention and Control for Hospital Personnel

- List the OSHA guidelines that were established to protect employees.

  a. _____

  b. _____

  c. _____

  d. _____

  e. _____

Client Education

- List six topics the nurse needs to discuss with the client in relation to infection-control practices.

  a. _____

  b. _____

  c. _____

  d. _____

  e. _____

  f. _____

Surgical Asepsis

- List three teaching points that reduce the risk of client-associated contamination during sterile procedures or treatments.

  a. _____

  b. _____

  c. _____

- List the seven principles of surgical asepsis.

  a. _____

  b. _____

  c. _____

  d. _____

  e. _____

  f. _____

  g. _____

• List and briefly explain the nine steps of a sterile procedure.

a. _____

b. _____

c. _____

d. _____

e. _____

f. _____

g. _____

h. _____

i. _____

𝒩𝒫 Evaluation

• The success of infection-control techniques is measured by determining whether the goals for reducing or preventing infection are achieved.

• Two important skills in evaluation are the ability to correctly assess wounds for healing and the ability to conduct a physical assessment of body systems.

• A clear description of any signs and symptoms of systemic or local infection is necessary to give all nurses a baseline for comparative evaluation.

• List three expected outcomes for clients at risk for infection:

a. _____

b. _____

c. _____

Review Questions

The student should select the appropriate answer and cite the rationale for choosing that particular answer.

1. Of the following, which is not an element in the development or chain of infection?
   a. Infectious agent or pathogen
   b. Reservoir for pathogen growth
   c. Means of transmission
   d. Formation of immunoglobulin

   Answer: _____ Rationale: _____

   _____

   _____

2. Pathogenic organisms include all of the following except:
   a. Bacteria
   b. Leukocytes
   c. Viruses
   d. Fungi

   Answer: _____ Rationale: _____

   _____

   _____

3. The severity of a client's illness will depend on all of the following except:
   a. Extent of infection
   b. Pathogenicity of the microorganism
   c. Susceptibility of the host
   d. Incubation period

   Answer: _____ Rationale: _____

   _____

   _____

4. Which of thse following best describes an iatrogenic infection?
   a. It results from a diagnostic or therapeutic procedure.
   b. It occurs when clients are infected with their own organisms as a result of immunodeficiency.
   c. It involves an incubation period of 3 to 4 weeks before it can be detected.
   d. It results from an extended infection of the urinary tract.

Answer: _____ Rationale: _____

_____

_____

5. The nurse sets up a nonbarrier sterile field on the client's overbed table. In which of the following instances is the field contaminated?
   a. The nurse keeps the top of the table above his or her waist.
   b. Sterile saline solution is spilled on the field.
   c. Sterile objects are kept within a 1-inch border of the field.
   d. The nurse, who has a cold, wears a double mask.

Answer: _____ Rationale: _____

_____

_____

6. When a client on respiratory isolation must be transported to another part of the hospital, the nurse:
   a. Places a mask on the client before leaving the room
   b. Obtains a physician's order to prohibit the client from being transported
   c. Advises other health team members to wear masks and gowns when coming in contact with the client
   d. Instructs the client to cover her mouth and nose with a tissue when coughing or sneezing

Answer: _____ Rationale: _____

_____

_____

34

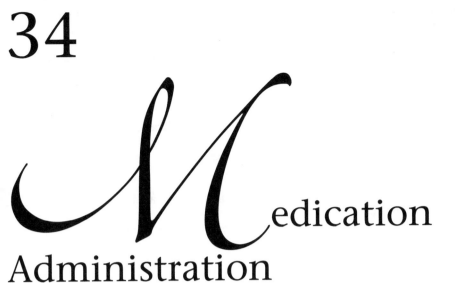

Medication Administration

*P*reliminary Reading

Chapter 34, pp. 821-909

*C*omprehensive Understanding

Scientific Knowledge Base

- The medications administered to clients are used to prevent, diagnose, or treat disease.

Pharmacological Concepts

- A single medication may have three different names. Define each one.

  a. *Chemical name:* _____

  _____

  b. *Generic name:* _____

  _____

  c. *Trade name:* _____

  _____

- A medication classification indicates: _____

  _____

  _____

- The form of the medication determines its: _____

  _____

  _____

Medication Legislation and Standards

- Briefly summarize the role of the federal government in regulation. _____

  _____

  _____

- Explain the Pure Food and Drug Act of 1906.

  _____

  _____

- The Food and Drug Administration (FDA) is responsible for: _____

  _____

  _____

- The USP and the National Formulary set standards for:

  _____

  _____

- Summarize the role of state and local regulation. _____

  _____

  _____

- Summarize the role of health care institutions.

  _____

  _____

- Nurse Practice Acts are responsible for: _____

  _____

  _____

Pharmacokinetics as the Basis of Medication Actions

- Pharmacokinetics is: _____

  _____

  _____

Absorption

- Define *absorption*. _____

  _____

  _____

- Briefly explain the following factors that influence drug absorption.

  a. Route of administration: _____

  _____

  _____

  b. Ability of a medication to dissolve: _____

  _____

  _____

  c. Blood flow to the area of absorption: _____

  _____

  _____

  d. Body surface area: _____

  _____

  _____

  e. Lipid solubility of a medication: _____

  _____

  _____

Distribution

- The rate and extent of distribution depend on the physical and chemical properties of the drug and on the physiological makeup of the person taking the drug.

- Explain how each of the following affect the rate and extent of medication distribution.

  a. Circulation: _____

  _____

  _____

  b. Membrane permeability: _____

  _____

  _____

  c. Protein binding: _____

  _____

  _____

Metabolism

- Define *biotransformation* and identify where it

  occurs. _____

  _____

  _____

Excretion

- After drugs are metabolized, they exit the body

  through the _____ ,

  _____ , _____ ,

  and _____ .

- Identify the primary organ for drug excretion
  and explain what happens if this organ func-

  tion declines. _____

  _____

  _____

Types of Medication Action

- Define the following predicted or unintended
  effects of drugs:

  a. Therapeutic effects: _____

  _____

  _____

  b. Side effects: _____

  _____

  _____

  c. Adverse effects: _____

  _____

  _____

  d. Toxic effects: _____

  _____

  _____

  e. Idiosyncratic reactions:

  _____

  _____

  f. Allergic reactions: _____

  _____

  _____

g. Anaphylactic reactions: _____

  _____

  _____

- A medication interaction is: _____

  _____

  _____

- A synergistic effect is: _____

  _____

  _____

Medication Dose Responses

- When a medication is prescribed, the goal is to
  achieve a constant blood level within a safe
  therapeutic range.

- Repeated doses are required to achieve a constant therapeutic concentration of a medication because a portion of a drug is always being
  excreted.

- Define.

  a. *Serum concentration:* _____

  _____

  _____

  b. *Serum half-life:* _____

  _____

  _____

- Explain the following time intervals of medication actions:

  a. Onset of drug action: _____

  _____

  b. Peak action: _____

  _____

  c. Trough: _____

  _____

  _____

d. Duration of action: _____

_____

_____

e. Plateau: _____

_____

_____

- Identify the route that is ideal for achieving a constant therapeutic drug level.

_____

_____

Routes of Administration

- The route prescribed for a drug's administration depends on its properties, the desired effect, and the client's physical and mental condition.

Oral Routes

- The oral route is the easiest and the most commonly used route.

- Identify the types of oral routes, explain how the oral routes are used, and identify the effects of using these routes.

_____

_____

_____

Parenteral Routes

- The parenteral route involves administering a drug through injection into body tissues.

- List the four major types of parenteral injections.

a. _____

b. _____

c. _____

d. _____

- Define the following advanced techniques of medication administration.

a. Epidural: _____

_____

b. Intrathecal: _____

_____

c. Intraosseous: _____

_____

d. Intraperitoneal: _____

_____

e. Intrapleural: _____

_____

f. Intra-arterial: _____

_____

Topical Administration

- Medications that are applied to the skin and mucous membranes principally have local effects.

- Identify five methods for applying medications to mucous membranes.

a. _____

b. _____

c. _____

d. _____

e. _____

Inhalation Route

- Explain the following types of inhalations.

a. Nasal: _____

_____

b. Oral: _____

_____

c. Endotracheal or tracheal: _____

_____

Intraocular Route

- Intraocular administration involves inserting a medication disk, similar to a contact lens, into the client's eye.

Systems of Medication Measurement

- The following are measurements used in drug therapy. Briefly explain their basic units.

  a. Metric system: _____

  _____

  b. Apothecary system: _____

  _____

  c. Household measurements: _____

  _____

Solutions

- A solution is: _____

  _____

  _____

Clinical Calculations

Conversions Within One System

- Indicate which direction the decimal point is moved for the following mathematical calculations in the metric system.

  a. Division: _____

  _____

  b. Multiplication: _____

  _____

Conversion Between Systems

- To make actual drug calculations, it is necessary to work with units in the same measurement system.

- Before making a conversion, the nurse compares the measurement system available with that which has been ordered.

- Complete the following measurement equivalents:

Metric	Apothecary	Household
1 ml	_____ minims	_____ drops
_____ ml	_____ fluid drams	1 tablespoon
30 ml	_____ fluid ounce(s)	_____ tablespoon
_____ ml	_____ fluid ounce(s)	1 cup
_____ ml	1 pint	_____ pint
_____ ml	_____ quart	1 quart

- Complete the following conversions:

  a. 100 mg = _____ g

  b. 2.5 L = _____ ml

  c. 500 ml = _____ L

  d. 15 mg = _____ gr

  e. 30 gtt = _____ ml

  f. gr 1/6 = _____ mg

Dosage Calculations

- Write out the formula used to determine the correct dose when preparing solid or liquid forms of medications.

- Define the following.

  a. *Dose ordered:* _____

  _____

  b. *Dose on hand:* _____

  _____

  c. *Amount on hand:* _____

  _____

Chapter 34: Medication Administration   199

Pediatric Dosages

- Write out the formula applied to accurately cal culate pediatric dosages. _____

_____

_____

Administering Medications

- The nurse who is administering the medications is accountable for: _____

_____

_____

Prescriber's Role

- Identify the primary responsibilities of the prescriber in giving medications to clients.

_____

_____

Types of Orders in Acute Care Agencies

- Briefly explain the four common types of medication orders.

    a. Standing or routine: _____

    _____

    b. PRN: _____

    _____

    c. Single (one-time): _____

    _____

    d. STAT: _____

    _____

- List the five parts of a prescription.

    a. _____

    b. _____

    c. _____

    d. _____

    e. _____

    f. _____

- Identify the primary responsibility of the pharmacist in the administration of medications.

_____

_____

- List the three medication distribution systems and identify the advantages and disadvantages of each.

    a. _____

    b. _____

    c. _____

- Summarize the nurse's primary responsibilities when administering medications. _____

_____

_____

Critical Thinking in Medication Administration

- Summarize the knowledge needed from other disciplines to safely administer medications.

_____

_____

_____

- Psychomotor skills, the client's attitudes, knowledge, physical and mental status, and responses can make medication administration a complex experience.

- Accountability for the nurse in administering medications is: _____

_____

- A medication error is: _____

_____

Standards

- List the "six rights" of medication administration and briefly explain each one.

    a. _____

    b. _____

    c. _____

    d. _____

    e. _____

    f. _____

Maintaining Client's Rights

- Briefly summarize the Patient Care Partnership related to drug administration.

  _____

  _____

  _____

Nursing Process and Medication Administration

Assessment

- Explain the following factors to assess.

  a. History: _____

  _____

  b. History of allergies: _____

  _____

  c. Medication data: _____

  _____

  d. Diet history: _____

  _____

  e. Client's perceptual or coordination problems: _____

  _____

  f. Client's current condition: _____

  _____

  g. Client's attitude about medication use: ____

  _____

  h. Client's knowledge and understanding of medication therapy: _____

  _____

  i. Client's learning needs: _____

  _____

Nursing Diagnosis

- Assessment provides data on the client's condition, his or her ability to self-administer medications, and medication use patterns. This information can be used to determine actual or potential problems with medication therapy.

Planning

- The nurse organizes care activities to ensure the safe administration of medications.

- Identify the four goals that the nurse or client needs to meet before administration of medications.

  a. _____

  b. _____

  c. _____

  d. _____

Implementation

Health Promotion

- Identify factors that can influence the client's compliance with the medication regimen.

  _____

  _____

- Explain information that needs to be taught to the client and family in relation to medications. _____

  _____

  _____

Acute Care

- Explain why the following interventions are essential for safe and effective medication administration.

  a. Receiving medication orders: _____

  _____

  _____

  _____

  b. Correct transcription and communication of orders: _____

  _____

  _____

  _____

Chapter 34: Medication Administration   201

c. Accurate dose calculation and measurement: _____

_____

_____

d. Correct administration: _____

_____

_____

e. Recording medication administration: _____

_____

_____

Restorative Care

- Regardless of the type of medication activity, the nurse is responsible for: _____

_____

_____

Special Considerations for Administering Medications to Specific Age Groups

Infants and Children

- Identify the appropriate nursing action used in administering medications to an infant or child. _____

_____

_____

Older Adults

- List the five behavioral patterns of medication use characteristic of the older adult and briefly explain each one.

    a. _____

    _____

    b. _____

    _____

    c. _____

    _____

    d. _____

    _____

e. _____

_____

Evaluation

- The nurse must know the therapeutic action and common side effects of each medication in order to monitor a client's response to that medication.

- Many different evaluation measures can be used in the context of medication administration. Name some of them. _____

_____

- The most common type of measurement is:

_____

_____

Oral Administration

- The easiest and most desirable way to administer medications is by mouth.

- The primary contraindication to giving oral medications is: _____

_____

_____

- To protect the client against possible aspiration, the nurse: _____

_____

_____

Topical Medication Applications

- Topical medications are applied most often to intact skin. They can also be applied to mucous membranes.

Skin Applications
- Explain the procedure for administering the following skin applications.

    a. Ointment: _____

    _____

    b. Lotion: _____

    _____

c. Powder: _____

_____

Nasal Instillation
• Summarize the rationale for nasal instillations.

_____

_____

_____

Eye Instillation
• List four principles for administering eye instillations.

a. _____

_____

b. _____

_____

c. _____

_____

d. _____

_____

Ear Instillation
• Explain the procedure for administering ear instillations.

a. Adult: _____

_____

_____

b. Children: _____

_____

_____

Vaginal Instillation
• Vaginal medications are available as _____

_____, _____,

_____, or

_____

Rectal Instillation
• Explain the differences between vaginal and rectal suppositories and the reason for these differences. _____

_____

Administering Medications by Inhalation
• To maximize the effect of metered dose inhalers, the nurse advises the client to: _____

_____

Administering Medications by Irrigations
• Identify the principles the nurse follows when performing irrigations. _____

_____

_____

Parenteral Administration of Medications
• Each type of injection requires certain skills to ensure that the drug reaches the proper location.

• When medications are administered parenterally, it is an invasive procedure that must be performed using aseptic techniques.

Equipment
• Identify the three major types of syringes.

a. _____

_____

b. _____

_____

c. _____

_____

• Identify three factors that must be considered when selecting a needle for an injection.

a. _____

_____

b. _____

_____

c. _____

_____

- Identify the advantages of using the Tubex or Carpuject injection systems. _____

_____

_____

Preparing an Injection from an Ampule
- An ampule is: _____

_____

_____

- The procedure for withdrawing medications from ampules is outlined in Procedure 34-7.

Preparing an Injection from a Vial
- A vial is a: _____

_____

_____

- The vial is a closed system, and air must be injected into it to permit easy withdrawal of the solution.

- The procedure for withdrawal of medications from vials is outlined in Procedure 34-7.

Mixing Medications
- It is possible to mix two drugs together into one injection if the total dosage is within accepted limits.

- List the three principles to follow when mixing medications from two vials:

  a. _____

  _____

  b. _____

  _____

  c. _____

  _____

- When mixing medications from an ampule and a vial, which medication should be prepared first? _____

_____

Insulin Preparation
- Insulin is: _____

_____

_____

- Explain why insulin must be administered by injection: _____

_____

_____

- Insulin is classified by: _____

_____

_____

- _____
  is the only insulin used for sliding scales.

- Identify the simple guidelines for mixing two kinds of insulin in the same syringe.

  _____

  _____

Administering Injections
- The characteristics of the tissues injected influence the: _____

_____

_____

- List the techniques used to minimize client discomfort that is associated with injections.

  a. _____

  _____

  b. _____

  _____

  c. _____

  _____

  d. _____

  _____

  e. _____

  _____

f. _____

_____

g. _____

_____

Subcutaneous Injections

- Subcutaneous injections involve placing the medications into the loose connective tissue under the dermis.

- Explain the differences in absorption between a subcutaneous and an intramuscular injection.

- The best sites for SQ injections include

_____, _____,

and _____.

- The site most frequently recommended for

heparin injection is _____

_____

- The site chosen should be free of _____

_____, _____,

and _____.

- Identify the maximum amount of water-soluble medication given by the SQ route.

_____

_____

- State the rule that may be followed to determine if a SQ injection should be given at a 90-

or 45-degree angle. _____

_____

_____

Intramuscular Injections

- Identify the major risk of using the IM route.

_____

_____

- The angle of insertion for an IM injection is

degrees.

- Indicate the maximum volume of medication for IM injection in each of the following groups.

a. Well-developed adult: _____

_____

b. Older children, older adults, or thin adults:

_____

c. Older infants and small children: _____

_____

Sites

- List the assessment criteria for selecting an IM site.

a. _____

_____

b. _____

_____

c. _____

_____

d. _____

_____

- Describe the advantages and disadvantages of the following injection sites.

a. Vastus lateralis: _____

_____

_____

b. Ventrogluteal: _____

_____

c. Dorsogluteal: _____

_____

_____

d. Deltoid: _____

_____

_____

Chapter 34: Medication Administration   205

Special Techniques in IM Injections

- Explain the rationale for administering an intramuscular injection using the air-lock technique. _____

  _____

  _____

- Explain the rationale for using the Z-track method of injection. _____

  _____

  _____

Intradermal Injections

- Explain the rationale for administering an intradermal injection. _____

  _____

  _____

Safety in Administering Medications by Injection

- Explain the rationale for each of the following.

  a. Needleless device: _____

  _____

  _____

  b. One-handed needle recapping technique:

  _____

  _____

Intravenous Administration

- The nurse administers medications intravenously by the following methods. _____

  _____

  _____

- Identify the advantage and disadvantage of the large-volume infusion method.

  _____

  _____

- Explain the advantage and disadvantage of the IV bolus route of administration.

  _____

  _____

  _____

- List the advantages of using volume-controlled infusions.

  a. _____

  _____

  b. _____

  _____

  c. _____

  _____

- Piggyback sets are: _____

  _____

- A tandem setup is: _____

  _____

- Volume-control administration sets are:

  _____

- A miniinfusor pump is: _____

  _____

- List the three advantages of using intermittent venous access devices.

  a. _____

  _____

  b. _____

  _____

  c. _____

  _____

Administration of Intravenous Therapy in the Home

- When receiving home intravenous therapy, client education should include: _____

  _____

  _____

Review Questions

The student should select the appropriate answer and cite the rationale for choosing that particular answer.

1. The study of how drugs enter the body, reach their sites of action, are metabolized, and exit from the body is called:
   a. Pharmacology
   b. Pharmacokinetics
   c. Pharmacopoeia
   d. Biopharmaceutica

Answer: _____ Rationale: _____

_____

_____

2. Which statement correctly characterizes drug absorption?
   a. Most drugs must enter the systemic circulation to have a therapeutic effect.
   b. Mucous membranes are relatively impermeable to chemicals, making absorption slow.
   c. Oral medications are absorbed more quickly when administered with meals.
   d. Drugs administered subcutaneously are absorbed more quickly than those injected intramuscularly.

Answer: _____ Rationale: _____

_____

_____

3. The onset of drug action is the time it takes for a drug to:
   a. Produce a response
   b. Accelerate the cellular process
   c. Reach its highest effective concentration
   d. Produce blood serum concentration and maintenance

Answer: _____ Rationale: _____

_____

_____

4. Which of the following is not a parenteral route of administration?
   a. Buccal
   b. Subcutaneous
   c. Intramuscular
   d. Intradermal

Answer: _____ Rationale: _____

_____

_____

5. Using the body surface area formula, what dose of drug X should a child who weighs 12 kg (body surface area = 0.54 m^2) receive if the normal adult dose of drug X is 300 mg?
   a. 50 mg
   b. 90 mg
   c. 100 mg
   d. 200 mg

Answer: _____ Rationale: _____

_____

_____

6. The nurse is preparing an insulin injection in which both regular and modified insulin will be mixed. Into which vial should the nurse inject air first?
   a. The vial of modified insulin
   b. The vial of regular insulin
   c. Either vial, as long as modified insulin is drawn up first
   d. Neither vial; it is not necessary to put air into vials before withdrawing medication

Answer: _____ Rationale: _____

_____

_____

35

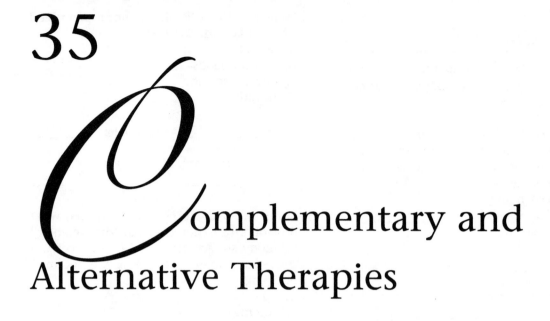

Complementary and Alternative Therapies

Preliminary Reading

Chapter 35, pp. 910-926

Comprehensive Understanding

• Describe the difference between the following terms.

a. Complementary therapies: _____

_____

_____

b. Alternative therapies: _____

_____

_____

• Explain the following traditional and ethnomedicine therapies and give an example of each.

a. Acupuncture: _____

_____

b. Ayurveda: _____

_____

c. Homeopathic medicine: _____

_____

d. Latin American practices: _____

_____

e. Naturopathic medicine: _____
_____

f. Traditional Chinese medicine: _____
_____

• Describe integrative medical programs: _____
_____

Nursing-Accessible Therapies

Relaxation Therapy
• Define *stress response*. _____
_____
_____

• Chronic stress is: _____
_____
_____

• Relaxation is: _____
_____
_____

• Progressive relaxation training helps to: _____
_____
_____

• Passive relaxation involves teaching: _____
_____
_____

• Relaxation techniques are effective in _____
_____, _____, _____,
and _____

• The type of relaxation intervention should be matched to: _____
_____

• Identify the limitations of relaxation therapy.
_____
_____

Meditation and Breathing
• Meditation is: _____
_____

• Identify the clinical applications of meditation. _____
_____

• Identify the limitations of meditation. _____
_____
_____
_____

Imagery
• Imagery is: _____
_____

• Creative visualization is: _____
_____

• Identify the clinical applications of imagery.
_____
_____
_____

• Identify the limitations of imagery. _____
_____
_____

Trained-Specific Therapies

Biofeedback
• Biofeedback is: _____
_____

• Identify the clinical applications of biofeedback. _____
_____

• Identify the limitations of biofeedback. _____
_____
_____

Therapeutic Touch

- Therapeutic touch is: _____

  _____

  _____

- Therapeutic touch consists of five phases. Explain each one.

  a. Centering: _____

  _____

  b. Assessment: _____

  _____

  c. Unruffling: _____

  _____

  d. Treatment: _____

  _____

  e. Evaluation: _____

  _____

- Identify the physiological indicators of energy

  imbalance. _____

  _____

- Identify the clinical applications for therapeu-

  tic touch. _____

  _____

- Identify the limitations of therapeutic touch.

  _____

Chiropractic Therapy

- Chiropractic therapy is: _____

  _____

- Describe the clinical applications of chiroprac-

  tic therapy. _____

  _____

  _____

- Identify the limitations of chiropractic

  therapy. _____

  _____

  _____

_____

Traditional and Ethnomedicine Therapies

Traditional Chinese Medicine

- Traditional Chinese Medicine (TCM) is: _____

  _____

  _____

  _____

- Explain the concept of Yin and Yang. _____

  _____

  _____

  _____

- Qi is: _____

  _____

  _____

- Traditional Chinese medicine classifies disease into three categories. State the influences of each:

  a. External causes: _____

  _____

  b. Internal causes: _____

  _____

  c. Nonexternal causes: _____

  _____

- Define *meridians*. _____

  _____

  _____

Acupuncture

- Acupuncture is: _____

  _____

  _____

- Describe the clinical applications of acupunc-

  ture. _____

  _____

  _____

- Identify the limitations of acupuncture. _____

_____

_____

_____

Herbal Therapies

- Herbal therapy is: _____

_____

_____

- The goal of herbal therapy is: _____

_____

_____

- Describe the clinical applications of herbal

therapy. _____

_____

_____

- Identify the limitations of herbal therapy. ____

_____

_____

_____

- Herbal products should be used cautiously

with: _____

_____

_____

Nursing Role in Complementary and Alternative Therapies

- Summarize the role of the nurse in relation to providing recommendations regarding complementary and alternative medicine

therapies. _____

_____

_____

_____

_____

Review Questions

The student should select the appropriate answer and cite the rationale for choosing that particular answer.

1. Patients choose to use unconventional therapy because:
   a. They are willing to pay more to feel better.
   b. It is now widely accepted by the Food and Drug Administration.
   c. They are dissatisfied with conventional medicine.
   d. They want religious approval for the remedies they use.

Answer: _____ Rationale: _____

_____

_____

2. The Dietary Supplement and Health Education Act states that:
   a. Herbs, vitamins, and minerals may be sold with their therapeutic advantages listed on the label.
   b. The Food and Drug Administration must evaluate all herbal therapies.
   c. Herbs, vitamins, and minerals may be sold as long as no therapeutic claims are made on the label.
   d. In conjunction with the Food and Drug Administration, all supplements are considered safe for use.

Answer: _____ Rationale: _____

_____

_____

3. Nurses can best assess their patient's use of alternative therapies by:
   a. Asking the patient true/false questions about their health
   b. Asking for a thorough medical history
   c. Reviewing laboratory studies that assess levels of certain herbs
   d. Asking open-ended questions on alternative therapies

Answer: _____ Rationale: _____

_____

_____

4. Which of the following steps should nurses take to be better informed about alternative therapies?
   a. Read current books and magazines on alternative therapies.
   b. Familiarize themselves with recent case studies on alternative therapies.
   c. Familiarize themselves with general principles of phytotherapy.
   d. Review herb manufacturer's literature on specific herbs.

Answer: _____ Rationale: _____

_____

_____

36

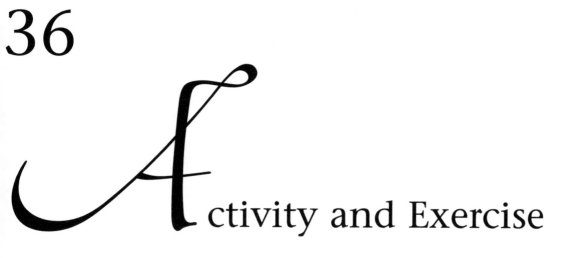

$\mathcal{A}$ctivity and Exercise

$\mathcal{P}$reliminary Reading

Chapter 36, pp. 929-958

$\mathcal{C}$omprehensive Understanding

Scientific Knowledge Base

• Body mechanics include: _____

_____

_____

Overview of Body Mechanics, Exercise, and Activity

• The coordinated efforts of the musculoskeletal and nervous systems maintain _____,

_____, and

during lifting, bending, moving, and performing _____ provide the foundation for

body mechanics.

• Define *body alignment*. _____

_____

_____

• Body balance is achieved when a _____,

_____, and

_____.

- Proper body alignment and posture are maintained by using two simple techniques. Name them.

  a. _____

  b. _____

- Define *center of gravity*. _____

  _____

  _____

- Coordinated body movement is the result of

  _____, _____,

  and _____.

- Define *friction*. _____

  _____

  _____

- List two techniques that minimize friction.

  a. _____

  b. _____

- Activity tolerance is: _____

  _____

  _____

- There are three categories of exercises. Briefly explain each one and give an example of each.

  a. Isotonic contraction: _____

  _____

  _____

  b. Isometric contraction: _____

  _____

  _____

Regulation of Movement
- List three systems responsible for coordinating body movements.

  a. _____

  b. _____

  c. _____

- List five functions of the skeletal system.

  a. _____

  b. _____

  c. _____

  d. _____

  e. _____

- Describe the following.

  a. Joints: _____

  _____

  b. Cartilaginous joint: _____

  _____

  c. Fibrous joint: _____

  _____

  d. Synovial joint: _____

  _____

  e. Ligaments: _____

  _____

  f. Cartilage: _____

  _____

  g. Tendons: _____

  _____

- Briefly describe how skeletal muscles affect movement. _____

  _____

  _____

- Briefly explain the muscles concerned with:

  a. Movement: _____

  _____

  b. Posture: _____

  _____

- Coordination and regulation of different muscle groups depend on the following. Briefly explain each.

  a. Antagonistic muscles: _____

  _____

  _____

b. Synergistic muscles: _____

_____

_____

c. Antigravity muscles: _____

_____

_____

• Briefly describe how movement and posture are regulated by the nervous system. _____

_____

_____

• Define *proprioception.* _____

_____

_____

• Balance is the ability to: _____

_____

_____

Principles of Body Mechanics

• Identify the physiological and pathological influences on body alignment and mobility.

_____

_____

_____

Pathological Influences on Body Mechanics

• Briefly explain how the following pathological conditions affect body alignment and mobility.

a. Congenital abnormalities: _____

_____

_____

b. Disorders of bones, joints, and muscles:

_____

_____

c. Central nervous system damage: _____

_____

_____

d. Musculoskeletal trauma: _____

_____

_____

Nursing Knowledge Base

• _____, _____,

_____, _____,

and _____
are important aspects of an individual and must be incorporated into the plan.

Developmental Changes

• The greatest change and impact on the maturational process is observed in _____

and _____.

• Identify the descriptive characteristics of body alignment and mobility related to the following developmental changes.

a. Infants: _____

_____

_____

b. Toddlers: _____

_____

_____

c. Adolescence: _____

_____

_____

d. Young to middle adults: _____

_____

_____

e. Older adults: _____

_____

_____

Behavioral Aspects

• Nurses need to take into consideration the client's _____,

_____, and _____.

• Clients are more open to developing an exercise program if they are at the stage of readiness to change their behavior.

Chapter 36: Activity and Exercise   215

Environmental Issues
- Explain the issues related to the following sites.

  a. Worksite: _____

  _____

  b. Schools: _____

  _____

  c. Community: _____

  _____

Cultural and Ethnic Influences
- The nurse must consider what motivates and what is deemed appropriate and enjoyable when developing a physical fitness program for culturally diverse populations.

Family and Social Support
- Briefly explain how a family may be a motivational tool in regard to physical fitness._____

  _____

  _____

  _____

Nursing Process

𝒩𝒫 Assessment

- Throughout the assessment, the nurse will be able to determine _____,

  _____, and _____.

- Briefly explain how assessment of body alignment and posture is carried out.

  a. Standing: _____

  _____

  b. Sitting: _____

  _____

  c. Recumbent: _____

  _____

- There are three components to assess in regard to mobility. Explain each.

  a. Range of motion: _____

  _____

  b. Gait: _____

  _____

  c. Exercise: _____

  _____

- Identify some factors that affect activity tolerance. _____

  _____

𝒩𝒫 Nursing Diagnosis

- Assessment of the _____,

  _____, _____,

  and _____

  provides clusters of data or defining characteristics that lead the nurse to identify nursing diagnoses. Give five examples.

  a. _____

  b. _____

  c. _____

  d. _____

  e. _____

𝒩𝒫 Planning

- The plan should include consideration of:

  a. _____

  b. _____

  c. _____

  d. _____

  e. _____

𝒩𝒫 Implementation

Health Promotion Activities

• List the five recommendations for exercise.

  a. _____

  b. _____

  c. _____

  d. _____

  e. _____

• Explain how to calculate the client's maximum heart rate (MHR)._____

  _____

  _____

• An exercise program can consist of the following. Explain each one.

  a. Aerobic exercise: _____

  _____

  _____

  b. Stretching and flexibility exercises: _____

  _____

  _____

  c. Resistance training: _____

  _____

  _____

• Briefly explain proper lifting techniques._____

  _____

  _____

Acute Care

• The musculoskeletal system can be maintained by encouraging the use of stretching and isometric-type exercises.

• Briefly explain the technique of stretching exercises: _____

  _____

  _____

• Explain how the nurse would maintain or improve joint mobility._____

  _____

  _____

• Explain how walking affects joint mobility.___

  _____

  _____

• Explain how the nurse would assist the client to walk._____

  _____

  _____

Restorative and Continuing Care

• The nurse, in collaboration with others, promotes activity and exercise by teaching the use of assistive devices most appropriate for a client's condition. Briefly explain.

  a. Canes: _____

  _____

  b. Crutches: _____

  _____

  c. Crutch gait: _____

  _____

• Explain the following gaits.

  a. Four-point: _____

  _____

  b Three-point: _____

  _____

  c. Two-point: _____

  _____

  d. Swing-through: _____

  _____

- Explain how the nurse would instruct the client in each of the following.
  a. Crutch walking on stairs: _____
  _____
  _____
  b. Sitting in the chair with crutches: _____
  _____
  _____

- Explain how the nurse would implement a plan of care to increase activity and exercise in the following specific disease conditions:
  a. Coronary heart disease (CHD): _____
  _____
  _____
  b. Hypertension: _____
  _____
  _____
  c. Chronic obstructive pulmonary disease:
  _____
  _____
  d. Diabetes mellitus: _____
  _____
  _____

𝒩𝒫 Evaluation

Client Care

- This phase of the nursing process evaluates the actual care delivered by the health team based on the expected outcomes.

- Comparisons are made with baseline measures that include pulse, blood pressure, strength, endurance, and physical well-being.

Client Expectations

- The nurse needs to know the client's expectations concerning activity and exercise.

𝓡eview Questions

The student should select the appropriate answer and cite the rationale for choosing that particular answer.

1. Which of the following is true of body mechanics?
   a. The narrower the base of support, the greater the stability of the nurse.
   b. The higher the center of gravity, the greater the stability of the nurse.
   c. When friction is reduced between the object to be moved and the surface on which it is moved, less force is required to move it.
   d. Rolling, turning, or pivoting requires more work than lifting.

Answer: _____ Rationale: _____
_____
_____

2. White, shiny, flexible bands of fibrous tissue binding joints together and connecting various bones and cartilage types are known as:
   a. Muscles
   b. Ligaments
   c. Joints
   d. Tendons

Answer: _____ Rationale: _____
_____
_____

3. The nurse would expect all of the following physiological effects of exercise on the body systems except:
   a. Decreased cardiac output
   b. Increased respiratory rate and depth
   c. Increased muscle tone, size, and strength
   d. Change in metabolic rate

Answer: _____ Rationale: _____
_____
_____

4. Which of the following is *not* appropriate in performing a three-person carry to transfer a client from bed to a stretcher?
   a. Use three nurses of a similar height.
   b. Place the stretcher parallel to the bed.
   c. Nurses roll the client to his or her chest.
   d. One nurse assumes the leadership role and directs the other two.

Answer: _____ Rationale: _____

_____

_____

5. Movements of the hip include all of the following except:
   a. Flexion
   b. Hyperextension
   c. Circumduction
   d. Opposition

Answer: _____ Rationale: _____

_____

_____

Critical Thinking for Nursing Care Plan for Activity Intolerance

Imagine that you are Mary, the nurse in the Care Plan on page 943 of your text. Complete the *Planning phase* of the critical thinking model by writing your answers in the appropriate boxes of the model shown. Think about the following:

- In developing Mrs. Swain's plan of care, what knowledge did Mary apply?

- In what way might Mary's previous experience assist in developing a plan of care for Mrs. Swain?

- When developing a plan of care, what intellectual or professional standards were applied to Mrs. Swain?

- What critical thinking attitudes might have been applied in developing Mrs. Swain plan?

- How will Mary accomplish her goals?

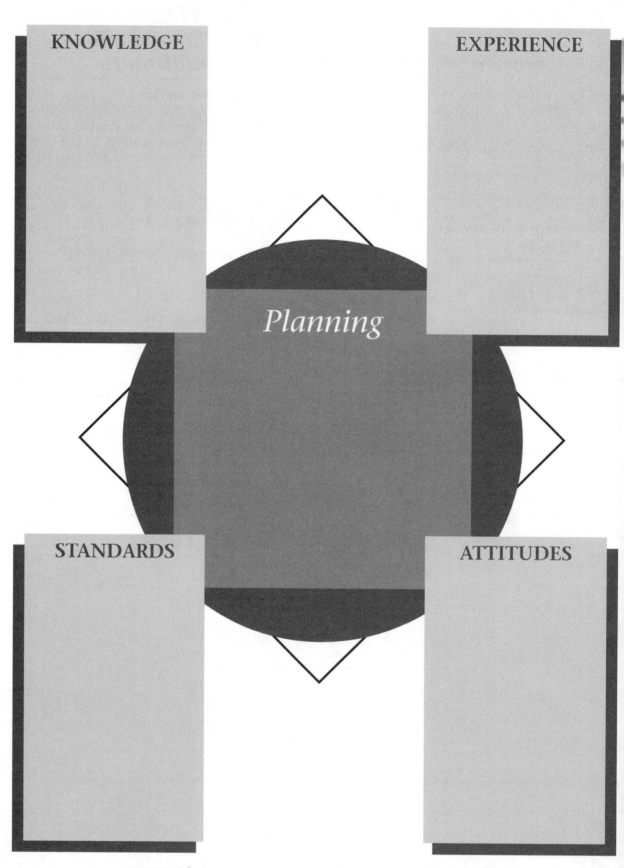

KNOWLEDGE

EXPERIENCE

Planning

STANDARDS

ATTITUDES

CHAPTER *36* Critical Thinking Model for Nursing Care Plan for *Activity Intolerance*

See answers on page 539.

37

Client Safety

Preliminary Reading

Chapter 37, pp. 959-1000

Comprehensive Understanding

Scientific Knowledge Base

Environmental Safety
- A client's environment includes: _____
_____
_____

- List the five characteristics of a safe environment.

  a. _____

  b. _____

  c. _____

  d. _____

  e. _____

- Give an example of the four basic physiological needs that influence a person's safety.

  a. Oxygen: _____
  _____

  b. Nutrition: _____
  _____

c. Temperature: _____

_____

d. Humidity: _____

_____

- Physical hazards in the community and health care settings place clients at risk for accidental injury and death. List the four physical hazards that contribute to falls.

  a. _____

  b. _____

  c. _____

  d. _____

- Define *pathogen*. _____

_____

_____

- Identify the most effective method for limiting the transmission of pathogens. _____

_____

_____

- Define *immunization*. _____

_____

_____

- Describe the two types of immunity.

  a. Active: _____

  _____

  b. Passive: _____

  _____

- Describe how the human immunodeficiency virus (HIV) is transmitted and who is at risk.

_____

_____

- A healthy environment is free from pollution. A pollutant is: _____

_____

_____

- Define the following types of pollution.

  a. *Air:* _____

  b. *Land:* _____

  c. *Water:* _____

  d. *Noise:* _____

- Define *bioterrorism* and the emergency management plan needed. _____

_____

_____

Nursing Knowledge Base

- In addition to being knowledgeable about the environment, nurses must be familiar with:

  a. _____

  b. _____

  c. _____

  d. _____

  e. _____

Risks at Developmental Stages
- Identify at least three threats to safety in the following developmental stages.

  a. Infant, toddler, preschooler: _____

  _____

  b. School-age: _____

  _____

  c. Adolescents: _____

  _____

  d. Adult: _____

  _____

  e. Older adult: _____

  _____

Individual Risk Factors
- Explain how the following risk factors can increase safety risks.

  a. Lifestyle: _____

  _____

  b. Impaired mobility: _____

  _____

c. Sensory or communication impairment: ____

_____

d. Lack of safety awareness: _____

_____

Risks in the Health Care Agency

- List the four major risks to client safety in the health care environment.

  a. _____

  b. _____

  c. _____

  d. _____

Safety and the Nursing Process

Assessment

- In order to conduct a thorough client assessment, the nurse will consider possible threats to the client's safety, including the client's immediate environment, as well as any individual risk factors.

- Identify the specific assessments a nurse needs to make in the following settings.

  a. Caring for a client in the home: _____

  _____

  b. Caring for a client in the health care facility:

  _____

  _____

- Explain the following health care environment risks:

  a. Risk for falls: _____

  b. Risk for medical errors: _____

  c. Bioterrorist attacks: _____

- Identify the seven features that should alert nurses to the possibility of a bioterrorism-related outbreak:

  a. _____

  b. _____

  c. _____

  d. _____

e. _____

f. _____

g. _____

Nursing Diagnosis

- Identify four actual or potential nursing diagnoses for safety risks.

  a. _____

  b. _____

  c. _____

  d. _____

Planning

- Identify common goals that focus on the client's need for safety.

  a. _____

  b. _____

  c. _____

Implementation

Health Promotion

- In order to promote an individual's health it is necessary for the individual to be in a safe environment and to practice a lifestyle that minimizes risk of injury.

- Identify at least four interventions for each of the following developmental age groups.

  a. Infant, toddler, preschooler: _____

  _____

  b. School-age: _____

  _____

  c. Adolescent: _____

  _____

  d. Adult: _____

  _____

  e. Older adult: _____

  _____

- Nursing interventions directed at eliminating environmental threats include _____, _____ , _____, and _____.

Acute Care

- List eight measures to prevent falls in the health care setting.

  a. _____

  b. _____

  c. _____

  d. _____

  e. _____

  f. _____

  g. _____

  h. _____

- A physical restraint is _____

  _____

  _____.

- The immobility imposed by restraining a client can lead to:

  a. Physical: _____

  _____

  b. Psychological: _____

  _____

- Use of restraints must meet the following objectives.

  a. _____

  b. _____

  c. _____

  d. _____

- Explain why an Ambularm is used. _____

  _____

  _____

- Explain the use of side rails. _____

  _____

  _____

- Describe four fire-containment guidelines.

  a. _____

  b. _____

  c. _____

  d. _____

- A poison is: _____

  _____

  _____

- List five teaching strategies for prevention of electrical hazards.

  a. _____

  b. _____

  c. _____

  d. _____

  e. _____

- A seizure is: _____

  _____

  _____

- Identify the measures with which the nurse must be familiar to reduce exposure to radiation.

  _____

  _____

  _____

  _____

- Briefly explain the four phases of the emergency management plan.

  a. Mitigation: _____

  _____

  b. Preparedness: _____

  _____

  c. Response: _____

  _____

224   Chapter 37: Client Safety

d. Recovery: _____

_____

Evaluation

Client Care

- The nurse continually assesses the client and family's need for additional support services

such as _____,

_____,

and _____

Client Expectations

- The expected outcomes include a _____

and _____.

eview Questions

The student should select the appropriate answer and cite the rationale for choosing that particular answer.

1. Which of the following would most threaten an individual's safety?
   a. 70% humidity
   b. Carbon dioxide
   c. Unrefrigerated fresh vegetables
   d. Lack of water supply

Answer: _____ Rationale: _____

_____

_____

2. The developmental stage that carries the highest risk of an injury from a fall is:
   a. Preschool
   b. School-age
   c. Adulthood
   d. Older adulthood

Answer: _____ Rationale: _____

_____

_____

3. Mrs. Field falls asleep while smoking in bed and drops the burning cigarette on her blanket. When she awakens, her bed is on fire, and she quickly calls the nurse. On observing the fire, the nurse should immediately:
   a. Report the fire
   b. Attempt to extinguish the fire
   c. Assist Mrs. Fields to a safe place
   d. Close all windows and doors to contain the fire

Answer: _____ Rationale: _____

_____

_____

4. Sixteen-year-old Jimmy is admitted to an adolescent unit with a diagnosis of substance abuse. The nurse examines Jimmy and finds that he has bloodshot eyes, slurred speech, and an unstable gait. He smells of alcohol and is unable to answer questions appropriately. The appropriate nursing diagnosis would be:
   a. Self-care deficit related to alcohol abuse
   b. Altered thought processes related to sensory overload
   c. Knowledge deficit related to alcohol abuse
   d. High risk for injury related to impaired sensory perception

Answer: _____ Rationale: _____

_____

_____

5. If a client receives an electric shock, the nurse's first action should be to:
   a. Assess the client's pulse
   b. Assess the client for thermal injury
   c. Notify the physician
   d. Notify the maintenance department

Answer: _____ Rationale: _____

_____

_____

Critical Thinking for Nursing Care Plan for Risk for Injury

Imagine that you are Mr. Key, the nurse in the Care Plan on page 974 of your text. Complete the *Assessment phase* of the critical thinking model by writing your answers in the appropriate boxes of the model shown. Think about the following:

- In developing Ms. Cohen's plan of care, what knowledge did Mr. Key apply?

- In what way might Mr. Key's previous experience assist in this case?

- What intellectual or professional standards were applied to Ms. Cohen?

- What critical thinking attitudes might have been applied in this case?

- As you review your assessment, what key areas did you cover?

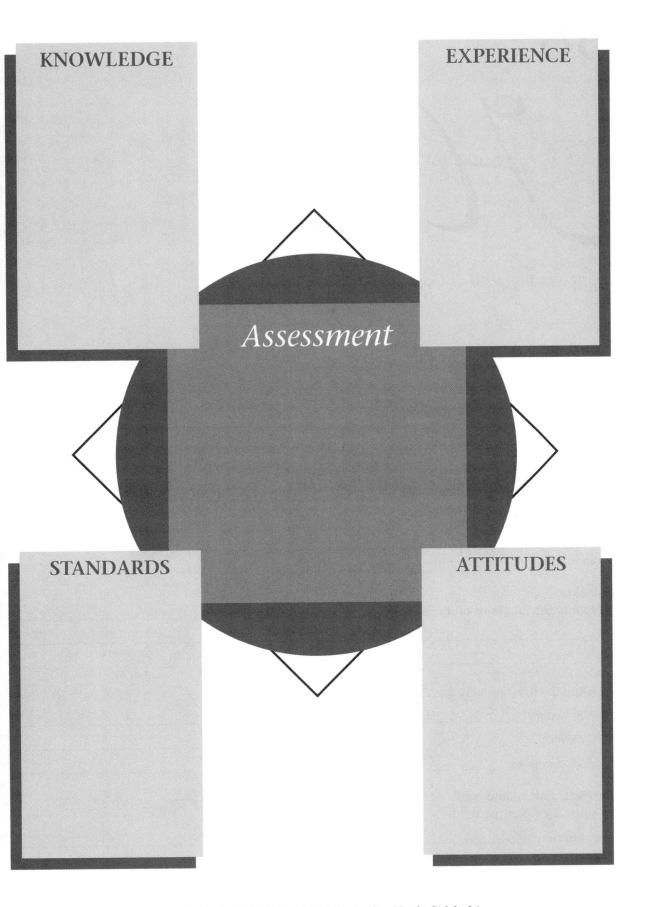

KNOWLEDGE

EXPERIENCE

Assessment

STANDARDS

ATTITUDES

CHAPTER *37* Critical Thinking Model for Nursing Care Plan for *Risk for Injury*

See answers on page 540.

38

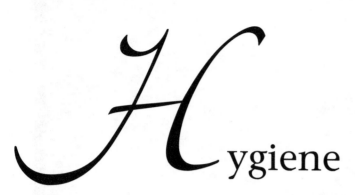

*H*ygiene

*P*reliminary Reading

Chapter 38, pp. 1001-1065

*C*omprehensive Understanding

Scientific Knowledge Base

- Proper hygienic care requires an understanding of the anatomy and physiology of the integument, oral cavity, eyes, ears, and nose.

The Skin
- Identify the functions of the skin. _____
_____
_____

- Define the three primary layers:
  a. *Epidermis:* _____
  b. *Dermis:* _____
  c. *Subcutaneous:* _____

The Feet, Hands, and Nails
- Define the following terms:
  a. *Cuticle:* _____
  b. *Lunula:* _____

The Oral Cavity

- There are three pairs of salivary glands that secrete about 1 liter of saliva a day.

- The buccal glands are: _____

  _____

  _____

- Teeth are responsible for: _____

  _____

  _____

- Regular oral hygiene is necessary to maintain the integrity of tooth surfaces and to prevent:

  _____

The Hair

- Identify the factors that can affect the hair's

  characteristics. _____

  _____

  _____

The Eyes, Ears, and Nose

- Cleansing of the sensitive sensory tissues should be done to prevent injury and client discomfort.

Nursing Knowledge Base

- Briefly explain each of the following.

  a. Social practices: _____

  _____

  _____

  b. Personal preferences: _____

  _____

  _____

  c. Body image: _____

  _____

  _____

  d. Socioeconomic status: _____

  _____

  _____

  e. Health beliefs and motivation: _____

  _____

  _____

f. Cultural variables: _____

  _____

  _____

g. Physical condition: _____

  _____

  _____

The Nursing Process

Assessment

Skin

- When inspecting the skin, the nurse examines

  _____, _____, _____,

  _____, _____,

  and _____.

- Common skin problems can affect how hygiene is administered. Describe the hygiene provided for the following.

  a. Dry skin: _____

  _____

  b. Acne: _____

  _____

  c. Skin rashes: _____

  _____

  d. Contact dermatitis: _____

  _____

  e. Abrasion: _____

  _____

- Briefly explain the six conditions that place clients at risk for impaired skin integrity.

  a. Immobilization: _____

  _____

  b. Reduced sensation: _____

  _____

  c. Nutrition and hydration: _____

  _____

  d. Secretions and excretions: _____

  _____

e. Vascular insufficiency: _____

_____

f. External devices: _____

_____

Feet and Nails

- Assessment of the feet involves a thorough examination of all skin surfaces, including the soles of the feet and the areas between the toes.

- Inspection of the feet for lesions includes:

_____

_____.

- Neuropathy is _____.
  Describe how the nurse would assess for this.

_____

_____

- Identify the characteristics of the following foot and nail problems.

  a. Calluses: _____

  _____

  b. Corns: _____

  _____

  c. Plantar warts: _____

  _____

  d. Tinea pedis: _____

  _____

  e. Ingrown nails: _____

  _____

  f. Ram's horn nails: _____

  _____

  g. Paronychia: _____

  _____

  h. Foot odors: _____

  _____

Oral Cavity

- The nurse inspects all areas of the oral cavity for _____, _____

  _____, and

  _____.

- _____ is a common symptom of gum disease and certain tooth disorders.

Hair

- Identify the characteristics of the following hair and scalp conditions.

  a. Dandruff: _____

  _____

  b. Ticks: _____

  _____

  c. Pediculosis: _____

  _____

  d. Pediculosis capitis: _____

  _____

  e. Pediculosis corporis: _____

  _____

  f. Pediculosis pubis: _____

  _____

  g. Alopecia: _____

  _____

Eyes, Ears, and Nose

- Identify the normal assessment findings for the following.

  a. Eyes: _____

  _____

  b. Nose: _____

  _____

  c. Ears: _____

  _____

Developmental Changes
Skin

- For each developmental stage, briefly describe normal conditions that create a high risk for impaired skin integrity.

  a. Neonate: _____

  _____

  _____

  b. Toddler: _____

  _____

  _____

  c. Adolescent: _____

  _____

  _____

  d. Older adult: _____

  _____

  _____

Feet and Nails

- Identify the common foot problems of the older adult. _____

  _____

  _____

The Mouth

- Identify the factors that can result in poor oral care: _____

  _____

  _____

Hair

- Throughout life, changes in the growth, distribution, and condition of hair influence hygiene. Explain. _____

  _____

  _____

Self-Care Ability

- Identify the factors that are assessed to determine a client's ability to perform routine hygiene._____

  _____

  _____

Hygienic Practices

- To assess the client's routine hygienic practices, the nurse would: _____

  _____.

Cultural Factors

- Culture plays a role in _____ and

  _____.

Clients at Risk for Hygiene Problems

- Give examples of clients at risk for the following.

  a. Oral problems: _____

  _____

  b. Skin problems: _____

  _____

  c. Foot problems: _____

  _____

  d. Eye care problems: _____

  _____

Special Considerations in Hygiene Assessment

- Explain briefly how footwear may predispose a client to foot and nail problems. _____

  _____

Nursing Diagnosis

- List five possible nursing diagnoses that apply to clients in need of hygienic care.

  a. _____

  b. _____

  c. _____

  d. _____

  e. _____

𝒩𝒫 Planning

- Identify some factors to consider when planning care. _____

_____

_____

𝒩𝒫 Implementation

Health Promotion

- The nurse educates clients about hygiene by:

_____

_____

- Summarize the goals for *Healthy People 2010*.

_____

_____

Acute and Restorative Care

Bathing and Skin Care

- A complete bed bath is: _____

_____

_____

- A partial bed bath involves: _____

_____

_____

- Identify guidelines the nurse should follow when assisting or providing a client with any type of bath. _____

_____

_____

- Explain bag baths and identify the advantages of this method. _____

_____

_____

- Define *perineal care* and identify the clients at risk for skin breakdown in the perineal area.

_____

_____

- A back rub promotes _____,

_____, _____,

_____, and _____

_____.

Foot and Nail Care

- Routine care involves _____,

_____, _____,

_____, and _____.

- List 16 guidelines to include when advising clients with peripheral neuropathy or vascular insufficiency about foot care.

  a. _____

  b. _____

  c. _____

  d. _____

  e. _____

  f. _____

  g. _____

  h. _____

  i _____

  j. _____

  k. _____

  l. _____

  m. _____

  n. _____

  o. _____

  p. _____

232   Chapter 38: Hygiene

Oral Hygiene

- Oral hygiene helps maintain: _____
_____
_____

- Briefly explain the following interventions in relation to oral hygiene.
  a. Diet: _____
  b. Brushing: _____
  c. Flossing: _____
  d. Denture care: _____

Hair and Scalp Care

- Briefly describe the rationale for the following interventions.
  a. Brushing and combing: _____
_____
  b. Shampooing: _____
_____
  c. Shaving: _____
_____
  d. Mustache and beard care: _____
_____

Care of the Eyes, Ears, and Nose

- Care focuses on preventing infection and maintaining normal sensory function.

- Describe basic eye care for a client. _____
_____
_____

- Describe the correct procedure for cleaning eyeglasses. _____
_____
_____

- Briefly describe proper contact lens care technique. _____
_____
_____

- Describe each of the following techniques necessary in caring for an artificial eye.
  a. Removal: _____
_____
  b. Cleansing: _____
_____
  c. Reinsertion: _____
_____
  d. Storage: _____
_____

Ear Care

- Describe the procedure for removing cerumen from the ear. _____
_____
_____

- Describe the following types of hearing aids.
  a. In-the-canal (ITC): _____
_____
  b. In-the-ear (ITE): _____
_____
  c. Behind-the-ear (BTE): _____
_____

Nasal Care

- Describe three interventions used to remove secretions from the nose.
  a. _____
  b. _____
  c. _____

Client's Room Environment

Maintaining Comfort

- Identify four factors the nurse can control to create a more comfortable environment.

  a. _____

  b. _____

  c. _____

  d. _____

Room Equipment

- A typical hospital room contains the following basic pieces of furniture: _____, _____, _____, _____, and _____ _____.

- Identify the points the nurse should remember when making a client's bed. _____ _____ _____

NP Evaluation

Client Care

- Client care evaluates the actual care delivered by the health care team based on the expected outcomes.

- The standards for evaluation are the expected outcomes established in the planning stage of the client's care.

Client Expectations

- A client expectation evaluates care from the client's perspective.

- The client's expectations are important guidelines in determining client satisfaction.

Review Questions

The student should select the appropriate answer and cite the rationale for choosing that particular answer.

1. Mr. Gray is a 19-year-old client in the rehabilitation unit. He is completely paralyzed below the neck. The most appropriate bath for Mr. Gray is a:
   a. Partial bed bath
   b. Complete bed bath
   c. Sitz bath
   d. Tepid bath

   Answer: _____ Rationale: _____
   _____
   _____

2. All of the following will help maintain skin integrity in the older adult except:
   a. Environmental air that is cold and dry
   b. Use of warm water and mild cleansing agents for bathing
   c. Bathing every other day
   d. Drinking 8 to 10 glasses of water a day

   Answer: _____ Rationale: _____
   _____
   _____

3. When preparing to give complete AM care to a client, what would the nurse do first?
   a. Gather the necessary equipment and supplies.
   b. Remove the client's gown or pajamas while maintaining privacy.
   c. Assess the client's preferences for bathing practices.
   d. Lower the side rails and assist the client to assume a comfortable position.

   Answer: _____ Rationale: _____
   _____
   _____

4. Mrs. Veech is a diabetic. Which intervention should be included in her teaching plan regarding foot care?
   a. Use a pumice stone to smooth corns and calluses
   b. File toenails straight across and square
   c. Apply powder to dry areas along the feet and between the toes
   d. Wear elastic stockings to improve circulation

Answer: _____ Rationale: _____

_____

_____

5. Assessment of the hair and scalp reveals that John has head lice. An appropriate intervention would be:
   a. Shave hair off the affected area
   b. Place oil on the hair and scalp until all of the lice are dead
   c. Shampoo with Kwell and repeat 12 to 24 hours later
   d. Shampoo with regular shampoo and dry with hairdryer set at the hottest setting

Answer: _____ Rationale: _____

_____

_____

Critical Thinking for Nursing Care Plan for Self-Care Deficit, Bathing/Hygiene

Imagine that you are Jeanette, the nurse in the Care Plan on page 1020 of your text. Complete the *Planning phase* of the critical thinking model by writing your answers in the appropriate boxes of the model shown. Think about the following:

- In developing Mrs. Wyatt's plan of care, what knowledge did Jeanette apply?

- In what way might Jeanette's previous experience assist in developing a plan of care for Mrs. Wyatt?

- When developing a plan of care, what intellectual and professional standards were applied?

- What critical thinking attitudes might have been applied in developing Mrs. Wyatt's plan of care?

- How will Jeanette accomplish the goals?

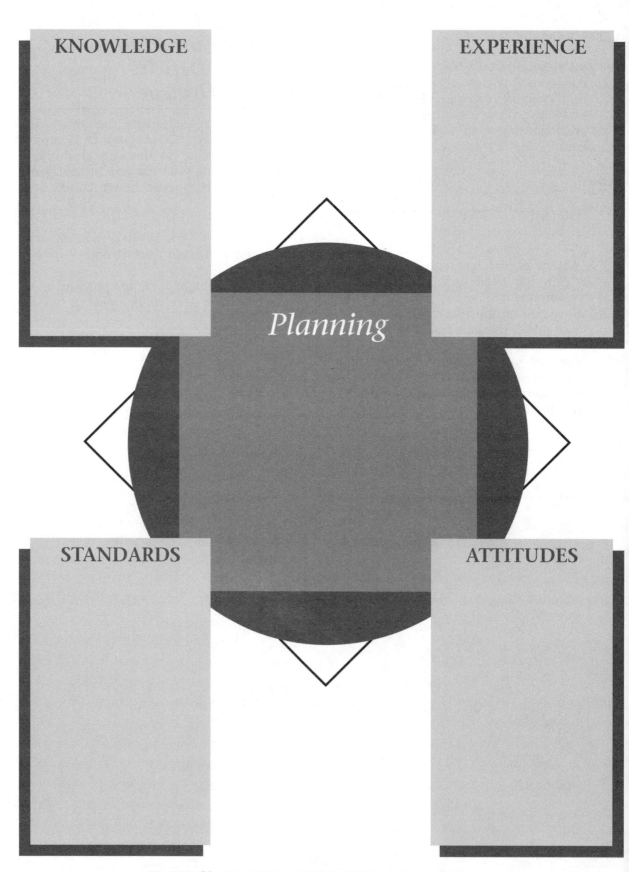

KNOWLEDGE

EXPERIENCE

Planning

STANDARDS

ATTITUDES

CHAPTER *38* Critical Thinking Model for *Self-Care Deficit, Bathing/Hygiene*

See answers on page 541.

39

$\mathcal{O}$xygenation

Chapter 39, pp. 1066-1133

$\mathcal{C}$omprehensive Understanding

Scientific Knowledge Base

- The cardiopulmonary physiology involves _____and

  _____.

Cardiovascular Physiology

- The function of the cardiac system is to deliver _____, _____,

  and other _____ and to remove the _____ through the _____,

  _____ and the _____.

- The right ventricle pumps blood through the _____ while the left ventricle pumps

  blood to the _____, supplying oxygen and nutrients to the tissues and removing
  wastes from the body.

- The chambers of the heart fill during _____ and empty during

  _____.

- Describe the Frank-Starling law of the heart. _____

  _____

  _____

- Briefly describe the flow of blood through the heart._____
  _____
  _____

- Describe the following types of circulation.

  a. Coronary artery: _____
  _____
  _____

  b. Systemic: _____
  _____
  _____

- Describe the following terms related to blood flow regulation.

  a. Cardiac output:_____
  _____
  _____
  _____

  b. Cardiac index:_____
  _____
  _____
  _____

  c. Stroke volume: _____
  _____
  _____
  _____

d. Preload: _____
  _____
  _____
  _____

e. Afterload: _____
  _____
  _____
  _____

f. Myocardial contractility: _____
  _____
  _____
  _____

- Describe how the following affect the conduction system of the heart.

  a. Sympathetic nerve fibers: _____
  _____
  _____
  _____

  b. Parasympathetic nerve fibers: _____
  _____
  _____
  _____

- Diagram and label the electrical conduction system of the heart in the box below.

- Diagram and label the components of the ECG waveform for normal sinus rhythm (NSR) in the box below.

Respiratory Physiology

- The three steps in the process of oxygenation

  are _____, _____

  and _____.

- The _____, _____,

  _____, _____, and _____

  _____, are essential for ventilation, perfusion, and exchange of respiratory gases.

- Define *ventilation.* _____
  _____
  _____

- Define the following terms related to the work of breathing.

  a. *Compliance:* _____
  _____
  _____
  _____

  b. *Surfactant:* _____
  _____
  _____
  _____

  c. *Airway resistance:* _____
  _____
  _____
  _____

  d. *Accessory muscles:* _____
  _____
  _____
  _____

- Spirometry is used to: _____
  _____
  _____

- Variations in lung volumes may be associated with health states such as _____,

  _____, _____,

  or _____.

- The amount of _____,

  _____, _____,

  and _____, can affect pressures and volumes within the lungs.

Chapter 39: Oxygenation   239

- The total lung capacity is: _____

  _____

  _____

  _____

- Gases are moved into and out of the lungs through pressure changes. Describe the changes that must occur to facilitate air into the lungs. _____

  _____

  _____

  _____

- Briefly describe the pulmonary circulation.

  _____

  _____

  _____

- Identify the normal distribution of pressures within the pulmonary circulation.

  _____

  _____

  _____

- Respiratory gases are exchanged in the _____

  and the _____

- Define *diffusion*. _____

  _____

- The rate of diffusion can be affected by: _____

  _____

- List four factors required for oxygen transport and delivery.

  a. _____

  b. _____

  c. _____

  d. _____

- Describe the breakdown of carbon dioxide as it is diffused into the red blood cells.

  _____

  _____

_____

_____

_____

_____

_____

- Explain the two regulators that control the process of respiration.

  a. Neural: _____

  _____

  b. Chemical: _____

  _____

Factors Affecting Oxygenation
- List the four factors that influence oxygenation.

  a. _____

  b. _____

  c. _____

  d. _____

- Explain the physiological process and give an example of each that affect a client's oxygenation.

  a. Decreased carrying capacity: _____

  _____

  _____

  _____

  b. Decreased inspired oxygen concentration:

  _____

  _____

  _____

  c. Hypovolemia: _____

  _____

  _____

  _____

d. Increased metabolic rate: _____

_____

_____

_____

• Explain how the following conditions affect chest wall movement.

a. Pregnancy: _____

_____

b. Obesity: _____

_____

c. Musculoskeletal abnormalities: _____

_____

d Trauma: _____

_____

e. Neuromuscular diseases: _____

_____

f. Central nervous system alterations: _____

_____

g. Influences of chronic disease: _____

_____

Alterations in Cardiac Functioning

• Alterations in cardiac functioning are caused by illnesses and conditions that affect _____

_____

and _____.

• Define *dysrhythmias*. _____

_____

_____

• Briefly describe the following dysrhythmias.

a. Sinus tachycardia: _____

_____

_____

b. Sinus bradycardia: _____

_____

_____

c. Sinus dysrhythmia: _____

_____

_____

d. PSVT: _____

_____

_____

e. PVCs: _____

_____

_____

f. Ventricular tachycardia:

_____

_____

_____

• Failure of the myocardium to eject sufficient volume to the systemic and pulmonary circulations can result in left-sided and right-sided heart failure. Complete the grid below.

Type of Failure	Clinical Findings
Left-sided	
Right-sided	

- Define each of the following.

  a. *Valvular heart disease:* _____

  _____

  b. *Stenosis:* _____

  _____

  c. *Regurgitation:* _____

  _____

  d. *Myocardial ischemia:* _____

  _____

  e. *Angina pectoris:* _____

  _____

  f. *Myocardial infarction:* _____

  _____

- Describe the chest pain associated with myocardial infarction. _____

  _____

  _____

  _____

- Briefly explain acute coronary syndrome (ACS).

  _____

  _____

  _____

  _____

Alterations in Respiratory Functioning

- The three primary alterations in respiratory function are _____,

  _____, _____,

  and _____.

- Complete the grid below.

Alterations	Causes	Signs and Symptoms
Hyperventilation		
Hypoventilation		
Hypoxia		

- Define the following terms.

  a. *Atelectasis:* _____

  _____

  b. *Cyanosis:* _____

  _____

Nursing Knowledge Base

Developmental Factors

- Identify at least one physiological factor influencing tissue oxygenation for each developmental level listed.

  a. Infants and toddlers: _____

  _____

  _____

  _____

b. School-age children and adolescents: _____

_____

_____

_____

c. Young and middle-age adults: _____

_____

_____

_____

d. Older adults: _____

_____

_____

_____/_____

Lifestyle Factors
- Briefly describe how the following lifestyle factors influence respiratory function.

a. Nutrition: _____

_____

_____

_____

b. Exercise: _____

_____

_____

_____

c. Cigarette smoking: _____

_____

_____

_____

d. Substance abuse: _____

_____

_____

_____

Environmental Factors
- List four occupational pollutants.

a. _____

b. _____

c. _____

d. _____

Stress/Anxiety
- Explain how stress and anxiety increase the oxygen demand.

_____

_____

_____

Nursing Process

Assessment

- The nursing assessment of a client's cardiopulmonary functioning should include data from the following areas. Briefly explain each.

a. Nursing history: _____

_____

_____

_____

_____

_____

b. Physical examination: _____

_____

_____

_____

_____

_____

c. Laboratory and diagnostic tests: _____

_____

_____

_____

_____

_____

- Define the following terms.

a. *Fatigue:* _____

_____

b. *Dyspnea:* _____

_____

c. *Orthopnea:* _____

_____

d. *Cough:* _____

e. *Productive cough:* _____

f. *Hemoptysis:* _____

g. *Wheezing:* _____

- Briefly explain the following techniques used during the physical examination to assess tissue oxygenation.

  a. Inspection: _____

  b. Palpation: _____

  c. Percussion: _____

  d. Auscultation: _____

- Describe the following diagnostic tests used to determine the adequacy of the cardiac conduction system.

  a. Electrocardiogram: _____

  b. Holter monitor: _____

  c. Exercise stress test: _____

  d. Thallium stress test: _____

  e. Electrophysiological studies (EPS): _____

- Describe the following tests that determine myocardial contraction and blood flow.

  a. Echocardiography: _____

b. Scintigraphy: _____

c. Cardiac catheterization and angiography:

- Describe the following tests used to measure the adequacy of ventilation and oxygenation.

  a. Pulmonary function tests: _____

  b. Peak expiratory flow rate (PEFR): _____

  c. Arterial blood gases: _____

  d. Oximetry: _____

  e. Complete blood count: _____

  f. Cardiac enzymes: _____

  g. Serum electrolytes: _____

244   Chapter 39: Oxygenation

h. Cholesterol: _____

_____

_____

_____

- Describe the following tests used to visualize structures of the respiratory system.

  a. Chest x-ray: _____

  _____

  _____

  _____

  b. Bronchoscopy: _____

  _____

  _____

  _____

  c. Lung scan: _____

  _____

  _____

  _____

- Describe the following tests used to determine abnormal cells or infection in the respiratory tract.

  a. Throat cultures: _____

  _____

  _____

  _____

  b. Sputum specimens: _____

  _____

  _____

  _____

Nursing Diagnosis

- Clients with an altered level of oxygenation can have nursing diagnoses that are primarily of a cardiovascular or pulmonary origin.

Planning

- List six goals appropriate for a client with actual or potential oxygenation needs.

  a. _____

  b. _____

  c. _____

  d. _____

  e. _____

  f. _____

Implementation

Health Promotion

- Describe the purpose of the influenza and pneumococcal vaccine and explain for whom the vaccines are recommended. _____

  _____

  _____

  _____

  _____

- Avoiding exposure to secondhand smoke is essential to maintaining optimal cardiopulmonary function.

- Identify some healthy lifestyle behaviors that decrease the risk of cardiopulmonary disease.

  _____

  _____

  _____

  _____

  _____

  _____

Acute Care

- Nursing interventions for the client with acute pulmonary illnesses are directed toward _____, _____, and

  _____.

- List five treatment modalities appropriate for a client with dyspnea.

  a. _____

  b. _____

  c. _____

  d. _____

  e. _____

Airway Maintenance

- Describe selected nursing interventions used to promote and maintain adequate oxygenation by completing the grid below. Include the purpose of the intervention.

Nursing Interventions	Purpose
Cascade cough	
Huff cough	
Quad cough	
Oropharyngeal and nasopharyngeal suctioning	
Tracheal suctioning	
Oral airway	
Tracheal airway	

Mobilization of Pulmonary Secretions

- Nursing interventions that promote mobilization of pulmonary secretions include the following. Briefly explain each one.

a. Hydration: _____

_____

_____

_____

b. Humidification: _____

_____

_____

c. Nebulization: _____

_____

_____

d. Chest physiotherapy (CPT): _____

_____

_____

_____

- Briefly describe the three activities involved in CPT.

a. Postural drainage: _____

_____

b. Chest percussion: _____

_____

c. Vibration: _____

_____

Briefly explain the following types of suctioning techniques.

a. Oropharyngeal: _____

_____

_____

b. Nasopharyngeal: _____

_____

_____

c. Orotracheal: _____

_____

_____

d. Nasotracheal: _____

_____

_____

- Nursing interventions that maintain or promote lung expansion include the following noninvasive techniques. Briefly explain each one.

a. Positioning: _____

_____

b. Incentive spirometry: _____

_____

- Identify the three reasons for inserting chest tubes.

a. _____

b. _____

c. _____

- Define the following.

a. *Hemothorax:* _____

_____

b. *Pneumothorax:* _____

_____

- List the two types of drainage systems used with chest tubes.

a. _____

b. _____

- Identify five special considerations the nurse needs to address when dealing with chest tubes.

a. _____

b. _____

c. _____

d. _____

e. _____

- Promotion of lung expansion, mobilization of secretions, and maintenance of a patent airway assist the client in meeting oxygenation needs.

- Identify the goals of oxygen therapy. _____

  _____

  _____

  _____

  _____

- List four safety measures to institute when a client receives oxygen administration.

  a. _____

  b. _____

  c. _____

  d. _____

- Describe the following methods of oxygen delivery and identify the usual flow rates.

  a. Nasal cannula: _____

  _____

  b. Nasal catheter: _____

  _____

  c. Transtracheal oxygen: _____

  _____

  d. Face mask: _____

  _____

  e. Venturi mask: _____

  _____

- Identify the indications for a client to receive

  home oxygen therapy. _____

  _____

  _____

- Identify the teaching required by the client for

  use of home oxygen therapy. _____

  _____

  _____

  _____

- List the three goals of cardiopulmonary resuscitation (CPR).

  a. _____

  b. _____

  c. _____

Restorative Care

- Cardiopulmonary rehabilitation is: _____

  _____

  _____

  _____

- Briefly explain the following breathing exercises used to improve ventilation and oxygenation.

  a. Pursed-lip breathing: _____

  _____

  _____

  _____

  b. Diaphragmatic breathing: _____

  _____

  _____

  _____

Evaluation

Client Care

- Evaluates the actual care provided to the client by the health care team based on the expected outcomes.

- The client is the only person who can evaluate his or her degree of breathlessness.

- Evaluation of _____

  _____, _____

  _____, and

  provide the nurse with objective measurements of the success of therapies and treatments.

Client Expectations

- Evaluate the care from the client's perspective.

- Working closely with the client will enable the nurse to redefine those client expectations that can be realistically met within the limitations of the client's condition and treatment.

248   Chapter 39: Oxygenation

• List three evaluative criteria for a client with alterations in oxygenation.

a. _____

b. _____

c. _____

*R*eview Questions

The student should select the appropriate answer and cite the rationale for choosing that particular answer.

1. Ventilation, perfusion, and exchange of gases are the major purposes of:
   a. Respiration
   b. Circulation
   c. Aerobic metabolism
   d. Anaerobic metabolism

Answer: _____ Rationale: _____

_____

_____

2. *Afterload* refers to:
   a. The amount of blood ejected from the left ventricle each minute
   b. The amount of blood ejected from the left ventricle with each contraction
   c. The resistance to left ventricle ejection
   d. The amount of blood in the left ventricle at the end of diastole

Answer: _____ Rationale: _____

_____

_____

3. The movement of gases into and out of the lungs depends on the:
   a. 50% oxygen content in the atmospheric air
   b. Pressure gradient between the atmosphere and the alveoli
   c. Use of accessory muscles of respiration during expiration
   d. Amount of carbon dioxide dissolved in the fluid of the alveoli

Answer: _____ Rationale: _____

_____

_____

4. The client's ECG shows an abnormal rhythm that slows during inspiration and increases with expiration. The rate is 70 to 80 beats per minute. The P-wave, PR interval, and QRS complex are normal. This is referred to as:
   a. Sinus tachycardia
   b. Sinus dysrhythmia
   c. Supraventricular tachycardia
   d. Premature ventricular contractions

Answer: _____ Rationale: _____

_____

_____

5. Mr. Isaac comes to the ER complaining of difficulty breathing. An objective finding associated with his dyspnea might include:
   a. Statements about a sense of impending doom
   b. Complaints of shortness of breath
   c. Feelings of heaviness in the chest
   d. Use of accessory muscles of respiration

Answer: _____ Rationale: _____

_____

_____

6. The use of chest physiotherapy to mobilize pulmonary secretions involves the use of:
   a. Hydration
   b. Percussion
   c. Nebulization
   d. Humidification

Answer: _____ Rationale: _____

_____

_____

Critical Thinking for Nursing Care Plan for Ineffective Airway Clearance

Imagine that you are the student nurse in the Care Plan on page 1094 of your text. Complete the *Assessment phase* of the critical thinking model by writing your answers in the appropriate boxes of the model shown. Think about the following:

- What knowledge base was applied to Mr. Edwards?

- In what way might your previous experience apply in this case?

- What intellectual or professional standards were applied to Mr. Edwards?

- What critical thinking attitudes did you use in assessing Mr. Edwards?

- As you review your assessment, what key areas did you cover?

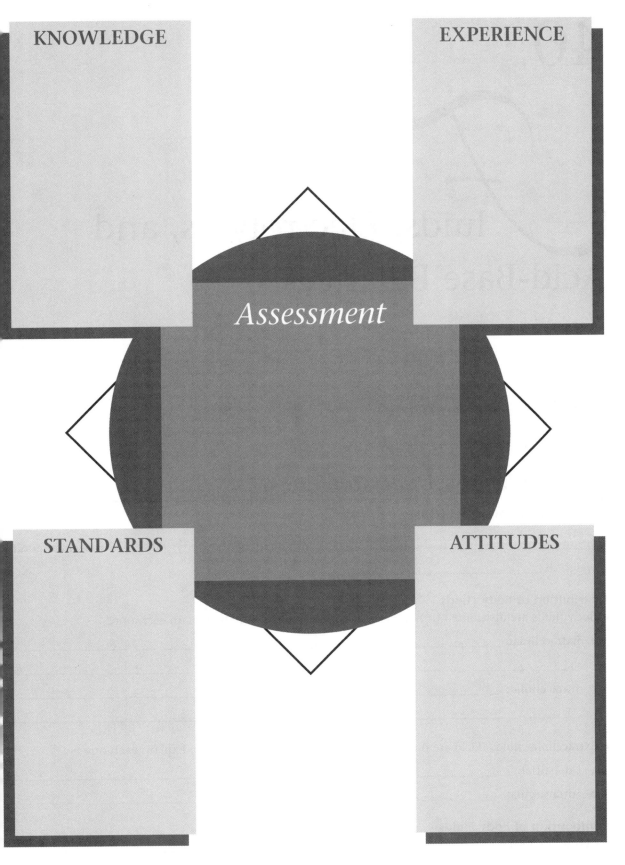

KNOWLEDGE

EXPERIENCE

Assessment

STANDARDS

ATTITUDES

CHAPTER *39* Critical Thinking Model for *Ineffective Airway Clearance*

See answers on page 542.

40

$\mathcal{F}$luids, Electrolytes, and Acid-Base Balances

$\mathcal{P}$reliminary Reading

Chapter 40, pp. 1134-1197

$\mathcal{C}$omprehensive Understanding

Scientific Knowledge Base

- _____ is the largest single component of the body; 60% of the average adult's weight is _____.

Distribution of Body Fluids
- Body fluids are distributed in two distinct compartments. Briefly explain each one.

    a. Extracellular: _____

    _____

    b. Intracellular: _____

    _____

- Extracellular fluids (ECF) are divided into two smaller compartments. Explain each one.

    a. Interstitial: _____

    b. Intravascular: _____

Composition of Body Fluids
- Define *electrolyte*. _____

    _____

    _____

• Define the following terms related to the composition of body fluids.

a. *Cations:* _____

b. *Anions:* _____

c. *mEq/L:* _____

d. *Solute:* _____

e. *Solvent:* _____

f. *Minerals:* _____

g. *Cells:* _____

Movement of Body Fluids

• Fluids and electrolytes shift from compartment to compartment to facilitate body processes.

• List and briefly describe the four factors responsible for movement of body fluids.

a. _____

b. _____

c. _____

d. _____

• Define the following terms related to osmosis.

a. *Osmotic pressure:* _____
_____

b. *Isotonic:* _____
_____

c. *Hypotonic:* _____
_____

d. *Hypertonic:* _____
_____

• Define *hydrostatic pressure.* _____
_____
_____

Regulation of Body Fluids

• Body fluids are regulated by _____,
_____, and _____.
This balance is termed _____.

• Briefly describe the physiological stimuli triggering the thirst mechanism. _____
_____
_____
_____
_____

• For each hormone, identify the stimuli for its release and its influence on fluid and electrolyte balance in the grid below.

Hormone	Stimuli	Action
ADH		
Aldosterone		
Glucocorticoids		

• Fluid output occurs through four organs. List and explain each one.

a. _____
_____

b. _____
_____

c. _____
_____

d. _____
_____

• Define.

a. *Insensible water loss:* _____
_____

b. *Sensible water loss:* _____
_____

Regulation of Electrolytes

• The major cations are _____
_____, _____
and _____. They are located in
the _____ and _____ fluid

• The major anions are _____
_____, and _____

• Give the normal values, function, and regulatory mechanisms for the major body electrolytes in the grid below.

Electrolyte	Values	Function	Regulatory Mechanism
Sodium			
Potassium			
Glucocorticoids			
Calcium			
Magnesium			
Chloride			
Bicarbonate			
Phosphate			

Physiological Regulation

- Identify and describe the acid-base regulatory mechanisms for each of the following buffering systems.

    a. Chemical regulation: _____

    _____

    _____

    _____

    _____

    b. Biological regulation: _____

    _____

    _____

    _____

_____

_____

- Describe the physiological mechanism through which the lungs regulate hydrogen ion concentration. _____

    _____

    _____

    _____

    _____

- For each electrolyte disturbance, identify the diagnostic laboratory finding, and list at least four characteristic signs and symptoms in the grid below.

Imbalance	Lab Finding	Signs and Symptoms
Hyponatremia		
Hypernatremia		
Hypokalemia		
Hyperkalemia		
Hypocalcemia		
Hypercalcemia		
Hypomagnesemia		
Hypermagnesemia		

- The basic types of fluid imbalances are _____ and _____.

- Isotonic deficit and excess exist when. _____
_____
_____.

- Osmolar imbalances are: _____
_____
_____.

- Complete the grid below giving the causes, signs, and symptoms of the listed fluid disturbances.

Fluid Disturbances	Causes	Signs and Symptoms
Fluid volume deficit (FVD)		
Fluid volume deficit (FVE)		
Third-space syndrome		
Hyperosmolar imbalance		
Hypoosmolar imbalance		

- Briefly explain the following components of the acid-base balance.

  a. pH: _____
  _____

  b. $PaCO_2$: _____
  _____

  c. PaO_2: _____
  _____

  d. Oxygen saturation: _____
  _____

  e. Base excess: _____
  _____

  f. Bicarbonate: _____
  _____

- The four primary types of acid-base imbalances are listed in the following grid. For each acid-base imbalance, identify the diagnostic laboratory finding and list the characteristic signs and symptoms.

256   Chapter 40: Fluids, Electrolytes, and Acid-Base Balances

Acid-Base Imbalance	Lab Findings	Signs and Symptoms
Respiratory acidosis		
Respiratory alkalosis		
Metabolic acidosis		
Metabolic alkalosis		

Nursing Knowledge Base

- List the five major risk factors that can affect fluid and electrolyte imbalances. Give two examples of each.

  a. _____

  _____

  b. _____

  _____

  c. _____

  _____

  d. _____

  _____

  e. _____

  _____

Nursing Process

𝒩𝓅 Assessment

- Briefly describe the fluid changes that are associated with aging and development.

  a. Infants: _____

  _____

  _____

  _____

  b. Children: _____

  _____

  _____

  _____

  c. Adolescents: _____

  _____

  _____

  _____

  d. Older adults: _____

  _____

  _____

  _____

- Explain how the following acute illnesses affect fluid, electrolyte, and acid-base balances.

  a. Surgery: _____

  _____

  _____

  _____

  b. Burns: _____

  _____

  _____

  _____

Chapter 40: Fluids, Electrolytes, and Acid-Base Balances   257

c. Respiratory disorders: _____

_____

_____

_____

d. Head injury: _____

_____

_____

_____

- Describe how the following chronic illnesses affect fluid, electrolyte, and acid-base imbalances.

    a. Cancer: _____

    _____

    _____

    _____

    b. Cardiovascular disease: _____

    _____

    _____

    _____

    c. Renal disorders: _____

    _____

    _____

    _____

    d. Gastrointestinal disturbances: _____

    _____

    _____

    _____

- Briefly explain how the following affect fluid, electrolyte, and acid-base imbalance.

    a. Diet: _____

    _____

    _____

    _____

    _____

b. Lifestyle factors: _____

_____

_____

_____

_____

_____

c. Medication: _____

_____

_____

_____

_____

._____

- Indicate the possible fluid, electrolyte, or acid-base imbalances associated with each physical finding.

    a. Weight loss of 6% to 9%: _____

    _____

    b. Irritability: _____

    _____

    c. Lethargy: _____

    _____

    d. Bulging fontanels (infant): _____

    _____

    e. Periorbital edema: _____

    _____

    f. Sticky, dry mucous membranes:

    _____

    g. Chvostek's sign: _____

    _____

    h. Distended neck veins: _____

    _____

    i. Dysrhythmias: _____

    _____

    j. Weak pulse: _____

    _____

    k. Low blood pressure: _____

    _____

l. Third heart sound: _____

_____

m. Increased respiratory rate: _____

_____

n. Crackles: _____

_____

o. Anorexia: _____

_____

p. Abdominal cramps: _____

_____

q. Poor skin turgor: _____

_____

r. Oliguria or anuria: _____

_____

s. Increased specific gravity: _____

_____

t. Muscle cramps, tetany: _____

_____

u. Hypertonicity of muscles on palpation: ____

_____

v. Decreased or absent deep tendon reflexes:

_____

w. Increased temperature: _____

_____

x. Distended abdomen: _____

_____

y. Cold, clammy skin: _____

_____

z. 2+ edema: _____

_____

- Recording intake and output (I&O) is essential for obtaining an accurate database. This information helps maintain an ongoing evaluation of hydration status to prevent severe imbalances.

- Explain the rationale for each of the following laboratory tests.

a. Serum electrolytes: _____

_____

b. CBC: _____

_____

c. Creatinine: _____

_____

d. BUN: _____

_____

e. Serum osmolality: _____

_____

f. Urine specific gravity: _____

_____

- Arterial blood gas levels (ABGs) provide information on the status of acid-base balance. Give the normal value for each.

a. pH: _____

_____

b. $PaCO_2$: _____

_____

c. PaO_2: _____

_____

d. SaO_2: _____

_____

e. HCO_3: _____

_____

Nursing Diagnosis

- List five potential or actual nursing diagnoses for a client with fluid, electrolyte, or acid-base imbalances.

a. _____

_____

b. _____

_____

c. _____

_____

d. _____

_____

e. _____

_____

𝒩𝒫 Planning

- List three goals that are appropriate for a client with altered fluid, electrolyte, or acid-base imbalances.

  a. _____

  _____

  b. _____

  _____

  c. _____

  _____

𝒩𝒫 Implementation

Health Promotion

- Identify some common risk factors for imbalances for which the caregiver may implement appropriate preventive measures.

  _____

  _____

  _____

Acute Care

- When implementing specific measures to increase or decrease fluid, two interventions are necessary. Explain each one.

  a. Daily weights: _____

  _____

  b. I&O: _____

  _____

- List and briefly describe the enteral replacement of fluids.

  a. _____

  _____

  b. _____

  _____

- Briefly explain the need for a restricted fluid intake and how the nurse would implement the restriction. _____

  _____

  _____

  _____

  _____

- List the three methods of parenteral replacement.

  a. _____

  _____

  b. _____

  _____

  c. _____

  _____

- Vascular assist devices are: _____

  _____

  _____.

- Total parenteral nutrition (TPN) is: _____

  _____

  _____

  _____

  _____.

- Identify the primary goal of IV fluid replacement. _____

  _____

  _____.

- Define the following types of electrolyte solutions.

  a. *Isotonic:* _____

  _____

  b. *Hypotonic:* _____

  _____

  c. *Hypertonic:* _____

  _____

- List two major purposes of infusion pumps.

  a. _____

  _____

  b. _____

  _____

- List three groups of clients for whom venipunctures may be difficult.

  a. _____

  b. _____

  c. _____

- List four factors that may affect IV flow rates.

  a. _____

  b. _____

  c. _____

  d. _____

- List four interventions that can reduce the risk of infusion-related infections.

  a. _____

  b. _____

  c. _____

  d. _____

- Indicate the sequence to be followed when changing the gown of a client with an IV line.

  a. _____

  b. _____

  c. _____

  d. _____

  e. _____

  f. _____

- Complete the grid below describing complications of IV therapy.

Complication	Assessment Finding	Nursing Action
Infiltration		
Phlebitis		
Fluid overload		
Bleeding		

- Briefly summarize the procedure for discontinuing intravenous infusions. _____

  _____

  _____

  _____

  _____

  _____

  _____

- List three objectives for blood transfusion.

  a. _____

  _____

  b. _____

  _____

  c. _____

  _____

- Complete the grid below describing the major blood groups.

	A	**B**	**O**	**AB**
Antigens present				
Antibodies present				

- Define *autotransfusion*. _____

  _____

  _____

- Identify the five nursing interventions associated with blood transfusions and give the rationale for each.

  a. _____

  _____

  b. _____

  _____

  c. _____

  _____

  d. _____

  _____

  e. _____

  _____

- Define *transfusion reaction* and identify its cause.

  _____

  _____

  _____

  _____

- List the five signs and symptoms most commonly associated with transfusion reactions.

  a. _____

  b. _____

  c. _____

  d. _____

  e. _____

- Define the following risks associated with blood transfusions.

  a. *Hyperkalemia:* _____

  _____

b. *Hypocalcemia:* _____

_____

c. *Iron overload (hemosiderosis):* _____

_____

d. *Circulatory overload:* _____

_____

- List the nine steps the nurse should follow if a transfusion reaction is suspected.

  a. _____

  b. _____

  c. _____

  d. _____

  e. _____

  f. _____

  g. _____

  h. _____

  i _____

- Identify three nursing interventions to correct acid-base imbalances and give the rationale for each.

  a. _____

  b. _____

  c. _____

Restorative Care

- Older adults and the chronically ill require special considerations to prevent complications from developing. Briefly summarize the following.

  a. Home intravenous therapy: _____

  _____

  _____

  b. Nutritional support: _____

  _____

  _____

  _____

c. Medication safety: _____

_____

_____

_____

Evaluation

Client Care

- Evaluates the actual care delivered by the health care team based on the expected outcomes.

- The nurse integrates what he or she knows about the health alterations, the effects of medications and fluids, and the client's presenting clinical status.

Client Expectations

- Evaluation of care from the client's perspective.

- Often the client's level of satisfaction with care also depends on the nurse's success in involving friends and family.

Review Questions

The student should select the appropriate answer and cite the rationale for choosing that particular answer.

1. The body fluids comprising the interstitial fluid and blood plasma are:
   a. Intracellular
   b. Extracellular
   c. Hypotonic
   d. Hypertonic

   Answer: _____ Rationale: _____

   _____

   _____

2. Which of the following statements is true with regard to the lungs' regulation of acid-base balance?
   a. The lungs serve a minor role in the physiological buffering of H ions.
   b. It takes several days for the lungs to restore pH to a normal level.
   c. The lungs correct imbalances by altering the rate and depth of respiration.
   d. The lungs maintain normal pH by either retaining or excreting bicarbonate.

   Answer: _____ Rationale: _____

   _____

   _____

3. Mrs. Green's arterial blood gas results are as follows: pH, 7.32; $PaCO_2$, 52; PaO_2, 78; HCO_3, 24. Mrs. Green has:
   a. Respiratory acidosis
   b. Respiratory alkalosis
   c. Metabolic acidosis
   d. Metabolic alkalosis

   Answer: _____ Rationale: _____

   _____

   _____

4. Mr. Frank is an 82-year-old client who has had a 3-day history of vomiting and diarrhea. Which symptom would you expect to find on a physical examination?
   a. Neck vein distention
   b. Crackles in the lungs
   c. Tachycardia
   d. Hypertension

   Answer: _____ Rationale: _____

   _____

   _____

5. Which of the following is most likely to result in respiratory alkalosis?
   a. Fad dieting
   b. Hyperventilation
   c. Chronic alcoholism
   d. Steroid use

   Answer: _____ Rationale: _____

   _____

   _____

Critical Thinking for Ineffective Airway Clearance/Risk for Fluid Volume Deficit

Imagine that you are the student nurse in the Care Plan on page 1156 of your text. Complete the *Planning phase* of the critical thinking model by writing your answers in the appropriate boxes of the model shown. Think about the following:

- In developing Mrs. Bottomly's plan of care, what knowledge did you apply?

- In what way might your previous experience assist you in developing a plan of care for Mrs. Bottomly?

- When developing a plan of care, what intellectual and professional standards were applied?

- What critical thinking attitudes might have been applied to developing Mrs. Bottomly's care?

- How will you accomplish your goals?

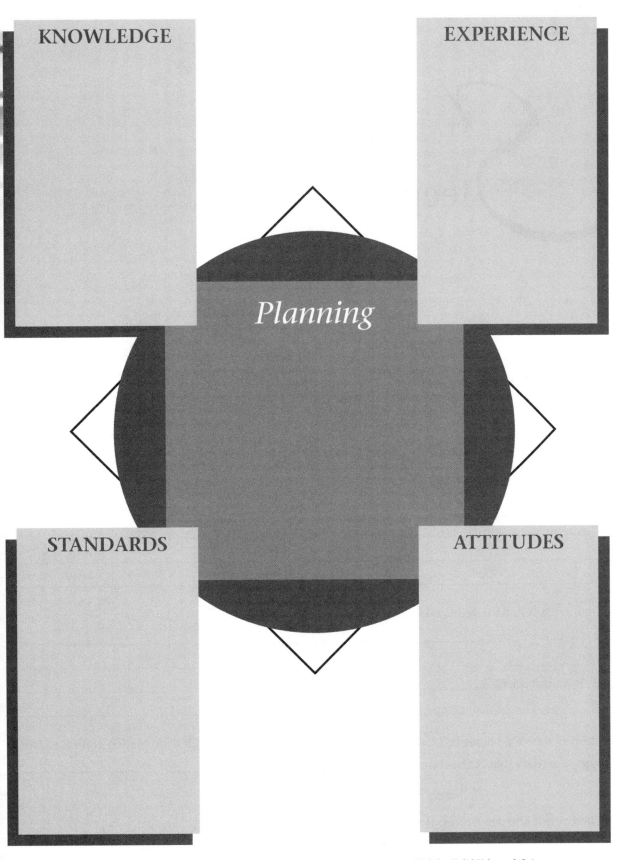

KNOWLEDGE

EXPERIENCE

Planning

STANDARDS

ATTITUDES

CHAPTER *40* Critical Thinking Model for *Ineffective Airway Clearance/Risk for Fulid Volume deficit*

See answers on page 543.

41

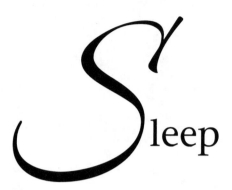

*S*leep

*P*reliminary Reading

Chapter 41, pp. 1198-1227

*C*omprehensive Understanding

Scientific Knowledge Base

Physiology of Sleep
• Define *sleep.*_____

_____

_____

• Define the following terms related to sleep.

   a. *Circadian rhythm:* _____

   _____

   b. *Biological clocks:* _____

   _____

• Sleep involves a sequence of physiological states maintained by highly integrated central nervous system activity that is associated with changes in the _____, _____, _____, and _____ systems.

• The control and regulation of sleep depends on the interrelationship between two cerebral mechanisms that intermittently activate and suppress the brain's higher centers to control sleep and wakefulness.

- Summarize the function of the reticular activating system (RAS). _____
_____
_____

- The area of the brain called the *bulbar synchronizing region* (BSR) is responsible for:
_____
_____

- Explain the two stages of sleep.

  a. NREM: _____
  _____
  _____
  _____

  b. REM: _____
  _____
  _____
  _____

- Describe the characteristics of the following cycles of sleep.

  a. Stage 1: _____
  _____

  b. Stage 2: _____
  _____

  c. Stage 3: _____
  _____

  d. Stage 4: _____
  _____

  e. REM: _____
  _____

- Explain briefly the functions of sleep: _____
_____
_____
_____
_____

Physical Illness

- Explain how the following conditions affect sleep.

  a. Discomfort: _____
  _____

  b. Respiratory disease: _____
  _____

  c. Coronary artery disease: _____
  _____

  d. Hypertension: _____
  _____

  e. Hypothyroidism: _____
  _____

  f. Hyperthyroidism: _____
  _____

  g. Nocturia: _____
  _____

  h. Restless legs syndrome: _____
  _____

Sleep Disorders

- Briefly describe the following categories of sleep disorders.

  a. Dyssomnias: _____
  _____
  _____
  _____

  b. Parasomnias: _____
  _____
  _____
  _____

- Define *insomnia*. _____
_____
_____
_____

- List two conditions that are associated with insomnia.

  a. _____

  b. _____

- Define *sleep apnea.* _____
  _____
  _____

- Define the following types of apnea.

  a. *Central apnea:* _____
  _____

  b. *Obstructive apnea:* _____
  _____

- Briefly explain excessive daytime sleepiness (EDS). _____
  _____
  _____
  _____

- Define *narcolepsy.* _____
  _____
  _____
  _____

- Define the following terms related to narcolepsy.

  a. *Cataplexy:* _____
  _____

  b. *Hypnagogic hallucinations:* _____
  _____

- Identify the developmental stage in which narcolepsy symptoms first develop._____
  _____
  _____

- Identify the treatment modalities for a client with narcolepsy._____
  _____
  _____

- Sleep deprivation is: _____
  _____
  _____

- List the physiological and psychological manifestations of sleep deprivation in the grid below.

Physiological Symptoms	Psychological Symptoms

- Explain the following parasomnias.

  a. Somnambulism: _____

  _____

  b. Nocturnal enuresis: _____

  _____

  c. Bruxism: _____

  _____

Nursing Knowledge Base

Sleep and Rest
- Define.

  a. *Rest:* _____

  _____

  b. *Sleep:* _____

  _____

Normal Sleep Requirements and Patterns
- Complete the grid below listing the normal sleep patterns and rituals for the following developmental stages.

Developmental Stage	Sleep Patterns	Usual Rituals
Neonates		
Infants		
Toddlers		
Preschoolers		
School-age children		
Adolescents		
Young adults		
Middle adults		
Older adults		

Factors Affecting Sleep

- A number of factors affect the quantity and quality of sleep.

- Sleepiness and sleep deprivation are common side effects of medications. Describe how each of the following affects sleep and give an example of each.

    a. Drugs and substances: _____

    _____

    b. Lifestyle: _____

    _____

- List four alterations in routine that can disrupt sleep patterns.

    a. _____

    b. _____

    c. _____

    d. _____

- Explain how emotional stress affects sleep.

    _____

    _____

- List and briefly describe three environmental factors that affect sleep.

    a. _____

    b. _____

    c. _____

- Explain how exercise promotes sleep._____

    _____

    _____

- List and briefly describe five foods that affect sleep and why.

    a. _____

    b. _____

    c. _____

    d. _____

    e. _____

Nursing Process

Assessment

- Sleep is a subjective experience.

- Assessment is aimed at understanding the characteristics of any sleep problem and the client's usual sleep habits so that ways for promoting sleep can be incorporated into the nursing care.

- Identify three sources for sleep assessment.

    a. _____

    b. _____

    c. _____

- List the 10 components of a sleep history.

    a. _____

    b. _____

    c. _____

    d. _____

    e. _____

    f. _____

    g. _____

    h. _____

    i. _____

- List and briefly describe the six areas to assess with a client who has a sleeping problem.

    a. _____

    b. _____

    c. _____

    d. _____

    e. _____

    f. _____

- Identify the questions a nurse would ask to determine the client's usual sleep pattern.

    _____

    _____

    _____

    _____

    _____

- Briefly explain how the following factors interfere with sleep.

  a. Physical and psychological illness: _____

  _____

  _____

  _____

  b. Current life events: _____

  _____

  _____

  _____

  c. Bedtime routines: _____

  _____

  _____

  _____

  d. Bedtime environment: _____

  _____

  _____

  _____

- List four behaviors a client may manifest with sleep deprivation.

  a. _____

  b. _____

  c. _____

  d. _____

Nursing Diagnosis

- If a sleep pattern disturbance is identified, the nurse specifies the condition.

- Assessment should also identify the related factor or probable cause of the sleep disturbance.

Planning

- It is important for the plan of care to include strategies that are appropriate for the client's environment and lifestyle.

- List four goals appropriate for a client needing rest or sleep.

  a. _____

  b. _____

  c. _____

  d. _____

Implementation

- Nursing interventions designed to improve the quality of a person's sleep are largely focused on health promotion.

Health Promotion

- Many factors affect the ability to gain adequate rest and sleep. Briefly give examples of each of the following.

  a. Environmental control: _____

  _____

  _____

  _____

  b. Promoting bedtime routines: _____

  _____

  _____

  _____

  c. Comfort: _____

  _____

  _____

  _____

  d. Periods of rest and sleep: _____

  _____

  _____

  _____

  e. Stress reduction: _____

  _____

  _____

  _____

  f. Bedtime snacks: _____

  _____

  _____

  _____

g. Pharmacological approaches: _____

_____

_____

_____

Acute Care

- For each of the following situations, give two examples of nursing measures that will promote sleep.

  a. Environmental control:

     1. _____

     2. _____

  b. Promoting comfort:

     1. _____

     2. _____

  c. Establishing periods of rest and sleep:

     1. _____

     2. _____

  d. Stress reduction:

     1. _____

     2. _____

Restorative or Continuing Care

- Give an example of the following interventions that are implemented in restorative environment.

  a. Promoting comfort: _____

     _____

     _____

     _____

  b. Controlling physiological disturbances: ___

     _____

     _____

     _____

  c. Pharmacological approaches: _____

     _____

     _____

     _____

- Briefly describe the effect of benzodiazepines in promoting sleep._____

     _____

     _____

- Identify three types of clients who should not use benzodiazepines and explain why.

  a. _____

  b. _____

  c. _____

- The regular use of sleeping medication can lead to: _____

     _____

     _____

N𝑝 Evaluation

Client Care

- With regard to sleep disturbances, the client is the source for outcomes evaluation. List three outcomes for a client with a sleep disturbance.

  a. _____

  b. _____

  c. _____

Client Expectations

- Client expectations evaluate care from the client's perspective. Identify some subtle behaviors a client may exhibit that indicate satisfaction. _____

     _____

     _____

     _____

Review Questions

The student should select the appropriate answer and cite the rationale for choosing that particular answer.

1. The 24-hour day-night cycle is known as:
   a. Circadian rhythm
   b. Infradium rhythm
   c. Ultradian rhythm
   d. Non-REM rhythm

Answer: _____ Rationale: _____

_____

_____

2. Which of the following substances will promote normal sleep patterns?
   a. l-tryptophan
   b. Beta-blockers
   c. Alcohol
   d. Narcotics

Answer: _____ Rationale: _____

_____

_____

3. All of the following are symptoms of sleep deprivation except:
   a. Hyperactivity
   b. Irritability
   c. Rise in body temperature
   d. Decreased motivation

Answer: _____ Rationale: _____

_____

_____

4. Mrs. Peterson complains of difficulty falling asleep, awakening earlier than desired, and not feeling rested. She attributes these problems to leg pain that is secondary to her arthritis. What would be the appropriate nursing diagnosis for her?
   a. *Sleep pattern disturbances related to arthritis*
   b. *Fatigue related to leg pain*
   c. *Knowledge deficit related to sleep hygiene measures*
   d. *Sleep pattern disturbances related to chronic leg pain*

Answer: _____ Rationale: _____

_____

_____

5. A nursing care plan for a client with sleep problems has been implemented. All of the following would be expected outcomes except:
   a. Client reports no episodes of awakening during the night.
   b. Client falls asleep within 1 hour of going to bed.
   c. Client reports satisfaction with amount of sleep.
   d. Client rates sleep as an 8 or above on the visual analog scale.

Answer: _____ Rationale: _____

_____

_____

Critical Thinking for Nursing Care Plan for Sleep Pattern Disturbance

Imagine that you are the nurse in the Care Plan on page 1216 of your text. Complete the *Evaluation phase* of the critical thinking model by writing your answers in the appropriate boxes of the model shown. Think about the following:

- What knowledge did you apply in evaluating Julie's care?

- In what way might your previous experience influence your evaluation of Julie's care?

- During evaluation, what intellectual and professional standards were applied to Julie's care?

- In what way do critical thinking attitudes play a role in how you approach the evaluation of Julie's plan?

- How might you evaluate Julie's plan of care?

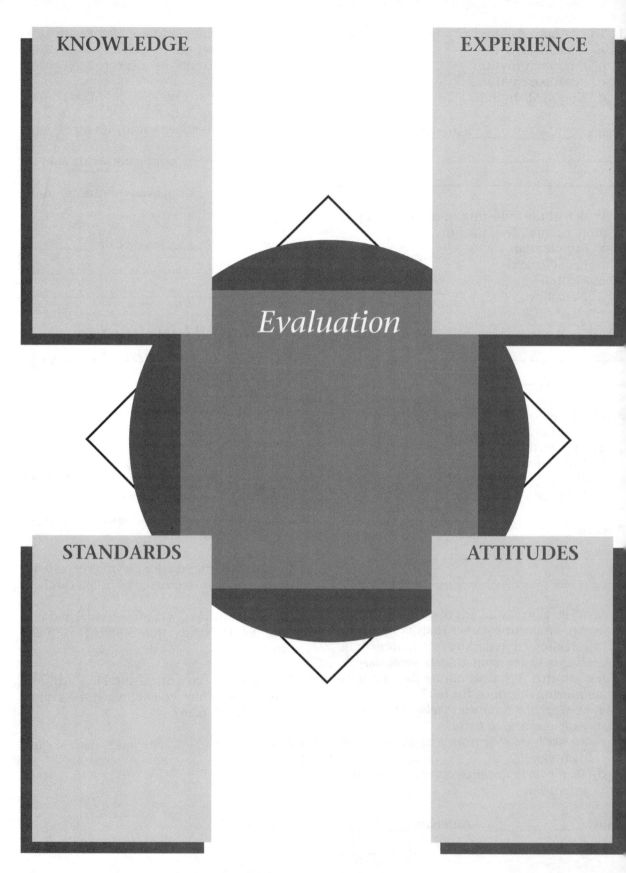

KNOWLEDGE

EXPERIENCE

Evaluation

STANDARDS

ATTITUDES

CHAPTER *41* Critical Thinking Model for *Sleep Pattern Disturbance*

See answers on page 544.

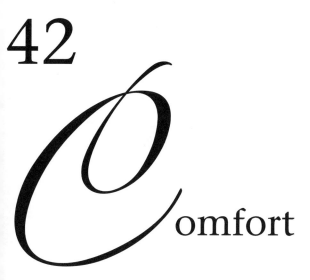

42

$\mathcal{C}$omfort

$\mathcal{P}$reliminary Reading

Chapter 42, pp. 1228-1270

$\mathcal{C}$omprehensive Understanding

- Pain is subjective; no two persons experience pain in the same way, and no two painful events create identical responses or feelings in a person.

- The context of comfort is the umbrella under which pain and pain management options are viewed.

- Providing pain relief is considered a basic human right and is incorporated into *A Patient's Bill of Rights*.

Scientific Knowledge Base

Nature of Pain
- Define *pain*. _____
  _____
  _____

Physiology of Pain
- Explain the four processes of nociceptive pain. _____
  a. Transduction _____
     _____
     _____
     _____

b. Transmission: _____

_____

_____

_____

c. Perception: _____

_____

_____

_____

d. Modulation: _____

_____

_____

_____

- Neuroregulators are: _____

_____

_____

_____

- Explain the two types of neuroregulators.

  a. Neurotransmitters: _____

  _____

  _____

  _____

  b. Neuromodulators: _____

  _____

  _____

  _____

- Identify the neurophysiological function of the following neuroregulators.

  a. Substance P: _____

  _____

  _____

  _____

  b. Prostaglandins: _____

  _____

  _____

  _____

c. Serotonin: _____

_____

_____

_____

d. Endorphins: _____

_____

_____

_____

e. Bradykinin: _____

_____

_____

_____

- Perception is the point at which: _____

_____

_____

- Explain the gate-control theory of pain:

  a. Sympathetic stimulation:

  1. _____

  2. _____

  3. _____

  4. _____

  5. _____

  b. Parasympathetic stimulation:

  1. _____

  2. _____

  3. _____

  4. _____

  5. _____

- Identify four behavioral changes that characterize a client experiencing pain.

  a. _____

  b. _____

  c. _____

  d. _____

- List four characteristics of acute pain.

  a. _____

  b. _____

  c. _____

  d. _____

Nursing Knowledge Base

Knowledge, Attitudes, and Beliefs
- The medical model of illness describes pain as:

  _____

  _____

- Identify common biases and misconceptions about pain. _____

  _____

  _____

  _____

  _____

  _____

  _____

  _____

  _____

  _____

Factors Influencing Pain
- Explain the developmental differences of client's reaction to pain.

  a. Young children: _____

  _____

  _____

  _____

  b. Toddlers and preschoolers: _____

  _____

  _____

  _____

  c. Older adults: _____

  _____

  _____

  _____

- Identify five reasons why older clients may not report pain.

  a. _____

  b. _____

  c. _____

  d. _____

  e. _____

- Fatigue heightens the perception of pain. Explain. _____

  _____

  _____

- Explain how a client's neurological function can influence pain: _____

  _____

  _____

- Give an example how the following influence pain.

  a. Social factors: _____

  _____

  b. Previous experience: _____

  _____

  c. Family and social support: _____

  _____

  d. Spiritual factors: _____

  _____

- Explain how the following physiological factors affect pain:

  a. Anxiety: _____

  _____

  b. Coping style: _____

  _____

- Explain how the following cultural factors affect pain:

  a. Meaning of pain: _____

  _____

  _____

b. Ethnicity: _____

_____

_____

Nursing Process and Pain

- Pain management extends beyond pain relief, encompassing the client's _____, _____, and _____.

𝒩𝒫 Assessment

- For clients with acute pain, the nurse primarily assesses _____,

_____,

and _____.

- For clients with chronic pain, assessment should be focused on _____,

_____, and _____, dimensions of the pain experience and on its history and context.

- Pain assessment and management "ABCDE"

    A: _____

    _____

    B: _____

    _____

    C: _____

    _____

    D: _____

    _____

    _____

    E: _____

    _____

- Identify examples of nonverbal expressions of pain. _____

_____

_____

_____

- Cognitively impaired clients require simple assessment approaches involving close observation of behavior changes.

- Briefly explain the common characteristics of pain.

    a. Onset and duration: _____

    _____

    _____

    _____

    b. Location: _____

    _____

    _____

    _____

    c. Intensity: _____

    _____

    _____

    _____

- Describe the following descriptive scales for measuring the severity of pain.

    a. Verbal descriptor scale (VDS): _____

    _____

    _____

    _____

    b. Visual analog scale (VAS): _____

    _____

    _____

    _____

    c. Faces scale: _____

    _____

    _____

    _____

- Identify some terms a client can use to describe the quality of pain. _____

_____

_____

_____

- Identify some measures a client may use to relieve pain. _____

_____

_____

- Identify some concomitant symptoms that occur with pain. _____

_____

_____

- Summarize how pain affects the psychological well-being of the client. _____

_____

_____

- Give examples of the following behavioral indicators of pain.

   a. Vocalizations: _____

   _____

   b. Facial expressions: _____

   _____

   c. Body movement: _____

   _____

   d. Social interaction: _____

   _____

- Explain how pain can influence activities of daily living in regard to the following.

   a. Sleep: _____

   _____

   _____

   _____

   b. Hygiene: _____

   _____

   _____

   _____

   c. Sexual relations: _____

   _____

   _____

   _____

   d. Employment: _____

   _____

   _____

   _____

   e. Social activities: _____

   _____

   _____

   _____

Nursing Diagnosis

- The nursing diagnosis should focus on the specific nature of the pain to help the nurse identify the most useful types of interventions for alleviating pain and minimizing its effect on the client's lifestyle and function.

- List five potential or actual nursing diagnoses related to a client in pain.

   a. _____
   b. _____
   c. _____
   d. _____
   e. _____

Planning

- An intervention that works for one client will not work for all clients.

- When developing a plan of care, the nurse selects priorities based on the client's level of pain and its effect on the client's condition.

- List the client outcomes appropriate for the client experiencing pain.

  a. _____

  b. _____

  c. _____

  d. _____

  e. _____

_NP_ Implementation

Health Promotion

- Teaching clients about the pain experience reduces anxiety and helps clients achieve a sense of control.

- Describe how you would teach a child about a painful procedure. _____

  _____

  _____

- Define the holistic health approach to pain control: _____

  _____

  _____

- The Agency for Healthcare Research and Quality (AHRQ) guidelines for acute pain management cite nonpharmacological interventions appropriate for clients who meet certain criteria. List those criteria.

  a. _____

  b. _____

  c. _____

  d. _____

  e. _____

- Nonpharmacological interventions such as the following lesson pain. Briefly explain each one.

  a. Relaxation: _____

  _____

  _____

  _____

- b. Guided imagery: _____

  _____

  _____

  _____

- Briefly explain how the nurse would lead a client through guided imagery. _____

  _____

  _____

  _____

- Briefly explain how the nurse would guide a client through progressive relaxation exercises.

  _____

  _____

  _____

- Define _distraction_, and list one disadvantage and advantage of using distraction.

  _____

  _____

  _____

- Describe the effects of using music as a distraction to control pain. _____

  _____

  _____

  _____

- Define the following pain-relief measures and the rationale for their use.

  a. Biofeedback: _____

  _____

  _____

  _____

  b. Cutaneous stimulation: _____

  _____

  _____

  _____

c. Herbals: _____

_____

_____

_____

d. Reducing pain perception: _____

_____

_____

_____

- What is TENS, and how is it believed to reduce pain? _____

_____

_____

_____

Acute Care

Pharmacological Pain-Relief Interventions

- Analgesics are the most common method of pain relief.

- Identify the three types of analgesics and explain the conditions for which they are generally prescribed.

a. _____

_____

b. _____

_____

c. _____

_____

- List the seven characteristics of an ideal analgesic.

a. _____

b. _____

c. _____

d. _____

e. _____

f. _____

g. _____

- Describe four major principles for analgesic administration.

a. _____

b. _____

c. _____

d. _____

- Explain the benefits of patient-controlled analgesia (PCA). _____

_____

_____

_____

- Describe what a local anesthetic is and give its physiological properties. _____

_____

_____

_____

- Identify four types of local anesthetics and the level of anesthesia they provide.

a. _____

_____

b. _____

_____

c. _____

_____

d. _____

_____

- List the seven advantages of an epidural analgesia.

a. _____

b. _____

c. _____

d. _____

e. _____

f. _____

g. _____

Chapter 42: Comfort   281

- List four goals for the care of a client with epidural infusions. Describe one action for each goal.

  a. _____

  _____

  b. _____

  _____

  c. _____

  _____

  d. _____

  _____

- Explain the following surgical interventions for pain.

  a. Dorsal rhizotomy: _____

  _____

  b. Chordotomy: _____

  _____

- Identify the three-step approach to cancer pain management recommended by the World Health Organization (1990).

  a. _____

  _____

  b. _____

  _____

  c. _____

  _____

- Identify clients who are candidates for continuous infusions.

  a. _____

  b. _____

  c. _____

  d. _____

- List four guidelines for safe administration of morphine sulfate via ambulatory infusion pumps.

  a. _____

  _____

b. _____

_____

c. _____

_____

d. _____

_____

Restorative Care

- Explain hospice programs. _____

  _____

  _____

  _____

Evaluation

Client Care

- Client care evaluates the actual care delivered by the health care team based on the expected outcomes.

- The nurse needs to know what responses to anticipate on the basis of the type of pain, the intervention, the timing of the intervention, the physiological nature of the injury or disease, and the client's previous responses.

Client Expectations

- The client, if able, is the best resource for evaluating the effectiveness of pain-relief measures.

- The family often is another valuable resource, particularly in the case of the client with cancer who may not be able to express discomfort during the latter stages of terminal illness.

Review Questions

The student should select the appropriate answer and cite the rationale for choosing that particular answer.

1. Pain is a protective mechanism warning of tissue injury and is largely a (an):
   a. Symptom of a severe illness or disease
   b. Subjective experience
   c. Objective experience
   d. Acute symptom of short duration

Answer: _____ Rationale: _____

_____

_____

2. A substance that can cause analgesia when it attaches to opiate receptors in the brain is:
   a. Substance P
   b. Serotonin
   c. Prostaglandin
   d. Endorphin

Answer: _____ Rationale: _____

_____

_____

3. To adequately assess the quality of a client's pain, which question would be appropriate?
   a. "Tell me what your pain feels like."
   b. "Is your pain a crushing sensation?"
   c. "How long have you had this pain?"
   d. "Is it a sharp pain or a dull pain?"

Answer: _____ Rationale: _____

_____

_____

4. The use of client distraction in pain control is based on the principle that:
   a. Small C fibers transmit impulses via the spinothalamic tract.
   b. The reticular formation can send inhibitory signals to gating mechanisms.
   c. Large A fibers compete with pain impulses to close gates to painful stimuli.
   d. Transmission of pain impulses from the spinal cord to the cerebral cortex can be inhibited.

Answer: _____ Rationale: _____

_____

_____

5. Teaching a child about painful procedures is best achieved by:
   a. Early warnings of the anticipated pain
   b. Storytelling about the upcoming procedure
   c. Relevant play directed toward procedure activities
   d. Avoiding explanations until the pain is experienced

Answer: _____ Rationale: _____

_____

_____

Critical Thinking for Nursing Care Plan for Acute Pain

Imagine that you are the student nurse in the Care Plan on page 1249 of your text. Complete the *Assessment phase* of the critical thinking model by writing your answers in the appropriate boxes of the model shown. Think about the following:

- What knowledge base was applied to Mrs. Mays?

- In what way might previous experience assist you in this case?

- What intellectual or professional standards were applied to the care of Mrs. Mays?

- What critical thinking attitudes did you use in assessing Mrs. Mays?

- As you review your assessment, what key areas did you cover?

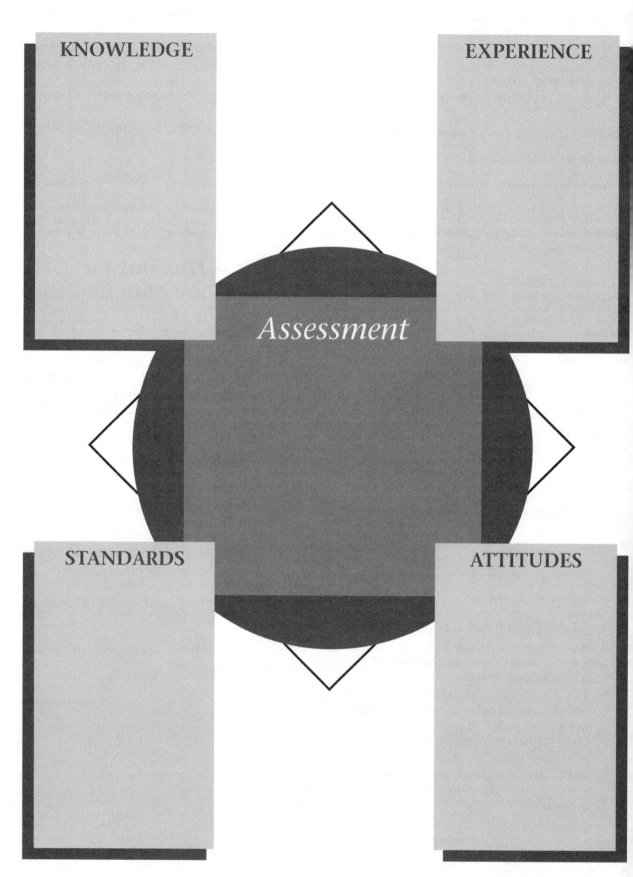

KNOWLEDGE

EXPERIENCE

Assessment

STANDARDS

ATTITUDES

CHAPTER 42   Critical Thinking Model for *Acute Pain*

See answers on page 545.

43

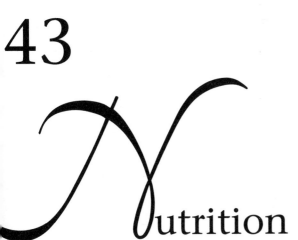

utrition

Preliminary Reading

Chapter 43, pp. 1271-1321

Comprehensive Understanding

Scientific Knowledge Base

Nutrients: The Biochemical Units of Nutrition
- The body requires fuel to provide energy for _____, _____, _____, and _____.

- Define the following terms.

  a. *Basal metabolic rate (BMR):* _____

  b. *Resting energy expenditure (REE):* _____

  c. *Nutrients:* _____

  d. *Nutrient density:* _____

- List the six categories of nutrients.

  a. _____

  b. _____

  c. _____

  d. _____

  e. _____

  f. _____

- Each gram of carbohydrate produces _____ kilocalories (kcal).

- Identify the three classifications of carbohydrates.

  a. _____

  b. _____

  c. _____

- Proteins provide a source of energy _____ kcal/g and are essential for _____.

- The simplest form of protein is: _____

  _____

  _____

- Explain the two forms of protein.

  a. Essential amino acids: _____

  _____

  _____

  b. Nonessential amino acids: _____

  _____

  _____

- Define the following terms.

  a. *Complete protein:* _____

  _____

  b. *Complementary proteins:* _____

  _____

  c. *Nitrogen balance:* _____

  _____

- Lipids (fats) are the most calorically dense nutrient, providing _____ kcal per gram.

- Describe the following composition of fats.

  a. Triglycerides: _____

  _____

  b. Fatty acids: _____

  _____

- Lipogenesis is: _____

  _____

  _____

- Define the following types of fats and give an example of each.

  a. *Saturated:* _____

  _____

  b. *Unsaturated:* _____

  _____

  c. *Monounsaturated:* _____

  _____

  d. *Polyunsaturated:* _____

  _____

- Deficiencies occur when fat intake falls below _____ of daily nutrition.

- Briefly explain how Olestra (a fat replacer) works. _____

  _____

  _____

- Water composes _____ of total body weight.

- _____ have the greatest percentage of total body weight as water, and _____ people have the least.

- Fluid needs are met by _____ and by water produced during _____.

- Vitamins are: _____

  _____

  _____

- Identify the water-soluble vitamins. _____

  _____

  _____

- Identify the fat-soluble vitamins. _____

  _____

  _____

- Minerals are: _____
  _____
  _____

- Minerals are classified as _____ when the daily requirement is 100 mg or more; and _____ when less than 100 mg is needed daily.

Anatomy and Physiology of Digestive System

- Digestion of food consists of the mechanical breakdown and chemical reactions by which food is reduced to its simplest form.

- Enzymes are: _____
  _____
  _____

- The following activities of digestion are interdependent. Explain each one.

  a. Mechanical: _____
  _____

  b. Chemical: _____
  _____

  c. Hormonal: _____
  _____

- The major portion of digestion occurs in the:
  _____
  _____

- Define the terms related to digestion.

  a. *Peristalsis:* _____
  _____

  b. *Dysphagia:* _____
  _____

  c. *Chyme:* _____
  _____

- The primary site of absorption is the: _____
  _____
  _____

- Absorption of water is the main function of the:
  _____
  _____
  _____

- In addition to water, electrolytes and minerals are absorbed, and bacteria in the colon synthesize _____ vitamins.

- Metabolism refers to: _____
  _____
  _____

- Describe the two types of metabolism.

  a. Anabolism: _____
  _____
  _____
  _____

  b. Catabolism: _____
  _____
  _____
  _____

- The body's major form of stored energy is _____, which is stored as _____.

- Glycogen is: _____
  _____
  _____

- Nutrient metabolism consists of three main processes. Explain each one.

  a. Glycogenolysis: _____
  _____

  b. Glycogenesis: _____
  _____

  c. Gluconeogenesis: _____
  _____

- Feces contain: _____
  _____
  _____

Dietary Guidelines

- Explain the Dietary Reference Intakes (DRIs) format. _____ _____ _____ _____ _____

- The estimated average requirement (EAR) serves as a _____ _____ _____ _____

- The tolerable upper intake level (UL) is: _____ _____ _____

- Using the space below, diagram and label the food guide pyramid developed by the U.S. Department of Agriculture (USDA).

- List the seven dietary guidelines for Americans issued by the USDA and the Department of Health and Human Services.

  a. _____

  b. _____

  c. _____

  d. _____

  e. _____

  f. _____

  g. _____

- Summarize the rationale for daily values on food labels. _____ _____ _____ _____

- Summarize *Healthy People 2010* goals. _____ _____ _____ _____

Nursing Knowledge Base

Nutrition During Human Growth and Development

Infants

- An energy intake of approximately _____ kcal/kg is needed in the first half of infancy, and an intake of _____ kcal/kg is needed in the second half.

- A full-term newborn is able to digest and absorb _____.

- Infants need _____ ml/kg/day of fluid.

- List at least four benefits for breast-feeding an infant.

  a. _____

  b. _____

  c. _____

  d. _____

- Explain why the following should not be used in infant formula.

  a. Cow's milk: _____

  _____

  b. Honey and corn syrup: _____

  _____

- List four indications of an infant's readiness to begin solid foods.

  a. _____

  b. _____

  c. _____

  d. _____

Toddlers and Preschoolers

- The toddler needs _____ calories but an increased amount of _____ in relation to body weight.

School-Age Children

- School-age children's diets should be assessed for: _____

  _____

- Explain some reasons for the increase in childhood obesity. _____

  _____

Adolescents

- Identify the common deficiencies in the following adolescent population.

  a. Girls: _____

  _____

  b. Boys: _____

  _____

  c. Those who eat fast-food: _____

  _____

  d. Those involved in intense exercise: _____

  _____

  e. Pregnant: _____

  _____

- Identify the diagnostic criteria for the following eating disorders:

  a. Anorexia nervosa: _____

  _____

  _____

  _____

  _____

  _____

  b. Bulimia nervosa: _____

  _____

  _____

  _____

  _____

  _____

Young and Middle Adults

- Obesity becomes a problem because of: _____

  _____

  _____

- Adult women who use oral contraceptives need extra _____

  _____.

Chapter 43: Nutrition   289

- The energy requirements of pregnancy are related to _____ _____.

- Explain the increased amounts of the following items that are required for pregnancy and lactation.

  a. Pregnancy

  1. Calories: _____ _____

  2. Calcium: _____ _____

  3. Iron: _____ _____

  4. Vitamins: _____ _____

  5. Fluids: _____ _____

  b. Lactation

  1. Calories: _____ _____

  2. Protein: _____ _____

  3. Calcium: _____ _____

  4. Vitamins: _____ _____

  5. Fluids: _____ _____

Older Adults

- List four factors that influence the nutritional status of the older adult. Using an asterisk, identify the one factor that is considered the most important.

  a. _____

  b. _____

  c. _____

  d. _____

Alternative Food Patterns

- A common alternative dietary pattern is the vegetarian diet. Describe briefly.

  _____

  _____

  _____

  _____

  _____

Nursing Process and Nutrition

- Close daily contact with clients and their families enables nurses to make observations about their physical status, food intake, weight gain or loss, and responses to therapy.

Assessment

- List the five components of a nutritional assessment.

  a. _____

  b. _____

  c. _____

  d. _____

  e. _____

- Define.

  a. *Anthropometry:* _____ _____

  b. *Body mass index (BMI):* _____ _____

  c. *Ideal body weight (IBW):* _____ _____

  d. *Bioelectrical impedance analysis (BIA):* _____ _____

- Identify the common laboratory tests used to study the nutritional status of a client.

  _____

  _____

  _____

  _____

- List the five factors on which a dietary history focuses.

  a. _____

  b. _____

  c. _____

  d. _____

  e. _____

- List seven factors that influence dietary patterns.

  a. _____

  b. _____

  c. _____

  d. _____

  e. _____

  f. _____

  g. _____

- For each assessment area, list at least two signs of good and poor nutrition.

  a. General appearance

     1. _____

     2. _____

  b. General vitality

     1. _____

     2. _____

  c. Weight

     1. _____

     2. _____

  d. Hair

     1. _____

     2. _____

  e. Skin

     1. _____

     2. _____

  f. Mouth

     1. _____

     2. _____

  g. Eyes

     1. _____

     2. _____

  h. Gastrointestinal function

     1. _____

     2. _____

  i. Cardiovascular function

     1. _____

     2. _____

  j. Neurological function

     1. _____

     2. _____

  k. Musculoskeletal function

     1. _____

     2. _____

Nursing Diagnosis

- List three potential or actual nursing diagnoses for altered nutritional status.

  a. _____

  b. _____

  c. _____

Planning

- Explain why the clients in the following situations are considered at risk for nutritional problems.

  a. Oral and throat surgery: _____

     _____

  b. GI surgery: _____

     _____

  c. Immobilization: _____

     _____

- List four goals for a client with nutritional problems.

  a. _____

  b. _____

  c. _____

  d. _____

𝒩𝒫 Implementation

- List three situations that occur in the hospital setting that influence nutritional intake.

  a. _____

  b. _____

  c. _____

- List five ways that a nurse can stimulate the client's appetite.

  a. _____

  b. _____

  c. _____

  d. _____

  e. _____

Health Promotion

- Clients can prevent the development of many diseases by incorporating a knowledge of nutrition into their lifestyle.

- Summarize meal planning and identify the factors that should be considered. _____

  _____

  _____

  _____

  _____

Acute Care

- Clients who are NPO and only receive standard IV fluids for more than 7 days are at nutritional risk.

- Define *enteral nutrition (EN)*. _____

  _____

- Explain the beneficial effect of enteral feedings as compared to parenteral nutrition.

  _____

  _____

  _____

  _____

  _____

  _____

  _____

  _____

- Explain aspiration and the physiological changes that occur in the client. _____

  _____

  _____

  _____

- Identify the clients who are suitable for the following types of formulas.

  a. Polymeric: _____

  _____

  b. Modular: _____

  _____

  c. Elemental: _____

  _____

  d. Specialty: _____

  _____

- Describe the following types of feeding tubes.

  a. Nasogastric: _____

  _____

  b. Gastrostomy: _____

  _____

  c. PEG: _____

  _____

- Identify the tube type preferred for enteral tube feedings. _____

  _____

- The most reliable method for testing the placement of a small bore feeding tube is: _____

  _____

  _____

- Describe a method that the nurse may use to test the placement of a small-bore feeding tube. _____

  _____

  _____

  _____

  _____

- List the five major complications of enteral feedings.

  a. _____

  b. _____

  c. _____

  d. _____

  e. _____

- List the three factors on which safe administration of parenteral nutrition (PN) depends.

  a. _____

  b. _____

  c. _____

- Lipid emulsions are: _____

  _____

- The adverse reactions to lipid emulsion include: _____

  _____

- Briefly describe the rationale for each action associated with the initiation and maintenance of total parenteral nutrition.

  a. Chest x-ray: _____

  _____

  b. Beginning an infusion: _____

  _____

- c. Infusion flow rate: _____

  _____

- List six potential complications of parenteral nutrition and identify the symptoms of each.

  a. _____

  b. _____

  c. _____

  d. _____

  e. _____

  f. _____

- Explain the goal of transition from PN to EN and/or oral feeding. _____

  _____

  _____

  _____

Restorative and Continuing Care

- Medical nutrition therapy (MNT) is: _____

  _____

  _____

  _____

- Restorative care includes both immediate post-surgical care and routine medical care and includes hospitalized and home care clients.

- Identify the nutritional interventions for the following common disease states:

  a. Peptic ulcers

     1. Inflammatory bowel disease: _____

        _____

     2. Malabsorption syndromes: _____

        _____

     3. Diverticulitis: _____

        _____

  b. Diabetes mellitus (DM)

     1. Type 1: _____

        _____

2. Type 2: _____

_____

c. Cardiovascular: _____

_____

d. Cancer: _____

_____

e. HIV: _____

_____

Evaluation

- Multidisciplinary collaboration remains essential in the provision of nutritional support.

Client Care

- The effectiveness of nutritional interventions delivered by the health care team is based on the expected outcomes.

- The client's ability to incorporate dietary changes into his or her lifestyle with the least amount of stress or disruption will ensure that outcome measures are successfully met.

Client Expectations

- Clients expect competent and accurate care. The plan of care must be altered if the outcomes aren't being met.

Review Questions

The student should select the appropriate answer and cite the rationale for choosing that particular answer.

1. Which nutrient is the body's most preferred energy source?
   a. Protein
   b. Fat
   c. Carbohydrate
   d. Vitamin

Answer: _____ Rationale: _____

_____

_____

2. Positive nitrogen balance would occur in which condition?
   a. Infection
   b. Starvation
   c. Burn injury
   d. Pregnancy

Answer: _____ Rationale: _____

_____

_____

3. Mrs. Nelson is talking with the nurse about the dietary needs of her 23-month-old daughter, Laura. Which of the following responses by the nurse would be appropriate?
   a. "Use skim milk to cut down on the fat in Laura's diet."
   b. "Laura should be drinking at least 1 quart of milk per day."
   c. "Laura needs fewer calories in relation to her body weight now than she did as an infant."
   d. "Laura needs less protein in her diet now because she isn't growing as fast."

Answer: _____ Rationale: _____

_____

_____

4. All of the following clients are at risk for alteration in nutrition except:
   a. Client J, who is 86 years old, lives alone, and has poorly fitting dentures
   b. Client K, who has been NPO for 7 days following bowel surgery and is receiving 3000 ml of 10% dextrose per day
   c. Client L, whose weight is 10% above his ideal body weight
   d. Client M, a 17-year-old girl who weighs 90 lb and frequently complains about her baby fat

Answer: _____ Rationale: _____

_____

_____

5. Which of the following is the most accurate method of bedside confirmation of placement of a small-bore nasogastric tube?
   a. Auscultate the epigastrium for gurgling or bubbling
   b. Test the pH of withdrawn gastric contents
   c. Assess the client's ability to speak
   d. Assess the length of the tube that is outside the client's nose

Answer: _____ Rationale: _____

_____

_____

6. A client who has been hospitalized after experiencing a heart attack will most likely receive a diet consisting of:
   a. Low fat, low sodium, and high carbohydrates
   b. Low fat, high protein, and high carbohydrates
   c. Low fat, low sodium, and low carbohydrates
   d. Liquids for several days, progressing to a soft and then a regular diet

Answer: _____ Rationale: _____

_____

_____

Critical Thinking for Nursing Care Plan for Altered Nutrition: Less Than Body Requirements

Imagine that you are Marie, the nurse in the Care Plan on page 1294 of your text. Complete the *Planning phase* of the critical thinking model by writing your answers in the appropriate boxes of the model shown. Think about the following:

- In developing Mrs. Cooper's plan of care, what knowledge did Marie apply?

- In what ways might Marie's previous experience assist in developing Mrs. Cooper's plan of care?

- When developing a plan of care for Mrs. Cooper, what intellectual and professional standards were applied?

- What critical thinking attitudes might have been applied in developing Mrs. Cooper's plan of care?

- How will Marie accomplish these goals?

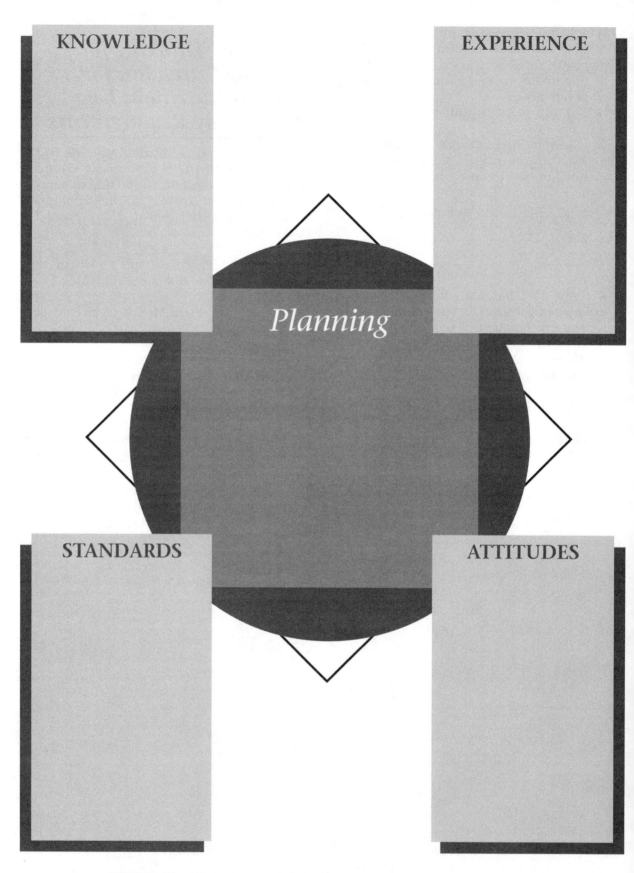

KNOWLEDGE

EXPERIENCE

Planning

STANDARDS

ATTITUDES

CHAPTER 43 Critical Thinking Model for *Imbalanced Nutrition: Less Than Body Requirements*

See answers on page 546.

44

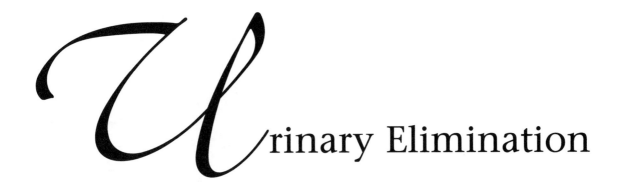

rinary Elimination

Preliminary Reading

Chapter 44, pp. 1322-1372

Comprehensive Understanding

Scientific Knowledge Base

• Summarize the function of each of the following organs in the urinary system.

a. Kidneys: _____

_____

b. Ureters: _____

_____

c. Bladder: _____

_____

d. Urethra: _____

_____

• Define the following terms related to urine elimination.

a. *Nephron:* _____

b. *Proteinuria:* _____

c. *Erythropoietin:* _____

d. *Renin:* _____

e. *Micturition:* _____

f. *Meatus:* _____

Act of Urination

- Number the steps describing the normal act of micturition in sequential order.

  _____ Parasympathetic impulses from the micturition center cause the detrusor muscle to begin contracting.

  _____ The external bladder sphincter relaxes.

  _____ Impulses travel to the cerebral cortex, making the person conscious of the need to void.

  _____ The detrusor muscle contracts.

  _____ The internal urethral sphincter relaxes, allowing urine to enter the urethra.

  _____ Urine passes through the urethral meatus.

  _____ Urine volume stretches the bladder walls, sending impulses to the spinal cord.

- Explain the following two alterations with elimination.

  a. Reflex bladder: _____

  _____

  b. Urinary retention: _____

  _____

- Problems related to the act of urination may be the result of cognitive, functional, or physical means and may result in incontinence, retention, or infection.

- Disease processes that primarily affect renal function (changes in urine volume or quality) are generally categorized as the following. Briefly explain.

  a. Prerenal: _____

  _____

  _____

  _____

  b. Renal: _____

  _____

  _____

  c. Postrenal: _____

  _____

  _____

- Define *oliguria*. _____

  _____

  _____

- Define *anuria*. _____

  _____

  _____

  _____

- List the characteristic signs of the uremic syndrome. _____

  _____

  _____

  _____

- Briefly describe the two methods of dialysis.

  a. Peritoneal: _____

  _____

  _____

  b. Hemodialysis: _____

  _____

  _____

- Identify some indications for dialysis. _____

  _____

  _____

  _____

- Briefly explain the following factors that influence urination.

    a. Sociocultural factors: _____

    _____

    _____

    b. Psychological factors: _____

    _____

    _____

    c. Muscle tone: _____

    _____

    _____

- Explain how the following affect the balance of urine excreted.

    a. Alcohol: _____

    _____

    _____

    _____

    b. Caffeine drinks: _____

    _____

    _____

    _____

    c. Fruits and vegetables: _____

    _____

    _____

    _____

    d. Febrile conditions: _____

    _____

    _____

    _____

- Briefly explain how the stress of surgery affects urine output. _____

    _____

    _____

    _____

    _____

    _____

- Briefly explain how anesthetics and narcotic analgesics affect urine output. _____

    _____

    _____

    _____

    _____

    _____

- A urinary diversion is: _____

    _____

- List five medications that affect urination.

    a. _____

    b. _____

    c. _____

    d. _____

    e. _____

- Explain what a cystoscopy is and how it may affect urination. _____

    _____

    _____

    _____

- Clients with urinary problems have disturbances in the act of micturition that involve a failure to store urine or a failure to empty urine. List the three most common.

    a. _____

    b. _____

    c. _____

- Define *urinary retention.* _____

    _____

    _____

- Define *retention with overflow.* _____

    _____

    _____

- List six signs or symptoms of urinary tract infections (UTIs).

  a. _____

  b. _____

  c. _____

  d. _____

  e. _____

  f. _____

- Identify the most common cause of UTIs. _____

  _____

  _____

- Identify the three common causes of UTIs in women.

  a. _____

  b. _____

  c. _____

- Define the following terms related to UTIs.

  a. *Bacteriuria:* _____

  _____

  b. *Dysuria:* _____

  _____

  c. *Hematuria:* _____

  _____

  d. *Pyelonephritis:* _____

  _____

- Define *urinary incontinence.* _____

  _____

- Briefly describe the five types of urinary incontinence.

  a. Functional: _____

  _____

  b. Overflow: _____

  _____

  c. Reflex: _____

  _____

  d. Stress: _____

  _____

  e. Urge: _____

  _____

- Identify some indications for urinary diversions.

  _____

  _____

- Briefly describe the following urinary diversions.

  a. Ileal loop or conduit: _____

  _____

  _____

  b. Ureterostomy: _____

  _____

  _____

  c. Nephrostomy: _____

  _____

  _____

Nursing Knowledge Base

- The nurse needs to know concepts other than anatomy and physiology, such as infection control, hygiene measures, growth and development, and psychosocial influences.

Infection Control and Hygiene

- Although the urinary tract is considered sterile, it is a common site for infections. Many UTIs are caused by: _____

  _____

- Hospital-acquired UTIs are related to _____,

  _____, or _____.

Developmental Considerations

- Briefly summarize the developmental changes that may influence urination.

  _____

  _____

  _____

  _____

Psychosocial Considerations

• Identify the psychosocial factors that may influence urination. _____

_____

_____

_____

_____

Nursing Process and Alterations in Urinary Function

𝒩𝒫 Assessment

Nursing History

• List the three major factors to be explored during a nursing history in regard to urinary elimination.

a. _____

b. _____

c. _____

• Describe the following symptoms of urinary alterations.

a. Urgency: _____

_____

b. Dysuria: _____

_____

c. Frequency: _____

_____

d. Hesitancy: _____

_____

e. Polyuria: _____

_____

f. Oliguria: _____

_____

g. Nocturia: _____

_____

h. Dribbling: _____

_____

i. Incontinence: _____

_____

j. Hematuria: _____

_____

k. Retention: _____

_____

l. Residual urine: _____

_____

• Briefly explain the organs that the nurse would assess to determine the presence and severity of urinary problems.

a. Skin and mucosal membranes: _____

_____

b. Kidneys: _____

_____

c. Bladder: _____

_____

d. Urethral meatus: _____

_____

• Assessment of urine involves _____

and _____.

• Describe the following characteristics of urine.

a. Color: _____

_____

_____

_____

b. Clarity: _____

_____

_____

_____

c. Odor: _____

_____

_____

_____

- Describe the following types of urine specimens collected for testing.

  a. Random: _____

  _____

  _____

  _____

  b. Clean-voided or midstream: _____

  _____

  _____

  _____

  c. Sterile: _____

  _____

  _____

  _____

  d. Timed urine: _____

  _____

  _____

  _____

- Common urine tests include the following. Briefly explain each.

  a. Urinalysis: _____

  _____

  _____

  _____

  b. Specific gravity: _____

  _____

  _____

  _____

  c. Urine culture: _____

  _____

  _____

  _____

- Briefly explain the following types of diagnostic examinations and give the nursing implications for each.

a. Abdominal roentgenogram: _____

_____

_____

_____

_____

_____

b. Intravenous pyelogram (IVP): _____

_____

_____

_____

_____

_____

c. Renal scan: _____

_____

_____

_____

_____

_____

d. CT scan: _____

_____

_____

_____

_____

_____

e. Ultrasound: _____

_____

_____

_____

_____

_____

_____

- List the three types of invasive procedures and the nursing implications.

  a. _____

  _____

  b. _____

  _____

c. _____

_____

𝒩𝒟 Nursing Diagnosis

- List six potential or actual nursing diagnoses related to urinary elimination.

  a. _____

  b. _____

  c. _____

  d. _____

  e. _____

  f. _____

𝒩𝒟 Planning

- List the six goals appropriate for a client with a urinary elimination problem.

  a. _____

  b. _____

  c. _____

  d. _____

  e. _____

  f. _____

𝒩𝒟 Implementation

Health Promotion

- List five techniques that may be used to stimulate the micturition reflex.

  a. _____

  b. _____

  c. _____

  d. _____

  e. _____

- Urine is normally acidic and tends to inhibit the growth of microorganisms. List four types of foods that increase urine acidity.

  a. _____

  b. _____

  c. _____

  d. _____

Acute Care

- Briefly explain how the nurse could help the hospitalized client maintain normal elimination habits. _____

  _____

  _____

  _____

- List and explain three types of medications that can be used to treat incontinence or retention.

  a. _____

  b. _____

  c. _____

- Briefly describe the following types of catheters.

  a. Straight single-use: _____

  _____

  _____

  _____

  b. Indwelling: _____

  _____

  _____

  _____

  c. Coudé: _____

  _____

  _____

  _____

- Explain the nursing measures taken to prevent infection and maintain an unobstructed flow of urine in catheterized clients.

  a. Fluid intake: _____

  _____

  _____

  _____

  b. Perineal hygiene: _____

  _____

  _____

  _____

Chapter 44: Urinary Elimination   303

c. Catheter care: _____

_____

_____

_____

- Briefly describe catheter irrigations and instillations. _____

_____

_____

_____

- Name two important principles to follow when removing an indwelling catheter.

a. _____

_____

b. _____

_____

- Briefly explain the two alternatives for urinary catheterization and give the nursing implications for each.

a. Suprapubic catheter: _____

_____

_____

_____

_____

_____

b. Condom catheter: _____

_____

_____

_____

_____

_____

- Name two precautions that should be taken to ensure client safety and comfort when using a condom catheter.

a. _____

b. _____

Restorative Care

- Define *pelvic floor exercises* (PFEs/Kegel exercises):

_____

_____

- Identify the goal of bladder retraining. _____

_____

_____

_____

_____

- List 11 measures the nurse can teach the incontinent client to gain control over urination.

a. _____

b. _____

c. _____

d. _____

e. _____

f. _____

g. _____

h. _____

i. _____

j. _____

k. _____

- A client with functional incontinence may benefit from habit training, which helps clients improve voluntary control over urination.

- List the nursing measures used to maintain skin integrity when urine comes in contact with the skin.

a. _____

b. _____

c. _____

d. _____

List two comfort measures for a client with the following sources of discomfort.

a. Incontinence

    1. _____

    2. _____

b. Dysuria

    1. _____

    2. _____

c. Painful distention

    1. _____

    2. _____

Evaluation

Client Care

Client care evaluates the actual care delivered by the health care team based on the expected outcomes.

- The nurse evaluates for change in the

_____, _____,

and _____.

Client Expectations

- Client expectations evaluate care from the client's perspective.

- The nurse can also assist the client in redefining unrealistic goals when an impairment is not likely to be altered as completely as the client might like.

Review Questions

The student should select the appropriate answer and cite the rationale for choosing that particular answer.

1. All of the following factors will influence the production of urine except:
   a. Anxiety
   b. Acute renal disease
   c. Febrile conditions
   d. Diuretic medications

   Answer: _____ Rationale: _____

   _____

   _____

2. Mrs. Rantz complains of leaking urine when she coughs or laughs. This is known as:
   a. Functional incontinence
   b. Stress incontinence
   c. Urge incontinence
   d. Reflex incontinence

   Answer: _____ Rationale: _____

   _____

   _____

3. Ms. Hathaway has a urinary tract infection. Which of the following symptoms would you expect her to exhibit?
   a. Proteinuria
   b. Dysuria
   c. Oliguria
   d. Polyuria

   Answer: _____ Rationale: _____

   _____

   _____

4. The nurse is working in the radiology department with a client who is having an intravenous pyelogram. Which of the following complaints by the client is an abnormal response?
   a. Shortness of breath and audible wheezing
   b. Feeling dizzy and warm with obvious facial flushing
   c. Thirst and feeling "worn out"
   d. Frequent, loose stools

   Answer: _____ Rationale: _____

   _____

   _____

5. The urinalysis of Ms. Hathaway reveals a high bacteria count. Ampicillin is prescribed for her urinary tract infection. The teaching plan for a UTI should include all of the following except: .
   a. Drink at least 2000 ml of fluid daily.
   b. Always wipe perineum from front to back.
   c. Explain the possible side effects of medication.
   d. Drink plenty of orange and grapefruit juices.

   Answer: _____ Rationale: _____

   _____

   _____

Critical Thinking for Nursing Care Plan for Functional Incontinence

Imagine that you are Judi, the student nurse in the Care Plan on page 1344 of your text. Complete the *Assessment phase* of the critical thinking model by writing your answers in the appropriate boxes of the model shown. Think about the following:

- What knowledge base was applied to the care of Judi's grandmother?

- In what way might Judi's previous experience assist in this case?

- What intellectual or professional standards were applied to Judi's grandmother?

- What critical thinking attitudes did you utilize in assessing Judi's grandmother?

- As you review the assessment, what key areas did Judi cover?

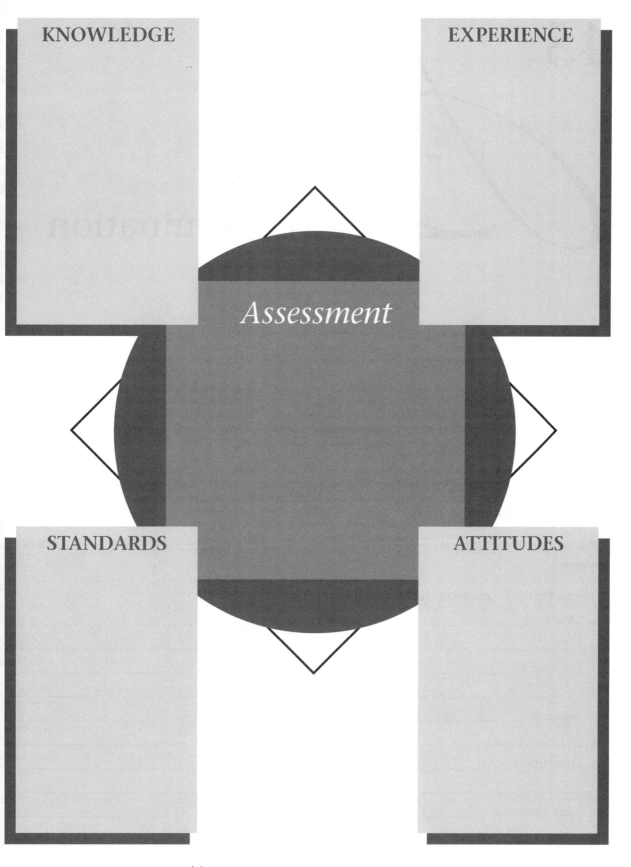

KNOWLEDGE

EXPERIENCE

Assessment

STANDARDS

ATTITUDES

CHAPTER 44   Critical Thinking Model for *Functional Urinary Incontinence*

See answers on page 547.

45

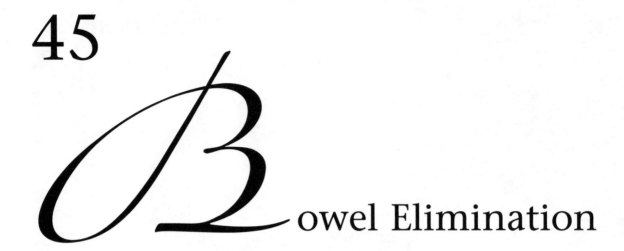

owel Elimination

Preliminary Reading

Chapter 45, pp. 1373-1417

Comprehensive Understanding

Scientific Knowledge Base

- The volume of fluids absorbed by the GI tract is high, making fluid balance a key function of the GI system.

- Summarize the functions of the following.

  a. Mouth: _____

  _____

  b Esophagus: _____

  _____

  c. Stomach: _____

  _____

  d. Small intestine: _____

  _____

  e. Large intestine: _____

  _____

- Define the following terms and identify the portion of the GI tract to which they relate.

  a. *Masticate:* _____

  _____

  b. *Bolus:* _____

  _____

  c. *Peristalsis:* _____

  _____

  d. *Flatus:* _____

  _____

  e. *Feces:* _____

  _____

- Indicate the correct sequence of mechanisms involved in normal defecation.

  _____ Increased intraabdominal pressure or Valsalva's maneuver occurs.

  _____ The external sphincter relaxes.

  _____ The internal sphincter relaxes and awareness of the need to defecate occurs.

  _____ The levator ani muscles relax.

  _____ Sensory nerves are stimulated via rectal distention.

Nursing Knowledge Base

Factors Affecting Bowel Elimination

- Briefly describe the normal elimination pattern of an infant. _____

  _____

  _____

  _____

- List six changes that occur in the GI system of the older adult that impair normal digestion and elimination.

  a. _____

  _____

  b. _____

  _____

  c. _____

  _____

d. _____

_____

e. _____

_____

f. _____

_____

- Identify the mechanisms that cause high-fiber diets to promote elimination. _____

  _____

  _____

  _____

  _____

  _____

- List five types of foods that are considered high in fiber (bulk).

  a. _____

  b. _____

  c. _____

  d. _____

  e. _____

- Define *lactose intolerance.* _____

  _____

- Summarize how an inadequate intake of fluids can affect the character of feces. _____

  _____

  _____

  _____

  _____

  _____

- Physical activity _____ peristalsis; immobilization _____ peristalsis.

- Weakened abdominal and pelvic floor muscles impair the ability to _____ and to _____.

- List two diseases of the GI tract that may be associated with stress.

  a. _____

  b. _____

- List four personal elimination habits that influence bowel function.

  a. _____

  b. _____

  c. _____

  d. _____

- Describe how the position of squatting facilitates defecation. _____

  _____

  _____

  _____

  _____

  _____

- List conditions that may result in painful defecation.

  a. _____

  b. _____

  c. _____

  d. _____

- Identify the common problems related to defecation that occur during pregnancy and explain why they occur. _____

  _____

  _____

  _____

- Summarize the effects of anesthetic agents and peristalsis on defecation. _____

  _____

  _____

  _____

- Describe the effect of each medication on elimination.

  a. Mineral oil: _____

  _____

  b. Dicyclomine HCl (Bentyl): _____

  _____

  c. Narcotics: _____

  _____

  d. Anticholinergics: _____

  _____

  e. Antibiotics: _____

  _____

  f. Histamines: _____

  _____

  g. NSAIDs: _____

  _____

- List three types of diagnostic tests for visualization of GI structures.

  a. _____

  b. _____

  c. _____

Common Bowel Elimination Problems
- List four factors that place a client at risk for elimination problems.

  a. _____

  b. _____

  c. _____

  d. _____

- Define *constipation*. _____

  _____

- List and briefly describe four causes of constipation.

  a. _____

  b. _____

  c. _____

  d. _____

- List three groups of clients in whom constipation could pose a significant health hazard.

  a. _____

  b. _____

  c. _____

- Define *fecal impaction*. _____
  _____

- List four signs and symptoms of fecal impaction.

  a. _____

  b. _____

  c. _____

  d. _____

- Define *diarrhea*. _____
  _____

- Name the two major complications associated with diarrhea.

  a. _____

  b. _____

- List five conditions and the physiological effects that cause diarrhea.

  a. _____

  b. _____

  c. _____

  d. _____

  e. _____

- Define *fecal incontinence*. _____
  _____

- Flatulence is _____.

  It is a common cause of _____,

  _____,

  and _____.

- Define *hemorrhoids*: _____
  _____

- List four conditions that cause hemorrhoids.

  a. _____

  b. _____

  c. _____

  d. _____

Bowel Diversions
- Define the following.

  a. *Stoma:* _____
  _____

  b. *Ileostomy:* _____
  _____

  c. *Colostomy:* _____
  _____

- The location of the ostomy determines the consistency of the stool.

- Briefly explain each of the following types of colostomy construction:

  a. Loop colostomy: _____
  _____

  b. End colostomy: _____
  _____

  c. Double-barrel colostomy: _____
  _____

- Briefly describe the following surgical procedures that provide continence for selected colectomy clients.

  a. Ileoanal pouch anastomosis: _____
  _____
  _____
  _____

  b. Kock continent ileostomy: _____
  _____
  _____
  _____

- Identify a major physiological concern of ostomy clients. _____

_____

_____

_____

Nursing Process and Bowel Elimination

𝒩𝒫 Assessment

- List 15 factors that affect elimination which need to be included in a nursing history for clients with altered elimination status.

  a. _____

  b. _____

  c. _____

  d. _____

  e. _____

  f. _____

  g. _____

  h. _____

  i. _____

  j. _____

  k. _____

  l. _____

  m. _____

  n. _____

  o. _____

- Summarize the following steps for assessing the abdomen.

  a. Inspection: _____

  _____

  _____

  b. Auscultation: _____

  _____

  _____

  _____

  c. Palpation: _____

  _____

  _____

  d. Percussion: _____

  _____

  _____

  _____

- Summarize the assessment of the rectum. _____

  _____

  _____

  _____

  _____

- Briefly describe the appropriate technique for collecting a fecal specimen. _____

  _____

  _____

  _____

  _____

  _____

  _____

- Define *guaiac test*. _____

  _____

- Describe the normal fecal characteristics.

  a. Color: _____

  _____

  b. Odor: _____

  _____

  c. Consistency: _____

  _____

  d. Frequency: _____

  _____

  e. Amount: _____

  _____

  f. Shape: _____

  _____

g. Constituents: _____

_____

- Indicate the possible cause for each of the following fecal characteristics.

    a. White or clay color: _____

    _____

    b. Black or tarry: _____

    _____

    c. Melena: _____

    _____

    d. Liquid consistency: _____

    _____

    e. Narrow, pencil-shaped: _____

    _____

Nursing Diagnosis

- List six potential or actual nursing diagnoses for a client with alteration in bowel elimination.

    a. _____

    b. _____

    c. _____

    d. _____

    e. _____

    f. _____

Planning

- List seven goals appropriate for clients with elimination problems.

    a. _____

    b. _____

    c. _____

    d. _____

    e. _____

    f. _____

    g. _____

Implementation

Health Promotion

- Explain how the following can assist the client to evacuate his or her bowels.

    a. Sitting position: _____

    _____

    b. Positioning on the bedpan: _____

    _____

- Explain the proper technique for positioning a client on a bedpan. _____

    _____

    _____

    _____

Acute Care

- Identify the primary action of the following.

    a. Cathartics: _____

    _____

    b. Laxatives: _____

    _____

    c. Antidiarrheals: _____

    _____

- The primary reason for an enema is: _____

    _____

- Briefly describe the following types of enemas.

    a. Tap water: _____

    _____

    b. Normal saline: _____

    _____

    c. Soapsuds solution: _____

    _____

    d. Hypertonic saline: _____

    _____

    e. Oil-retention: _____

    _____

    f. Carminative: _____

    _____

Chapter 45: Bowel Elimination   313

- Explain the physician's order, "Give enemas till clear." _____
  _____
  _____
  _____

- List three complications of digital removal of stool.
  a. _____
  b. _____
  c. _____

- List four reasons to insert a nasogastric tube for decompression.
  a. _____
  b. _____
  c. _____
  d. _____

- Explain how the Salem sump tube works. _____
  _____
  _____
  _____
  _____

- Explain how the nurse would provide comfort to a client with a NG tube. _____
  _____
  _____
  _____

- Explain how an NG tube can cause distention and how it can be prevented. _____
  _____
  _____
  _____

Restorative Care

Care of Ostomies

- List five factors to consider when selecting a pouching system for an ostomate.
  a. _____
  b. _____
  c. _____
  d. _____
  e. _____

- Summarize the goals of a bowel-training program. _____
  _____
  _____
  _____
  _____
  _____
  _____
  _____
  _____

- Summarize the nutritional considerations for ostomy clients. _____
  _____
  _____
  _____
  _____
  _____
  _____
  _____

- Briefly explain bowel training. _____
  _____
  _____
  _____
  _____
  _____
  _____

- Describe two nursing interventions that promote comfort for clients who experience the following:

    a. Hemorrhoids:

        1. _____

        2. _____

    b. Skin integrity:

        1. _____

        2. _____

Evaluation

Client Care

- Client care evaluates the actual care delivered by the health team based on expected outcomes.

- The client is the only one who is able to determine if the bowel elimination problems have been relieved and which therapies were the most effective.

Client Expectations

- Client expectations evaluate care from the client's perspective.

Review Questions

The student should select the appropriate answer and cite the rationale for choosing that particular answer.

1. Most nutrients and electrolytes are absorbed in the:
    a. Esophagus
    b. Small intestine
    c. Colon
    d. Stomach

Answer: _____ Rationale: _____

_____

_____

2. Which of the following should be included in the teaching plan for the client who is scheduled for a gastroscopy?
    a. Avoid eating and drinking for 2 to 4 hours after the test.
    b. A cleansing enema will be given the evening before the procedure.
    c. General anesthetic is usually used for the procedure.
    d. Moderate abdominal pain is common after the procedure.

Answer: _____ Rationale: _____

_____

_____

3. Mrs. Anthony is concerned about her breast-fed infant's stool, stating that it is yellow instead of brown. The nurse explains to Mrs. Anthony that:
    a. A change to formula may be necessary.
    b. Her infant is dehydrated and she should increase his fluid intake.
    c. The stool is normal for an infant.
    d. It will be necessary to send a stool specimen to the lab.

Answer: _____ Rationale: _____

_____

_____

4. After positioning a client on the bedpan, the nurse should:
    a. Leave the head of the bed flat
    b. Raise the head of the bed 30 degrees
    c. Raise the head of the bed to a 90-degree angle
    d. Raise the bed to the highest working level

Answer: _____ Rationale: _____

_____

_____

5. The physician has ordered a cleansing enema for 7-year-old Michael. The nurse realizes the maximum volume to be given would be:
   a. 100 to 150 ml
   b. 150 to 250 ml
   c. 300 to 500 ml
   d. 600 to 700 ml

Answer: _____ Rationale: _____

_____

_____

Critical Thinking for Nursing Care Plan for Constipation

Imagine that you are Javier, the nurse in the Care Plan on page 1393 of your text. Complete the *Planning phase* of the critical thinking model by writing your answers in the appropriate boxes of the model shown. Think about the following:

- In developing Larry's plan of care, what knowledge did Javier apply?

- In what way might Javier's previous experience assist in developing a plan of care for Larry?

- When developing a plan of care, what intellectual and professional standards were applied?

- What critical thinking attitudes might have been applied in developing a plan for Larry?

- How will Javier accomplish the goals?

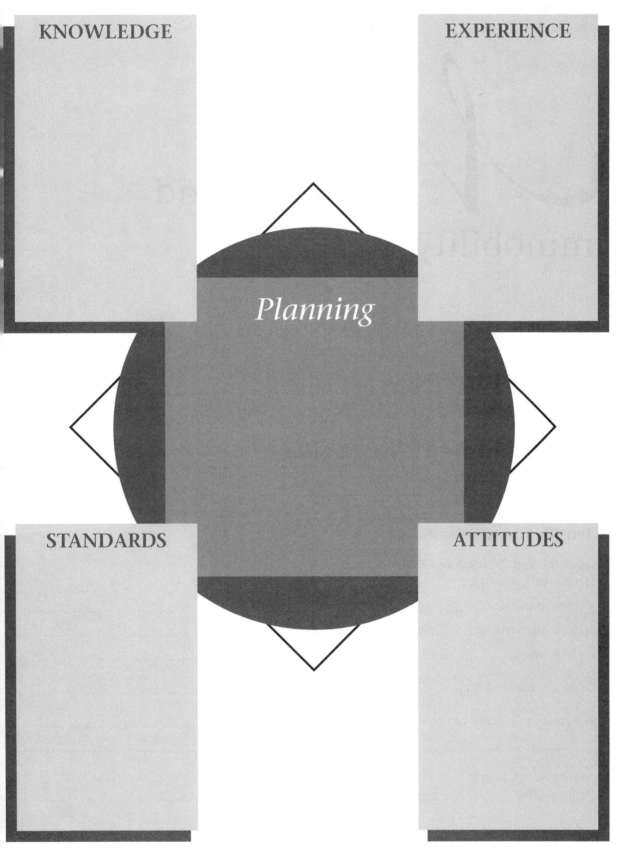

KNOWLEDGE

EXPERIENCE

Planning

STANDARDS

ATTITUDES

CHAPTER *45* Critical Thinking Model for *Constipation*

See answers on page 548.

46

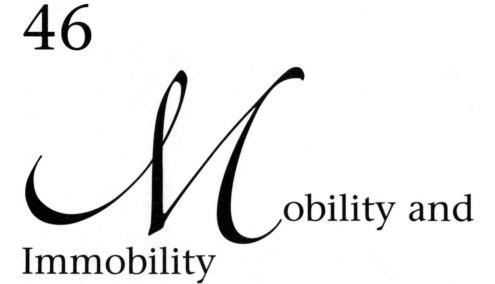

Mobility and Immobility

Preliminary Reading

Chapter 46, pp. 1420-1481

Comprehensive Understanding

- *Mobility* refers to: _____

Scientific Knowledge Base

Physiology and Principles of Body Mechanics
- Define the following.

  a. *Body mechanics:* _____

  b. *Body alignment:* _____

  c. *Body balance:* _____

- Balance is required for _____, _____, and _____.

- The ability to balance can be compromised by _____, _____,

  _____, and _____.

Gravity and Friction
- Define *friction.* _____

- List two techniques that minimize friction.

  a. _____

  b. _____

318   Chapter 46: Mobility and Immobility

Regulation of Movement

- List three systems responsible for coordinating body movements.

  a. _____

  b. _____

  c. _____

Skeletal System

- List four functions of the skeletal system.

  a. _____

  _____

  b. _____

  _____

  c. _____

  _____

  d. _____

  _____

- Describe what *pathological fractures* are. _____

  _____

- Describe the following types of joints and give an example of each.

  a. Synarthrotic joint: _____

  _____

  b. Cartilaginous joint: _____

  _____

  c. Fibrous joint: _____

  _____

  d. Synovial joint: _____

  _____

- Ligaments are: _____

  _____

- Tendons are: _____

  _____

- Cartilage is: _____

  _____

Skeletal Muscle

- Briefly describe how skeletal muscles affect movement. _____

  _____

  _____

  _____

- Briefly describe the two types of muscle contractions.

  a. Isotonic: _____

  _____

  b. Isometric: _____

  _____

- Define *leverage* and *posture*. _____

  _____

  _____

- Briefly explain how posture and movement are coordinated and regulated. _____

  _____

  _____

  _____

Nervous System

- Briefly describe how movement and posture are regulated by the nervous system. _____

  _____

  _____

  _____

  _____

Pathological Influences on Mobility

- Briefly explain how the following pathological conditions affect mobility.

  a. Postural abnormalities: _____

  _____

  _____

  _____

b. Impaired muscle development: _____

_____

_____

_____

c. Damage to the central nervous system: ___

_____

_____

_____

d. Direct trauma to the musculoskeletal system: _____

_____

_____

_____

Nursing Knowledge Base

Mobility-Immobility
- Define *bed rest.* _____

_____

- *Impaired physical mobility* is defined as: _____

_____

_____

Systemic Effects
- When there is an alteration in mobility, each body system is at risk. Identify at least two hazards of immobility for each area.

  a. Metabolic changes:

  1. _____

  _____

  2. _____

  _____

  b. Respiratory changes:

  1. _____

  _____

  2. _____

  _____

c. Cardiovascular changes:

  1. _____

  _____

  2. _____

  _____

d. Musculoskeletal changes:

  1. _____

  _____

  2. _____

  _____

e. Urinary elimination changes:

  1. _____

  _____

  2. _____

  _____

f. Integumentary changes:

  1. _____

  _____

  2. _____

  _____

Developmental Changes
- Identify the descriptive characteristics of body alignment and mobility related to the following developmental stages:

  a. Infants: _____

  _____

  _____

  _____

  b. Toddlers: _____

  _____

  _____

  _____

  c. Preschool children: _____

  _____

  _____

  _____

d. Adolescents: _____

_____

_____

_____

e. Adults: _____

_____

_____

_____

f. Older adults: _____

_____

_____

_____

Nursing Process for Impaired Body Alignment and Mobility

𝒩𝒫 Assessment

- Briefly describe the four major areas for assessment of client mobility.

  a. Range of motion: _____

  _____

  b. Gait: _____

  _____

  c. Exercise and activity tolerance: _____

  _____

  d. Body alignment: _____

  _____

- Briefly describe the physiological hazards of immobility in relation to the following systems:

  a. Metabolic: _____

  _____

  _____

  b. Respiratory: _____

  _____

  _____

  c. Cardiovascular: _____

  _____

  _____

  d. Musculoskeletal: _____

  _____

  _____

  e. Integumentary: _____

  _____

  _____

  f. Elimination: _____

  _____

  _____

𝒩𝒫 Nursing Diagnosis

- List six actual or potential nursing diagnoses related to an immobilized or partially immobilized client.

  a. _____

  b. _____

  c. _____

  d. _____

  e. _____

  f. _____

𝒩𝒫 Planning

- The nurse plans therapies according to severity of risks to the client, and the plan is individualized according to the client's

  _____, _____,

  and _____.

𝒩𝒫 Implementation

Health Promotion

- List the criteria the nurse needs to assess before lifting a client or object. _____

  _____

  _____

  _____

  _____

  _____

  _____

Chapter 46: Mobility and Immobility   321

Exercise

- Briefly explain the benefits of exercise. _____

_____

_____

_____

_____

_____

Acute Care

- Identify two nursing interventions to meet each of the following goals for the immobilized client.

  a. Maintain optimal nutritional (metabolic) state:

  1. _____

  _____

  2. _____

  _____

  b. Promote expansion of chest and lungs:

  1. _____

  _____

  2. _____

  _____

  c. Prevent stasis of pulmonary secretions:

  1. _____

  _____

  2. _____

  _____

  d. Maintain patent airway:

  1. _____

  _____

  2. _____

  _____

  e. Reduce orthostatic hypotension:

  1. _____

  _____

  2. _____

  _____

  f. Reduce cardiac workload:

  1. _____

  _____

  2. _____

  _____

  g. Prevent thrombus formation:

  1. _____

  _____

  2. _____

  _____

  h. Maintain muscle strength and joint mobility:

  1. _____

  _____

  2. _____

  _____

  i. Prevent pressure ulcers:

  1. _____

  _____

  2. _____

  _____

  j. Maintain normal elimination patterns:

  1. _____

  _____

  2. _____

  _____

  k. Maintain usual psychosocial state:

  1. _____

  _____

  2. _____

  _____

- Identify two nursing interventions for the following immobilized clients.

  a. Young child:

  1. _____

  _____

  2. _____

  _____

b. Older adult:

1. _____

   _____

2. _____

   _____

Positioning Techniques

- Indicate the correct use for each positioning device listed.

Device	Uses
Pillow	
Footboard	
Trochanter roll	
Sandbag	
Hand-wrist splints	
Trapeze bar	
Restraints	
Side rails	
Bed board	

- List four areas the nurse needs to consider in determining if assistance is required when moving a client in bed.

  a. _____

  b. _____

  c. _____

  d. _____

- List some general guidelines to apply in any transfer procedure. _____

  _____

  _____

  _____

Restorative Care

- The goal of restorative care is to: _____

  _____

- Instrumental activities of daily living (IADLs) are: _____

  _____

- List the common trouble areas for the clients in the following positions.

Positions (Give a brief of the Position)	Trouble Areas
Fowler's	a.
	b.
	c.
	d.
	e.
	f.
	g.
Supine	a.
	b.
	c.
	d.
	e.
	f.
	g.
	h.
Prone	a.
	b.
	c.
	d.
Side-lying	a.
	b.
	c.
	d.
	e.
Sims'	a.
	b.
	c.
	d.

Joint Mobility

- Indicate the type of joint and range-of-motion exercises for the body parts listed in the table below:

Body Part	Type of Joint	Type of Movement
Neck		
Shoulder		
Elbow		
Forearm		
Wrist		
Fingers and thumb		
Hip		
Knee		
Ankle and foot		
Toes		

Walking

- Identify the steps the nurse should take to prepare to assist a client to walk. _____

  _____

  _____

  _____

  _____

  _____

- Describe how the nurse would assist clients with the following:

  a. Hemiplegia: _____

  _____

  _____

  _____

  b. Hemiparesis: _____

  _____

  _____

  _____

Evaluation

Client Care

- Client care evaluates the actual care delivered by the health care team based on expected outcomes.

- The optimal outcomes are the client's ability to maintain or improve body alignment and joint mobility.

Client Expectations

- Client expectations evaluate care from the client's perspective.

Review Questions

The student should select the appropriate answer and cite the rationale for choosing that particular answer.

1. The nurse would expect all of the following physiological effects of exercise on the body systems except:
   a. Decreased cardiac output
   b. Increased respiratory rate and depth
   c. Increased muscle tone, size, and strength
   d. Change in metabolic rate

   Answer: _____ Rationale: _____

   _____

   _____

2. Which of the following is a potential hazard that the nurse should assess when the client is in the prone position?
   a. Unprotected pressure points at the sacrum and heels
   b. Internal rotation of the shoulder
   c. Increased cervical flexion
   d. Plantar flexion

   Answer: _____ Rationale: _____

   _____

   _____

3. Which of the following is a physiological effect of prolonged bed rest?
   a. A decrease in urinary excretion of nitrogen
   b. An increase in cardiac output
   c. A decrease in lean body mass
   d. A decrease in lung expansion

   Answer: _____ Rationale: _____

   _____

   _____

4. All of the following measures are used to assess for deep vein thrombosis except:
   a. Measuring the circumference of each leg daily, placing the tape measure at the midpoint of the knee
   b. Observing the dorsal aspect of lower extremities for redness, warmth, and tenderness
   c. Asking the client about the presence of calf pain
   d. Checking for a positive Homans' sign

Answer: _____ Rationale: _____

_____

_____

5. Which of the following is an appropriate intervention to maintain the respiratory system of the immobilized client?
   a. Turn the client every 4 hours
   b. Maintain a maximum fluid intake of 1500 ml per day
   c. Apply an abdominal binder continuously while in bed
   d. Encourage the use of an incentive spirometer

Answer: _____ Rationale: _____

_____

_____

Critical Thinking for Nursing Care Plan for Impaired Mobility

Imagine that you are the student nurse in the Care Plan on page 1446 of your text. Complete the *Evaluation phase* of the critical thinking model by writing your answers in the appropriate boxes of the model shown. Think about the following:

- What knowledge did you apply in evaluating Miss Adams' care?

- In what way might your previous experience influence your evaluation of Miss Adams?

- During evaluation, what intellectual and professional standards were applied to Miss Adams' care?

- In what ways do critical thinking attitudes play a role in how you approach evaluation of Miss Adams' care?

- How might you adjust Miss Adams' care?

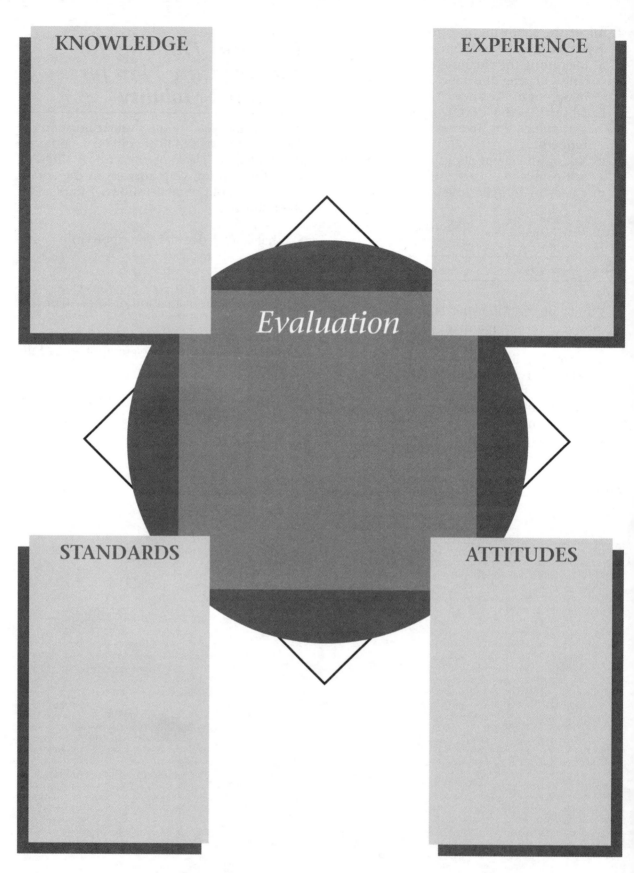

KNOWLEDGE

EXPERIENCE

Evaluation

STANDARDS

ATTITUDES

CHAPTER *46* Critical Thinking Model for Nursing Care Plan for *Impaired Mobility*

See answers on page 549.

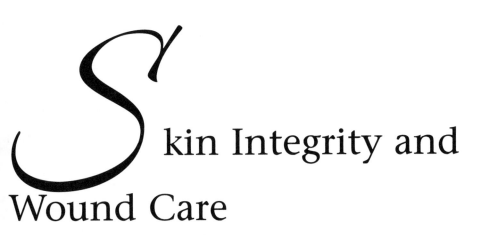

47

Skin Integrity and Wound Care

Preliminary Reading

Chapter 47, pp. 1482-1564

Comprehensive Understanding

Scientific Knowledge Base

Normal Integument
- Describe the function of each of the following.

  a. Epidermis: _____

  b. Dermis: _____

Pressure Ulcers
- Define *pressure ulcer.* _____

- Define the following terms that are related to the pathogenesis of pressure ulcers.

  a. *Tissue ischemia:* _____

  b. *Blanching:* _____

  c. *Capillary closing pressure:* _____

  d. *Normal reactive hyperemia:* _____

  e. *Nonblanching hyperemia:* _____

- Identify the two considerations with regard to the duration of pressure: _____

  _____

  _____

- Briefly explain how the following factors contribute to an increased risk for pressure ulcers.

  a. Impaired sensory perception: _____

  _____

  _____

  b. Impaired mobility: _____

  _____

  _____

  c. Alterations in level of consciousness: _____

  _____

  _____

  _____

  d. Shear: _____

  _____

  _____

  _____

  e. Friction: _____

  _____

  _____

  _____

  f. Moisture: _____

  _____

  _____

  _____

Classification of Pressure Ulcer Staging or Color

- Staging systems for pressure ulcers are based on the depth of tissue destroyed. Briefly describe each stage.

  I: _____

  _____

  II: _____

  _____

  III: _____

  _____

  IV: _____

  _____

- Describe the following wound classifications by color.

  a. Black wounds: _____

  _____

  b. Yellow wounds: _____

  _____

  c. Red wounds: _____

  _____

- Describe the physiological process involved with wound healing.

  a. Primary intention: _____

  _____

  _____

  _____

  b. Secondary intention: _____

  _____

  _____

  _____

- Explain the three components involved in the healing process of a partial-thickness wound:

  a. Inflammatory phase (reaction): _____

  _____

  _____

  _____

  b. Proliferative phase (regeneration): _____

  _____

  _____

  _____

  c. Maturation (remodeling): _____

  _____

  _____

  _____

- Briefly explain the following complications of wound healing.

  a. Hemorrhage: _____

  _____

  _____

  _____

b. Infection: _____
_____
_____

c. Dehiscence: _____
_____
_____

d. Evisceration: _____
_____
_____

e. Fistulas: _____
_____
_____

Nursing Knowledge Base

Prediction and Prevention of Pressure Ulcers
- Explain the following risk assessment scales.

  a. Norton scale: _____
  _____
  _____
  _____

  b. Braden scale: _____
  _____
  _____
  _____

Factors Influencing Pressure Ulcer Formation and Wound Healing
- Describe why each of the following factors increase the client's risk for pressure ulcer development.

  a. Nutrition: _____
  _____
  _____
  _____

b. Tissue perfusion: _____
_____
_____

c. Infection: _____
_____
_____
_____

d. Age: _____
_____
_____
_____

Psychosocial Impact of Wounds
- Identify the factors that may affect the client's perception of the wound.

_____
_____
_____
_____

Critical Thinking Synthesis Nursing Process

Assessment

- Identify the predictive strategies that should be implemented once a client has been identified as at risk:

  a. Mobility: _____
  _____

  b. Nutritional status: _____
  _____
  _____

  c. Body fluids: _____
  _____
  _____

  d. Pain: _____
  _____
  _____

- Briefly explain how the assessment differs under the following conditions.

  a. In the emergency setting: _____

  _____

  _____

  b. In the stable setting: _____

  _____

  _____

- Explain how the nurse assesses the following.

  a. Wound appearance: _____

  _____

  _____

  b. Drainage: _____

  _____

  _____

  c. Drains: _____

  _____

  _____

  d. Wound closures: _____

  _____

  _____

  e. Wound cultures: _____

  _____

  _____

𝒩𝒫 Nursing Diagnosis

- List three nursing diagnoses related to impaired skin integrity.

  a. _____

  b. _____

  c. _____

𝒩𝒫 Planning

- List six possible goals for the client at risk for pressure ulcers.

  a. _____

  b. _____

c. _____

d. _____

e. _____

f. _____

Implementation

𝒩𝒫 Health Promotion

- Briefly explain the following nursing interventions for the prevention of pressure ulcers.

  a. Topical skin care: _____

  _____

  _____

  _____

  b. Positioning: _____

  _____

  _____

  _____

  c. Support surfaces: _____

  _____

  _____

  _____

Acute Care

- Aspects of pressure ulcer treatment include local care of the wound and supportive measures. Briefly explain the principles of wound care in relation to debridement. _____

  _____

  _____

  _____

  _____

- Describe the three methods of debridement.

  a. _____

  _____

  b. _____

  _____

  c. _____

  _____

- Describe two nursing interventions that relate to nutritional status in the treatment of pressure ulcers.

  a. _____

  _____

  b. _____

  _____

- First aid for wounds includes the following. Briefly explain each one.

  a. Hemostasis: _____

  _____

  _____

  _____

  b. Cleansing: _____

  _____

  _____

  _____

  c. Protecting:

  _____

  _____

  _____

- List the purposes for dressings.

  a. _____

  _____

  b. _____

  _____

  c. _____

  _____

  d. _____

  _____

  e. _____

  _____

  f. _____

  _____

  g. _____

  _____

- List the clinical guidelines to use when selecting the appropriate dressing.

  a. _____

  _____

  b. _____

  _____

  c. _____

  _____

  d. _____

  _____

  e. _____

  _____

  f. _____

  _____

  g. _____

  _____

- Briefly describe the following types of dressings and their uses.

  a. Gauze: _____

  _____

  _____

  _____

  b. Wet-to-dry: _____

  _____

  _____

  _____

  c. Film: _____

  _____

  _____

  _____

  d. Hydrocolloid (HCD): _____

  _____

  _____

  _____

  e. Hydrogel: _____

  _____

  _____

  _____

f. Alginate: _____

_____

_____

_____

- To prepare for a dressing change, the nurse must know _____, _____, and _____.

- The physician's order for changing a dressing should indicate the _____, _____, and _____ to the wound.

- In relation to sterile versus clean dressing, the Agency for Healthcare Research and Quality (AHRQ) 1994 clinical practice guidelines recommend that _____ be used on pressure ulcers.

- The first step in packing a wound is to assess the _____, _____, and _____ of the wound.

- Summarize the principles of packing a wound.

_____

_____

_____

_____

_____

- Briefly describe how the wound vacuum-assisted closure device works. _____

_____

_____

_____

_____

- To secure the dressing, the nurse considers the _____, _____, _____, _____, and _____.

- Identify three principles that are important when cleaning an incision.

a. _____

_____

b. _____

_____

c. _____

_____

- Irrigation of a wound requires _____ technique.

- Irrigations are used for: _____

_____

- Summarize the nursing responsibilities for suture care. _____

_____

_____

_____

_____

_____

- The most important principle in suture removal is to: _____

_____

_____

_____

_____

_____

- Explain the purpose for drainage evacuation.

_____

_____

_____

- Explain the benefits of binders and bandages.

a. _____

_____

b. _____

_____

c. _____

_____

d. _____

_____

e. _____

_____

f. _____

_____

- List the nursing responsibilities when applying a bandage or binder.

a. _____

_____

b. _____

_____

c. _____

_____

d. _____

_____

- Describe the abdominal binder: _____

_____

_____

- Sling supports are used for: _____

_____

- Summarize the body's responses to heat and cold. _____

_____

_____

_____

_____

- Describe the physiologic responses to the following.

a. Heat applications: _____

_____

b. Cold applications: _____

_____

- List the factors that influence heat and cold tolerance.

a. _____

_____

b. _____

_____

c. _____

_____

d. _____

_____

e. _____

_____

f. _____

_____

- Prior to applying heat or cold therapies, the nurse assesses for temperature tolerance by:

_____

_____

_____

_____

_____

_____

- Cold therapy is contraindicated for: _____

_____

_____

- Heat and cold applications can be administered in _____ or _____ forms.

- Explain the following types of heat and cold applications, and give the nursing implications for each.

a. Moist or dry: _____

_____

_____

_____

Chapter 47: Skin Integrity and Wound Care   335

b. Warm, moist compresses: _____

_____

_____

_____

c. Warm soaks: _____

_____

_____

_____

d. Sitz baths: _____

_____

_____

_____

e. Aquathermia pads: _____

_____

_____

_____

f. Commercial hot packs: _____

_____

_____

_____

g. Cold, moist, and dry compresses: _____

_____

_____

_____

h. Cold soaks: _____

_____

_____

_____

i. Ice bags or collars: _____

_____

_____

_____

Evaluation

Client Care

- Client care evaluates the actual care delivered by the health care team based on the expected outcomes.

- The optimal outcomes are to _____, _____, and _____.

Client Expectations

- Client expectations evaluate care from the client's perspective.

- Clients with chronic wounds are often cared for in the home and have certain expectations about their level of _____, _____, _____, and _____.

Review Questions

The student should select the appropriate answer and cite the rationale for choosing that particular answer.

1. Ischemia is defined as:
   a. Increased tissue buildup during the healing process
   b. A deficiency of blood supply to a part
   c. Decreased fluid to the tissues
   d. Increased irritability of nerves

Answer: _____ Rationale: _____

_____

_____

2. Mr. Post is in a Fowler's position to improve his oxygenation status. The nurse notes that he frequently slides down in the bed and needs to be repositioned. Mr. Post is at risk for developing a pressure ulcer on his coccyx because of:
   a. Friction
   b. Shearing force
   c. Maceration
   d. Impaired peripheral circulation

Answer: _____   Rationale: _____
_____
_____

3. Which of the following is not a subscale on the Braden scale for predicting pressure ulcer risk?
   a. Age
   b. Sensory perception
   c. Moisture
   d. Activity

Answer: _____   Rationale: _____
_____
_____

4. Which of these clients has a nutritional risk for pressure ulcer development?
   a. Client A has an albumin level of 3.5.
   b. Client B has a hemoglobin level within normal limits.
   c. Client C has a protein intake of 0.5 gm per kilogram per day.
   d. Client D has a body weight that is 5% greater than his ideal weight.

Answer: _____   Rationale: _____
_____
_____

5. Mrs. Greer is an immobilized client. Which of the following will not increase her risk of pressure development?
   a. She has unrelieved pressure to her hip of greater than 32 mm Hg.
   b. She displays reactive hyperemia on her coccyx that lasts for 30 minutes after being turned to her side.

c. She has low-intensity pressure over a long period to her heels as a result of elastic stockings.
d. She is positioned so that she has an unequal distribution of body weight.

Answer: _____   Rationale: _____
_____
_____

6. Mr. Perkins has a stage II ulcer of his right heel. What would be the most appropriate treatment for this ulcer?
   a. Apply a thick layer of enzymatic ointment to the ulcer and the surrounding skin.
   b. Apply a calcium alginate dressing and change when strike-through is noted.
   c. Apply a heat lamp to the area for 20 minutes twice daily.
   d. Apply a hydrocolloid dressing and change it as necessary.

Answer: _____   Rationale: _____
_____
_____

Critical Thinking for Nursing Care Plan for Impaired Skin Integrity

Imagine that you are the student nurse in the Care Plan on page 1512 of your text. Complete the *Assessment phase* of the critical thinking model by writing your answers in the appropriate boxes of the model shown. Think about the following:

- What knowledge base was applied to Mrs. Stein?

- In what way might your previous experience assist you in this case?

- What intellectual or professional standards were applied to Mrs. Stein?

- What critical thinking attitudes did you use in assessing Mrs. Stein?

- As you review your assessment, what key areas did you cover?

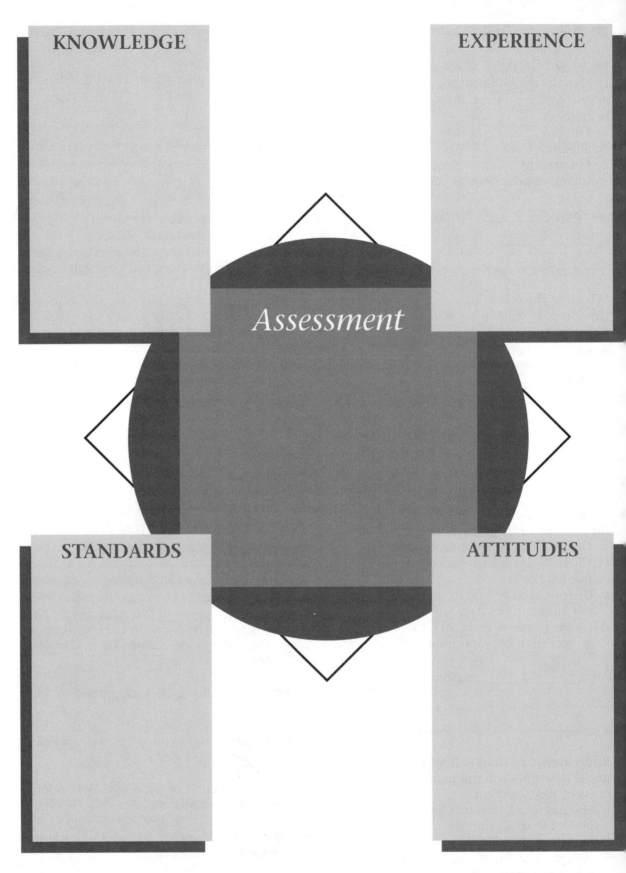

KNOWLEDGE

EXPERIENCE

Assessment

STANDARDS

ATTITUDES

CHAPTER 47   Critical Thinking Model for Nursing Care Plan for *Impaired Skin Integrity*

See answers on page 550.

48

$\mathcal{S}$ensory Alterations Care

$\mathcal{P}$reliminary Reading

Chapter 48, pp. 1565-1592

$\mathcal{C}$omprehensive Understanding

- Define *stereognosis*: _____

Scientific Knowledge Base

Normal Sensation
- List and briefly explain the three functional components necessary for any sensory experience.

  a. _____

  b. _____

  c. _____

Sensory Alterations
- The types of sensory alterations commonly seen by the nurse are _____,

  _____, and _____.

- When a client suffers from more than one sensory alteration, the ability to function and relate effectively within the environment is seriously impaired.

- List eight factors that influence sensory function and give an example of each.

  a. _____

  b. _____

  c. _____

  d. _____

e. _____

f. _____

g. _____

h. _____

- Define *sensory deficit*. _____

_____

- List the three major types of sensory deprivation and give an example of each.

  a. _____

  _____

  b. _____

  _____

  c. _____

  _____

- Define *sensory overload*. _____

_____

- Identify the behavioral changes that are associated with sensory overload. _____

_____

_____

_____

_____

Nursing Knowledge Base

Factors Affecting Sensory Function

- Explain how and why the following factors affect sensory function.

  a. Persons at risk: _____

  _____

  _____

  _____

  b. Meaningful stimuli: _____

  _____

  _____

  _____

c. Amount of stimuli: _____

_____

_____

_____

d. Social interaction: _____

_____

_____

_____

e. Environmental factors: _____

_____

_____

_____

f. Hazards: _____

_____

_____

_____

g. Family factors: _____

_____

_____

_____

h. Cultural factors: _____

_____

_____

_____

Critical Thinking Synthesis Nursing Process

Assessment

- The nurse collects a history that assesses the client's current sensory status and the degree to which a sensory deficit affects the client's

_____ , _____ ,

_____ , _____ ,

and _____ .

- When assessing the client's mental status the nurse needs to evaluate each of the following. Give an example of each.

  a. Physical appearance and behavior: _____

  _____

  _____

  _____

  b. Cognitive ability: _____

  _____

  _____

  _____

  c. Emotional stability: _____

  _____

  _____

  _____

- Complete the grid by describing at least one assessment technique for the identified sensory function and the behaviors for an adult and child that would indicate a sensory deficit.

Sense	Assessment Technique	Child Behavior	Adult Behavior
Vision			
Hearing			
Touch			
Smell			
Taste			
Position sense			

- Give an example of an assessment for the following.

  a. Ability to perform self-care: _____

  _____

  _____

  b. Health promotion habits: _____

  _____

  _____

  c. Hazards: _____

  _____

  _____

- Define the following types of aphasia.

  a. *Expressive:* _____

  _____

  b. *Receptive:* _____

  _____

Chapter 48: Sensory Alterations Care   341

Nursing Diagnosis

- List six actual or potential nursing diagnoses for a client with sensory alterations.

    a. _____

    b. _____

    c. _____

    d. _____

    e. _____

    f. _____

Planning

- List eight goals appropriate for clients with sensory alterations.

    a. _____

    b. _____

    c. _____

    d. _____

    e. _____

    f. _____

    g. _____

    h. _____

Implementation

Health Promotion

- List the three recommended screening interventions.

    a. _____

    b. _____

    c. _____

- The most common visual problem is: _____

    _____

    _____

- Explain how hearing loss occurs from loud noises. _____

    _____

    _____

    _____

    _____

    _____

- Identify the common trauma injuries that result in hearing or vision loss in both adults and children.

    a. Adults: _____

    _____

    _____

    _____

    b. Children: _____

    _____

    _____

    _____

- Explain the measures to take to maintain sensory function at the highest level with the use of assistive devices. _____

    _____

    _____

    _____

    _____

    _____

- Complete the grid by filling in the normal physiological changes that occur and cite how the nurse can minimize the loss.

Senses	Physiological Change	Interventions
Vision		
Hearing		
Taste and smell		
Touch		
Trachea		

- List three methods of establishing a safe environment with regard to the following adaptations:

a. Visual loss:

1. _____

2. _____

3. _____

b. Reduced hearing:

1. _____

2. _____

3. _____

c. Reduced olfaction:

1. _____

2. _____

3. _____

d. Reduced tactile sensation:

1. _____

2. _____

3. _____

- Describe six communication methods that are appropriate for clients with a hearing impairment.

a. _____

b. _____

c. _____

d. _____

e. _____

f. _____

Acute Care

- When clients enter acute care settings for therapeutic management of sensory deficits or as a result of traumatic injury, the following approaches are used to maximize sensory function. Briefly explain each.

  a. Orientation to the environment: _____

  _____

  _____

  _____

  _____

  b. Communication: _____

  _____

  _____

  _____

  _____

  c. Controlling sensory stimuli: _____

  _____

  _____

  _____

  _____

  d. Safety measures: _____

  _____

  _____

  _____

  _____

Restorative and Continuing Care

- After a client experiences a sensory loss, it becomes important to understand the implications of the loss and to make the adjustments needed to continue a normal lifestyle. Briefly explain.

  a. Understanding sensory loss: _____

  _____

  _____

  _____

  _____

  _____

  b. Socialization: _____

  _____

  _____

  _____

  _____

  c. Promoting self-care: _____

  _____

  _____

  _____

  _____

  _____

Evaluation

Client Care

- Client care evaluates the actual care delivered by the health care team based on expected outcomes.

- The client is the only one who will know if his or her sensory abilities are improved and which specific interventions or therapies are most successful in facilitating a change in performance.

Client Expectations

- Client expectations evaluate care from the client's perspective.

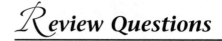

Review Questions

The student should select the appropriate answer and cite the rationale for choosing that particular answer.

1. All of the following are true of age-related factors that influence sensory function except:
   a. Refractive errors are the most common types of visual disorders in children.
   b. Visual changes in adulthood include presbyopia.
   c. Older adults hear high-pitched sounds best.
   d. Neonates are unable to discriminate sensory stimuli.

Answer: _____ Rationale: _____

_____

_____

2. Mr. Green, a 62-year-old farmer, has been hospitalized for 2 weeks for thrombophlebitis. He has no visitors, and the nurse notices that he appears bored, restless, and anxious. The type of alteration occurring because of sensory deprivation is:
   a. Affective
   b. Cognitive
   c. Perceptual
   d. Receptual

Answer: _____ Rationale: _____

_____

_____

3. Which of the following would not provide meaningful stimuli for a client?
   a. A clock or calendar with large numbers
   b. A television that is kept on all day at a low volume
   c. Family pictures and personal possessions
   d. Interesting magazines and books

Answer: _____ Rationale: _____

_____

_____

4. Clients with existing sensory loss must be protected from injury. What determines the safety precautions taken?
   a. The existing dangers in the environment
   b. The financial means to make needed safety changes
   c. The nature of the client's actual or potential sensory loss

d. The availability of a support system to enable the client to exist in his or her present environment

Answer: _____ Rationale: _____

_____

_____

5. A client who is unable to name common objects or express simple ideas in words or writing suffers from:
   a. Expressive aphasia
   b. Receptive aphasia
   c. Global aphasia
   d. Mental retardation

Answer: _____ Rationale: _____

_____

_____

Critical Thinking for Nursing Care Plan for Sensory Perceptual Alterations

Imagine that you are the community health nurse in the Care Plan on page 1579 of your text. Complete the *Planning phase* of the critical thinking model by writing your answers in the appropriate boxes of the model shown. Think about the following:

• In developing Judy's plan of care, what knowledge did you apply?

• In what way might your previous experience assist in developing a plan of care for Judy?

• When developing a plan of care, what intellectual and professional standards were applied?

• What critical thinking attitudes might have been applied in developing Judy's plan?

• How will you accomplish the goals?

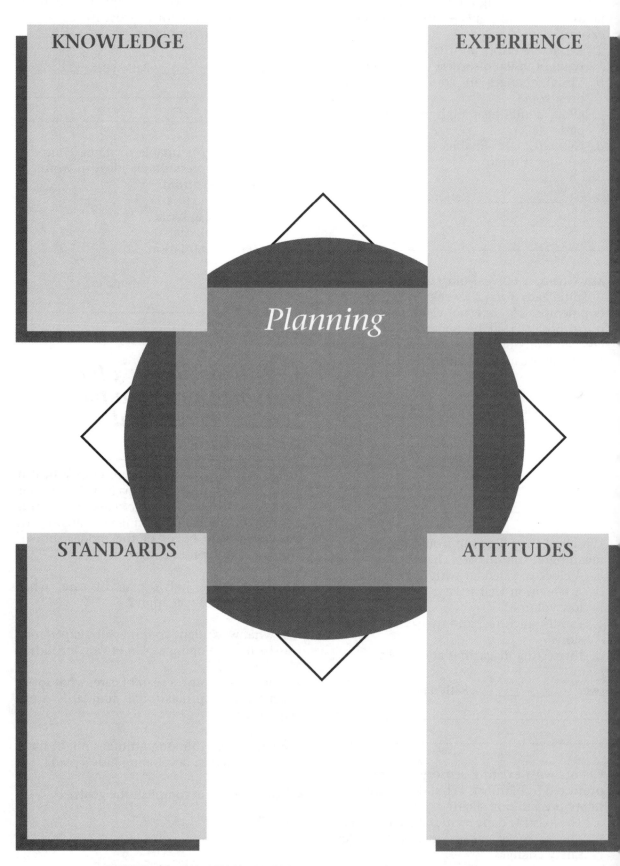

KNOWLEDGE

EXPERIENCE

Planning

STANDARDS

ATTITUDES

CHAPTER *48* Critical Thinking Model for Nursing Care Plan for *Sensory Perceptual Alterations*

See answers on page 551.

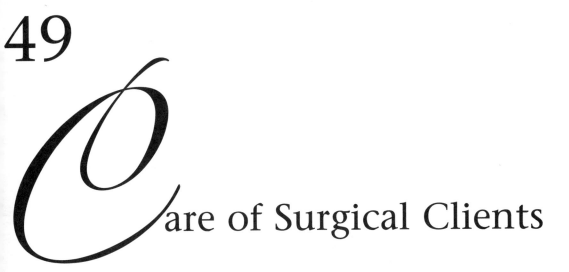

49

*C*are of Surgical Clients

*P*reliminary Reading

Chapter 49, pp. 1593-1641

*C*omprehensive Understanding

History of Surgical Nursing

- Summarize the historical changes that have occurred in surgical nursing. _____
  _____
  _____

Ambulatory Surgery
- List the benefits of ambulatory surgery.

  a._____

  b._____

  c._____

  d._____

Scientific Knowledge Base

Classification of Surgery
- Define the following surgical procedure classifications:

  a. *Palliative:* _____

  b. *Ablative:* _____

  c. *Emergency:* _____

d. *Minor:* _____

_____

e. *Urgent:* _____

_____

f. *Major:* _____

_____

g. *Reconstructive:* _____

_____

h. *Constructive:* _____

_____

i. *Elective:* _____

_____

j. *Transplant:* _____

_____

k. *Diagnostic:* _____

_____

Nursing Knowledge Base

The Nursing Process in the Preoperative Surgical Phase

🖊 Assessment

- Identify the data the nurse would collect from the client's medical history. _____

_____

_____

_____

_____

_____

- Briefly explain the following factors that increase the client's risk in surgery:

a. Age: _____

_____

_____

_____

_____

b. Nutrition: _____

_____

_____

_____

_____

c. Obesity: _____

_____

_____

_____

d. Immunocompetence: _____

_____

_____

_____

_____

_____

e. Fluid and electrolyte balance: _____

_____

_____

_____

_____

_____

f. Pregnancy: _____

_____

_____

_____

_____

g. Medication history: _____

_____

_____

_____

_____

_____

h. Allergies: _____

_____

_____

_____

_____

i. Smoking habits: _____

_____

_____

_____

_____

j. Alcohol ingestion and substance use and abuse: _____

_____

_____

_____

_____

_____

k. Family support: _____

_____

_____

_____

_____

_____

l. Occupation: _____

_____

_____

_____

_____

_____

- Explain the rationale for a preoperative pain assessment: _____

_____

_____

_____

_____

_____

- Briefly explain each of the following factors that need to be assessed in order to understand the impact of surgery on a client's and family's emotional health.

a. Self-concept: _____

_____

_____

_____

b. Body image: _____

_____

_____

_____

c. Coping resources: _____

_____

_____

_____

- Cultural differences influence the surgical experience. Give an example. _____

_____

_____

- Briefly describe the findings on which the nurse would focus related to the physical examination of the following body systems:

a. General survey: _____

_____

_____

_____

_____

b. Head and neck: _____

_____

_____

_____

_____

_____

Chapter 49: Care of Surgical Clients   349

c. Integument: _____

_____

_____

_____

d. Thorax and lungs: _____

_____

_____

_____

e. Heart and vascular system: _____

_____

_____

_____

_____

f. Abdomen: _____

_____

_____

_____

g. Neurological status: _____

_____

_____

_____

- Describe the following routine screening tests for surgical clients.

a. CBC: _____

_____

_____

b. Serum electrolytes: _____

_____

_____

c. Coagulation studies: _____

_____

_____

d. Serum creatinine: _____

_____

_____

e. Urinalysis: _____

_____

_____

_____

Nursing Diagnosis

- List 10 potential or actual nursing diagnoses appropriate for the preoperative client.

a. _____

b. _____

c. _____

d. _____

e. _____

f. _____

g. _____

h. _____

i _____

j. _____

Planning

- List eight goals of care for the perioperative client.

a. _____

b. _____

c. _____

d. _____

e. _____

f. _____

g. _____

h. _____

⚕ Implementation

- Surgery cannot be performed until a client understands the _____, _____, _____, and _____.

- Describe five ways in which structured preoperative teaching may influence a client's postoperative recovery.

  a. _____
     _____

  b. _____
     _____

  c. _____
     _____

  d. _____
     _____

  e. _____
     _____

- Describe the criteria developed by the Association of Operating Room Nurses (AORN) that may be used in determining the client's understanding of the surgical procedure.

  a. _____
     _____

  b. _____
     _____

  c. _____
     _____

  d. _____
     _____

e. _____
   _____

f. _____
   _____

g. _____
   _____

h. _____
   _____

Acute Care

- Briefly describe the following preoperative preparation.

  a. Maintenance of normal fluid and electrolyte balance: _____
     _____
     _____
     _____

  b. Reduction of risk of surgical wound infection: _____
     _____
     _____
     _____

  c. Prevention of bowel and bladder incontinence: _____
     _____
     _____
     _____

  d. Promotion of rest and comfort: _____
     _____
     _____
     _____

Day of Surgery

- List the nine responsibilities of a nurse caring for a client the morning of surgery.

  a. _____

  _____

  b. _____

  _____

  c. _____

  _____

  d. _____

  _____

  e. _____

  _____

  f. _____

  _____

  g. _____

  _____

  h. _____

  _____

  i. _____

  _____

- The signs and symptoms of a latex reaction are:

  _____

  _____

  _____

Np Evaluation

Client Care

- The admitting nurse and the nurse in the preoperative area are the sources to evaluate client outcomes.

- List three expected outcomes for a preoperative client.

  a. _____

  _____

  b. _____

  _____

c. _____

_____

Client Expectations

- Explain the difficulty in determining a client's expectations regarding preoperative teaching.

  _____

  _____

  _____

  _____

  _____

Transport to the Operating Room

- List 10 pieces of equipment that should be present in the postoperative bedside unit.

  a. _____

  b. _____

  c. _____

  d. _____

  e. _____

  f. _____

  g. _____

  h. _____

  i _____

  j. _____

Intraoperative Surgical Phase

Preoperative (Holding) Area

- In the holding areas, the nursing responsibilities include: _____

  _____

  _____

  _____

  _____

Admission to the Operating Room
- Describe the responsibilities of the nurse in the operating room. _____
_____
_____
_____
_____
_____

Introduction of Anesthesia
- Identify the risks of general anesthesia. _____
_____
_____
_____
_____
_____

- Regional anesthesia is: _____
_____

- Local anesthesia involves: _____
_____

- Define *conscious sedation* and identify its advantages. _____
_____
_____
_____
_____
_____

Positioning the Client for Surgery
- Explain the principles of positioning the client for surgery. _____
_____
_____
_____
_____
_____

- During the intraoperative phase, the nursing staff continues the preoperative plan. Documentation of intraoperative care provides useful data for the nurse who cares for the client postoperatively.

Postoperative Surgical Phase
- Identify the two phases of the postoperative period and describe the usual time frame for ambulatory and hospitalized clients.

  a. _____
  _____
  _____
  _____
  _____
  _____

  b. _____
  _____
  _____
  _____
  _____
  _____

Immediate Postoperative Recovery
- Describe the responsibilities of the nurse in the PACU. _____
_____
_____
_____
_____

Discharge from the PACU
- Identify the criteria for discharge from the PACU. _____
_____
_____
_____
_____
_____

Chapter 49: Care of Surgical Clients   353

Recovery in Ambulatory Surgery

- Describe the usual time spent by the client in the following phases of recovery and the reasons for it.

    a. Phase I: _____

    _____

    b. Phase II: _____

    _____

Postoperative Convalescence

- Identify the criteria for discharging ambulatory surgical clients. _____

    _____

    _____

    _____

    _____

The Nursing Process in Postoperative Care

NP Assessment

- Explain the frequency of assessments needed during the postoperative period. _____

    _____

    _____

    _____

    _____

    _____

- List three major causes of airway obstruction in the postoperative client.

    a. _____

    b. _____

    c. _____

- List four measures that will maintain airway patency.

    a. _____

    _____

    b. _____

    _____

c. _____

_____

d. _____

_____

- List four areas to assess in order to determine a postoperative client's circulatory status.

    a. _____

    _____

    b. _____

    _____

    c. _____

    _____

    d. _____

    _____

- Describe the characteristic findings associated with postoperative hemorrhage. _____

    _____

    _____

    _____

    _____

    _____

- Define the following terms related to temperature.

    a. Shivering: _____

    _____

    b. Malignant hyperthermia: _____

    _____

- List three areas the nurse assesses to determine fluid and electrolyte alterations.

    a. _____

    b. _____

    c. _____

- List the areas of assessment that help to determine a postoperative client's neurological status.

  a. _____

  b. _____

  c. _____

  d. _____

- The nurse assesses the condition of the skin for

  _____, _____,

  _____, and _____.

- Describe how the nurse would assess the amount of drainage from a wound. _____

  _____

  _____

  _____

  _____

  _____

- The client may regain voluntary control over urinary function in _____ hours after anesthesia.

- Normally during the immediate recovery phase, bowel sounds are auscultated in all four quadrants.

- Distention may occur in the client who develops a _____.

- List three nursing measures used to minimize nausea in the immediate postoperative period.

  a. _____

  _____

  b. _____

  _____

  c. _____

  _____

- Postoperative pain can be perceived when

  _____ is regained.

- Assessment of the client's discomfort and evaluation of pain relief therapies are essential nursing functions.

- Acute incisional pain causes clients to become

  _____ and _____.

Nursing Diagnosis

- Identify two actual or potential nursing diagnoses that are appropriate for a postoperative client.

  a. _____

  b. _____

Planning

- List the typical postoperative orders prescribed by surgeons.

  a. _____

  b. _____

  c. _____

  d. _____

  e. _____

  f. _____

  g. _____

  h. _____

  i _____

- Identify the goals of care for the postoperative client.

  a. _____

  b. _____

  c. _____

  d. _____

Implementation

- Complete the grid on the next page. Identify three nursing interventions for each area of need in the postoperative client.

Area of Need	Nursing Intervention
Maintaining respiratory function	
Preventing circulatory status	
Promoting normal bowel elimination	
Promoting adequate nutrition	
Promoting urinary elimination	
Promoting wound healing	
Promoting rest and comfort	
Maintaining self-concept	

Evaluation

Client Care

- The nurse evaluates the effectiveness of care provided to the surgical client on the basis of expected outcomes following nursing interventions.

- Describe how the nurse would evaluate the ambulatory surgical client. _____

_____

_____

_____

_____

_____

_____

Client Expectations

- With short hospital stays and ambulatory surgery, it is important to evaluate the client's expectations early in the postoperative process.

*R*eview Questions

The student should select the appropriate answer and cite the rationale for choosing that particular answer.

1. Mrs. Young, a 45-year-old diabetic client, is having a hysterectomy in the morning. Because of her history, the nurse would expect:
   a. An increased risk of hemorrhaging
   b. Fluid and electrolyte imbalances
   c. Altered elimination of anesthetic agents
   d. Impaired wound healing

   Answer: _____ Rationale: _____

   _____

   _____

2. The purposes of the nursing history for the client who is to have surgery include all of the following except:
   a. Identifying the client's perception and expectations about surgery
   b. Obtaining information about the client's past experience with surgery
   c. Deciding whether surgery is indicated
   d. Understanding the impact surgery has on the client's and family's emotional health

   Answer: _____ Rationale: _____

   _____

   _____

3. All of the following clients are at risk for developing serious fluid and electrolyte imbalances during and after surgery except:
   a. Client E, who is 81 years old and having emergency surgery for a bowel obstruction following 4 days of vomiting and diarrhea
   b. Client F, who is 1 year old and having a cleft palate repair
   c. Client G, who is 55 years old and has a history of chronic respiratory disease
   d. Client H, who is 79 years old and has a history of congestive heart failure

   Answer: _____ Rationale: _____

   _____

   _____

4. The purpose of postoperative leg exercises is to:
   a. Promote venous return
   b. Maintain muscle tone
   c. Assess range of motion
   d. Exercise fatigued muscles

   Answer: _____ Rationale: _____

   _____

   _____

5. The PACU nurse notices that the client is shivering. This is most commonly caused by:
   a. The use of a reflective blanket on the operating room table
   b. Side effects of certain anesthetic agents
   c. Cold irrigations used during surgery
   d. Malignant hyperthermia, a serious condition

   Answer: _____ Rationale: _____

   _____

   _____

Critical Thinking for Nursing Care Plan for Knowledge Deficit Related to Preoperative and Postoperative Care

Imagine that you are Joe, the nurse in the Care Plan on page 1609 of your text. Complete the *Evaluation phase* of the critical thinking model by writing your answers in the appropriate boxes of the model shown. Think about the following:

- What knowledge did Joe apply in evaluating Mrs. Campana's care?

- In what way might Joe's previous experience influence his evaluation of Mrs. Campana's care?

- During evaluation, what intellectual and professional standards were applied to Mrs. Campana's care?

- In what way do critical thinking attitudes play a role in how you approach evaluation of Mrs. Campana's care?

- How might Joe adjust Mrs. Campana's care?

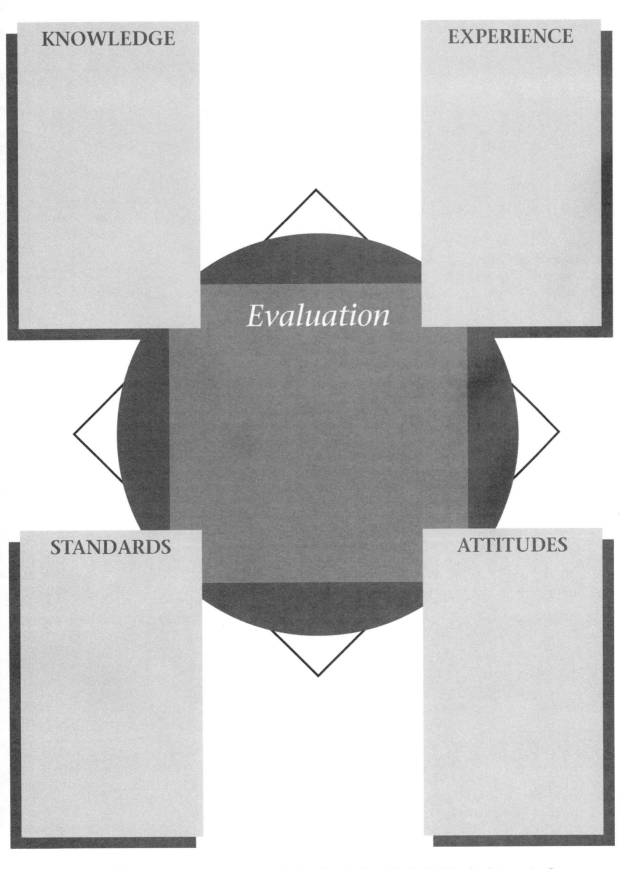

KNOWLEDGE

EXPERIENCE

Evaluation

STANDARDS

ATTITUDES

CHAPTER *49* Critical Thinking Model for Nursing Care Plan for *Knowledge Deficit Related to Perioperative Care*

See answers on page 552.

PROCEDURE PERFORMANCE CHECKLIST
Skill 31-1 Measuring Body Temperature

	S	U	NP	Comments
1. Assess for temperature alterations and factors that influence body temperature.	____	____	____	_____
2. Determine any activity that may interfere with accuracy of temperature measurement.	____	____	____	_____
3. Determine appropriate site and measurement device to be used.	____	____	____	_____
4. Explain to client how temperature will be taken and importance of maintaining proper position.	____	____	____	_____
5. Perform hand hygiene.	____	____	____	_____
6. Obtain temperature reading:				
A. Oral temperature measurement with electronic thermometer:				
(1) Apply disposable gloves (optional).	____	____	____	_____
(2) Remove thermometer pack from charging unit. Attach oral probe (blue tip) to thermometer unit. Grasp top of probe stem, being careful not to apply pressure on the ejection button.	____	____	____	_____
(3) Slide disposable plastic probe cover over thermometer probe until it locks in place.	____	____	____	_____
(4) Have client sit or lie in bed. Ask client to open mouth, then place thermometer probe under tongue in posterior sublingual pocket lateral to center of jaw.	____	____	____	_____
(5) Ask client to hold thermometer probe with lips closed.	____	____	____	_____
(6) Leave thermometer probe in place until audible signal occurs and temperature appears on digital display. Remove thermometer probe from client's mouth.	____	____	____	_____
(7) Push ejection button on thermometer stem to discard plastic probe cover into appropriate receptacle.	____	____	____	_____
(8) Return thermometer stem to storage well of recording unit.	____	____	____	_____
(9) If gloves were worn, remove and dispose of them in appropriate receptacle.	____	____	____	_____
(10) Return thermometer to charger.	____	____	____	_____

Continued

	S	U	NP	Comments

B. Rectal temperature measurement with electronic thermometer:

(1) Provide privacy and assist client to Sims' position. ___ ___ ___ _____

(2) Apply disposable gloves. ___ ___ ___ _____

(3) Remove thermometer pack from charging unit. Attach rectal probe (red tip) to thermometer unit. Grasp top of probe stem. ___ ___ ___ _____

(4) Slide disposable plastic probe cover over thermometer probe until it locks in place. ___ ___ ___ _____

(5) Lubricate 2.5 to 3.5 cm (1 – 1 1/2 in) of probe for an adult. ___ ___ ___ _____

(6) With nondominant hand, separate buttocks to expose anus. Ask client to breathe slowly and relax. ___ ___ ___ _____

(7) Gently insert thermometer 3.5 cm (1 1/2 in) for adult. ___ ___ ___ _____

(8) If resistance is felt, withdraw thermometer immediately. Never force thermometer. ___ ___ ___ _____

(9) Leave thermometer probe in place until audible signal occurs and temperature appears on digital display. Remove thermometer probe from client's anus. ___ ___ ___ _____

(10) Push ejection button on thermometer stem to discard plastic probe cover. ___ ___ ___ _____

(11) Return thermometer stem to storage well of recording unit. ___ ___ ___ _____

(12) Wipe client's anal area with soft tissue and discard tissue. Assist client to a comfortable position. ___ ___ ___ _____

(13) Remove and dispose of gloves. Perform hand hygiene. ___ ___ ___ _____

(14) Return thermometer to charger. ___ ___ ___ _____

C. Axillary temperature measurement with electronic thermometer:

(1) Provide privacy. ___ ___ ___ _____

(2) Assist client to supine or sitting position. ___ ___ ___ _____

(3) Move client's clothing or gown away from his or her shoulder and arm. ___ ___ ___ _____

(4) Remove thermometer pack from charging unit. Be sure oral probe (blue tip) is attached to thermometer unit. Grasp top of probe stem. ___ ___ ___ _____

Continued

	S	U	NP	Comments
(5) Slide disposable plastic probe cover over thermometer probe until it locks in place.	___	___	___	_____
(6) Raise client's arm away from torso and inspect for skin lesions and excessive perspiration. Insert probe into center of client's axilla, lower arm over probe, and place arm across chest.	___	___	___	_____
(7) Hold probe in place until audible signal occurs and temperature appears on digital display.	___	___	___	_____
(8) Remove probe from axilla.	___	___	___	_____
(9) Push ejection button on probe to discard plastic probe cover.	___	___	___	_____
(10) Return probe to storage well of recording unit.	___	___	___	_____
(11) Assist client to a comfortable position.	___	___	___	_____
(12) Perform hand hygiene.	___	___	___	_____
(13) Return thermometer to charger.	___	___	___	_____

D. Tympanic membrane temperature with electronic thermometer:

	S	U	NP	Comments
(1) Assist client to a comfortable position with head turned toward the side, away from nurse.	___	___	___	_____
(2) Note if there is obvious cerumen in the ear canal.	___	___	___	_____
(3) Remove handheld thermometer unit from charging base, being careful to not apply pressure on the ejection button.	___	___	___	_____
(4) Slide disposable speculum cover over tip until it locks into place.	___	___	___	_____
(5) Insert speculum into ear canal following manufacturer's instructions for tympanic probe positioning:				
(a) Pull ear pinna upward and back for adult.	___	___	___	_____
(b) Move thermometer in a figure-eight pattern.	___	___	___	_____
(c) Fit probe gently in ear canal and do not move it.	___	___	___	_____
(d) Point probe toward client's nose.	___	___	___	_____
(6) Depress scan button on handheld unit. Leave thermometer probe in place until audible signal occurs and client's temperature appears on digital display.	___	___	___	_____
(7) Carefully remove speculum from client's auditory canal.	___	___	___	_____

Continued

	S	U	NP	Comments
(8) Push ejection button on handheld unit to discard plastic probe cover.	____	____	____	_____
(9) If second reading is required, replace probe cover and wait 2 to 3 minutes.	____	____	____	_____
(10) Return handheld unit to charging base.	____	____	____	_____
7. Assist client to a comfortable position.	____	____	____	_____
8. Perform hand hygiene.	____	____	____	_____
9. Discuss findings with client as needed.	____	____	____	_____
10. If temperature is being assessed for the first time, establish temperature as baseline if within normal range.	____	____	____	_____
11. Compare temperature reading with previous baseline and normal temperature range for client's age group.	____	____	____	_____
12. Record temperature and report abnormal findings.	____	____	____	_____

PROCEDURE PERFORMANCE CHECKLIST
Skill 31-2 Assessing the Radial and Apical Pulses

	S	U	NP	Comments
1. Determine need to assess radial or apical pulse.	____	____	____	_____
2. Assess for factors that influence pulse rate.	____	____	____	_____
3. Determine previous baseline apical rate (if available) from client's record.	____	____	____	_____
4. Explain that pulse or heart rate is to be assessed. Encourage client to relax and not speak.	____	____	____	_____
5. Perform hand hygiene.	____	____	____	_____
6. Provide privacy.	____	____	____	_____
7. Obtain pulse measurement:				
A. Radial pulse:				
(1) Assist client to supine or sitting position.	____	____	____	_____
(2) If client is supine, place client's forearm straight alongside the body or across lower chest or upper abdomen with wrist extended straight. If client is sitting, bend client's elbow 90 degrees and support his or her lower arm on a chair or on your arm. Slightly flex client's wrist, with palm down.	____	____	____	_____
(3) Place tips of first two fingers of hand over groove along radial or thumb side of client's inner wrist.	____	____	____	_____
(4) Lightly compress against client's radius, obliterate pulse initially, then relax pressure.	____	____	____	_____
(5) Determine strength of pulse.	____	____	____	_____
(6) After pulse can be felt regularly, look at watch's second hand and begin to count rate.	____	____	____	_____
(7) If pulse is regular, count rate for 30 seconds and multiply total by 2.	____	____	____	_____
(8) If pulse is irregular, count rate for 60 seconds. Assess frequency and pattern of irregularity.	____	____	____	_____
B. Apical pulse:				
(1) Assist client to supine or sitting position. Expose client's sternum and left side of chest.	____	____	____	_____
(2) Locate anatomical landmarks to identify the point of maximal impulse.	____	____	____	_____

Continued

	S	U	NP	Comments

(3) Place diaphragm of stethoscope in palm of your hand for 5 to 10 seconds.

(4) Place diaphragm of stethoscope over point of maximal impulse at the fifth intercostal space at the left midclavicular line and auscultate for normal S_1 and S_2 heart sounds.

(5) When S_1 and S_2 are heard with regularity, look at watch's second hand and begin to count rate.

(6) If apical rate is regular, count for 30 seconds and multiply by 2.

(7) If rate is irregular or client is receiving cardiovascular medication, count for 60 seconds.

(8) Note regularity of any dysrhythmia.

(9) Replace client's gown and bed linen.

(10) Assist client in returning to a comfortable position.

(11) Clean earpieces and diaphragm of stethoscope with alcohol swab as needed.

8. Perform hand hygiene.

9. Discuss findings with client as needed.

10. Compare readings with client's previous baseline and/or acceptable range of heart rate for client's age group.

11. Compare peripheral pulse rate with apical rate and note discrepancy.

12. Compare radial pulse equality and note discrepancy.

13. Correlate pulse rate with data obtained from blood pressure and related signs and symptoms.

14. Record pulse rate with assessment site and report abnormal findings.

STUDENT: _____ DATE: _____

INSTRUCTOR: _____ DATE: _____

	S	U	NP	Comments
1. Determine need to assess client's respirations.	____	____	____	_____
2. Assess pertinent laboratory values.	____	____	____	_____
3. Determine previous baseline respiratory rate (if available) from client's record.	____	____	____	_____
4. Perform hand hygiene. Provide privacy.	____	____	____	_____
5. Assist client to a comfortable position, preferably sitting or lying with the head of the bed elevated 45 to 60 degrees. Be sure client's chest is visible. If necessary, move client's bed linen or gown.	____	____	____	_____
6. Place client's arm in relaxed position across the abdomen or lower chest, or place nurse's hand directly over client's upper abdomen.	____	____	____	_____
7. Observe complete respiratory cycle (one inspiration and one expiration).	____	____	____	_____
8. After cycle is observed, look at watch's second hand and begin to count rate.	____	____	____	_____
9. If rhythm is regular, count number of respirations in 30 seconds and multiply by 2. If rhythm is irregular, less than 2, or greater than 20, count respirations for 60 seconds.	____	____	____	_____
10. Note depth of respirations.	____	____	____	_____
11. Note rhythm of ventilatory cycle.	____	____	____	_____
12. Replace client's bed linen and gown.	____	____	____	_____
13. Perform hand hygiene.	____	____	____	_____
14. Discuss findings with client as needed.	____	____	____	_____
15. If respirations are being assessed for the first time, establish rate, rhythm, and depth as baseline if within normal range.	____	____	____	_____
16. Compare respirations with client's previous baseline and normal rate, rhythm, and depth.	____	____	____	_____
17. Record respiratory rate and character and any use of oxygen, and report abnormal findings.	____	____	____	_____

STUDENT: _____ DATE: _____

INSTRUCTOR: _____ DATE: _____

PROCEDURE PERFORMANCE CHECKLIST

Skill 31-4 Measuring Oxygen Saturation (Pulse Oximetry)

	S	U	NP	Comments
1. Determine need to measure client's oxygen saturation.	____	____	____	_____
2. Assess for factors that influence measurement of SpO_2.	____	____	____	_____
3. Review client's record for prescriber's order.	____	____	____	_____
4. Determine previous baseline SpO_2 (if available) from client's record.	____	____	____	_____
5. Explain purpose of procedure to client.	____	____	____	_____
6. Perform hand hygiene.	____	____	____	_____
7. Assess site for sensor probe placement.	____	____	____	_____
8. Assist client to a comfortable position. If client's finger is chosen as monitoring site, support client's lower arm.	____	____	____	_____
9. Instruct client to breathe normally.	____	____	____	_____
10. Use acetone to remove any fingernail polish from digit to be assessed.	____	____	____	_____
11. Attach sensor probe to monitoring site. Tell client that clip-on probe will feel like a clothespin on the finger and will not hurt.	____	____	____	_____
12. Turn on oximeter by activating power. Observe pulse waveform/intensity display and audible beep. Correlate oximeter pulse rate with client's radial pulse.	____	____	____	_____
13. Leave probe in place until oximeter readout reaches constant value and pulse display reaches full strength during each cardiac cycle. Read SpO_2 on digital display.	____	____	____	_____
14. Inform client that oximeter alarm will sound if probe falls off or is moved. Verify SpO_2 alarm limits and alarm volume for continuous monitoring. Verify that alarms are on. Assess skin integrity under sensor probe and relocate sensor probe at least every 4 hours.	____	____	____	_____
15. Assist client in returning to a comfortable position.	____	____	____	_____
16. Perform hand hygiene.	____	____	____	_____
17. Discuss findings with client as needed.	____	____	____	_____
18. Remove probe and turn oximeter power off after intermittent measurements. Store probe in appropriate location.	____	____	____	_____

Continued

	S	U	NP	Comments
19. Compare SpO$_2$ reading with client baseline and acceptable values.	____	____	____	_____
20. Correlate SpO$_2$ reading with SaO$_2$ reading obtained from arterial blood gas measurements, if available.	____	____	____	_____
21. Correlate SpO$_2$ reading with data obtained from respiratory assessment.	____	____	____	_____
22. Report and record SpO$_2$ readings, respiratory status, oxygen therapy, and client's responses.	____	____	____	_____

PROCEDURE PERFORMANCE CHECKLIST
Skill 31-5 Measuring Blood Pressure

	S	U	NP	Comments
1. Determine need to assess client's BP.	___	___	___	_____
2. Determine best site for BP assessment.	___	___	___	_____
3. Select appropriate cuff size.	___	___	___	_____
4. Determine previous baseline BP (if available) from client's record.	___	___	___	_____
5. Encourage client to avoid exercise and smoking for 30 minutes before assessment of BP.	___	___	___	_____
6. Perform hand hygiene. Assist client to sitting or lying position. Make sure room is warm, quiet, and relaxing.	___	___	___	_____
7. Explain to client that BP is to be assessed and have client rest at least 5 minutes before measurement is taken. Ask client not to speak while BP is being measured.	___	___	___	_____
8. With client sitting or lying, position client's forearm or thigh and provide support if needed.	___	___	___	_____
9. Expose extremity by removing constricting clothing.	___	___	___	_____
10. Palpate brachial artery or popliteal artery. Position cuff 2.5 cm above site of pulsation. Center bladder of cuff above artery. With cuff fully deflated, wrap cuff evenly and snugly around upper arm.	___	___	___	_____
11. Position manometer vertically at eye level, no more than 1 m away from client.	___	___	___	_____
12. To determine baseline BP (two-step method), palpate artery distal to cuff with fingertips of one hand while inflating cuff rapidly to pressure 30 mm Hg above point at which pulse disappears. Slowly deflate cuff and note point when pulse reappears. Deflate cuff fully and wait 30 seconds.	___	___	___	_____
13. Place stethoscope earpieces in ears.	___	___	___	_____
14. Relocate brachial or popliteal artery and place bell or diaphragm chestpiece of stethoscope over it.	___	___	___	_____
15. Close valve of pressure bulb clockwise until tight. Inflate cuff to 30 mm Hg above palpated systolic pressure.	___	___	___	_____
16. Slowly release valve and allow mercury to fall at rate of 2 to 3 mm Hg/sec.	___	___	___	_____
17. Note point on manometer when first clear sound is heard.	___	___	___	_____

Continued

	S	U	NP	Comments

18. Continue to deflate cuff, noting point at which muffled or dampened sound appears. ____ ____ ____ _____

19. Continue to deflate cuff gradually, noting point at which sound disappears. Note pressure to nearest 2 mm Hg. Listen to 10 to 20 mm Hg after the last sound, then allow remaining air to escape quickly. ____ ____ ____ _____

20. Deflate cuff rapidly and completely. Remove cuff from client's arm unless measurement must be repeated. If this is the first assessment of the client, repeat procedure on other arm. ____ ____ ____ _____

21. Assist client in returning to a comfortable position and cover upper arm if previously clothed. ____ ____ ____ _____

22. Perform hand hygiene. ____ ____ ____ _____

23. Discuss findings with client as needed. ____ ____ ____ _____

24. Compare reading with previous baseline and/or acceptable BP for client's age group. ____ ____ ____ _____

25. Compare BP in both of client's arms or legs. ____ ____ ____ _____

26. Correlate BP with data obtained from pulse assessment and related cardiovascular signs and symptoms. ____ ____ ____ _____

27. Inform client of value of and need for periodic reassessment of BP. ____ ____ ____ _____

28. Record BP and report abnormal findings. ____ ____ ____ _____

Note: One-step method begins with Step 13.

PROCEDURE PERFORMANCE CHECKLIST
Skill 33-1 Hand Hygiene

	S	U	NP	Comments
1. Inspect surfaces of hands for breaks or cuts in skin or cuticles. Report and cover lesions before providing client care.	____	____	____	_____
2. Inspect hands for heavy soiling.	____	____	____	_____
3. Inspect nails for length.	____	____	____	_____
4. Assess client's risk for or extent of infection.	____	____	____	_____
5. Push wristwatch and long uniform sleeves above wrists. Remove rings during washing.	____	____	____	_____
6. If hands are visibly dirty or contaminated with protein-containing material, use plain or antimicrobial soap and water:	____	____	____	_____
A. Stand in front of sink, keeping hands and uniform away from sink surface.	____	____	____	_____
B. Turn on water. Turn faucet on or push knee pedals laterally or press foot pedals to regulate water flow and temperature.	____	____	____	_____
C. Avoid splashing water onto uniform.	____	____	____	_____
D. Regulate flow of water so that temperature is warm.	____	____	____	_____
E. Wet hands and wrists thoroughly under running water. Keep hands and forearms lower than elbows during washing.	____	____	____	_____
F. Apply a small amount of soap, lathering thoroughly.	____	____	____	_____
G. Wash hands using plenty of lather and friction for at least 10 to 15 seconds. Interlace fingers and rub palms and back of hands with circular motion at least 5 times each. Keep fingertips down.	____	____	____	_____
H. Clean fingernails of both hands with additional soap or clean orangewood stick.	____	____	____	_____
I. Rinse hands and wrists thoroughly, keeping hands down and elbows up.	____	____	____	_____
J. Optional: Repeat steps 5 through 13 and extend period of washing if hands are heavily soiled.	____	____	____	_____
K. Dry hands thoroughly from fingers to wrists and forearms with paper towel, single-use cloth, or warm air dryer.	____	____	____	_____
L. Discard paper towel, if used, in proper receptacle.	____	____	____	_____

Continued

	S	U	NP	Comments

M. Turn off water with foot or knee pedals. To turn off hand faucet, use clean, dry paper towel. Avoid touching handles with hands.

N. If hands are dry or chapped, a small amount of lotion or barrier cream can be applied.

O. Inspect surfaces of hands for obvious signs of soil or other contaminants.

P. Inspect hands for dermatitis or cracked skin.

7. If hands are not visibly soiled, use an alcohol-based waterless antiseptic for routine decontamination:

A. Apply an ample amount of product to the palm of one hand.

B. Rub hands together, covering all surfaces.

C. Rub hands together until alcohol is dry. Allow hands to dry before applying gloves.

D. If hands are dry or chapped, a small amount of lotion or barrier cream can be applied.

STUDENT: _____ DATE: _____

INSTRUCTOR: _____ DATE: _____

PROCEDURE PERFORMANCE CHECKLIST
Skill 33-2 Preparation of a Sterile Field

	S	U	NP	Comments
1. Prepare sterile field just before planned procedure.	____	____	____	_____
2. Select clean work surface above waist level.	____	____	____	_____
3. Assemble equipment.	____	____	____	_____
4. Check dates on supplies.	____	____	____	_____
5. Perform hand hygiene.				
6. Place pack with sterile drape on work surface and open pack.	____	____	____	_____
7. Pick up folded top of drape with one hand; let it unfold. Discard outer cover of pack.	____	____	____	_____
8. Hold drape up and away from the body with both hands.	____	____	____	_____
9. Position bottom half of drape over work surface.	____	____	____	_____
10. Allow top half of drape to be placed over work surface last, positioning as needed.	____	____	____	_____
11. Add sterile items:				
A. Open sterile item.	____	____	____	_____
B. Peel wrapper; do not allow it to touch sterile field.	____	____	____	_____
C. Place item onto field at an angle. Do not hold arm over field.	____	____	____	_____
D. Dispose of wrapper.	____	____	____	_____
12. Perform procedure using sterile technique.	____	____	____	_____

STUDENT: _____ DATE: _____

INSTRUCTOR: _____ DATE: _____

Skill 33-3 Surgical Hand Washing: Preparing for Gowning

	S	U	NP	Comments
1. Consult institutional policy for length of time for hand washing.	____	____	____	_____
2. Keep fingernails short, clean, and healthy. Remove artificial nails.	____	____	____	_____
3. Inspect hands for presence of abrasions, cuts, or open lesions.	____	____	____	_____
4. Apply surgical shoe covers, cap or hood, face mask, and protective eyewear.	____	____	____	_____
5. Surgical hand washing:				
A. Turn on water using knee or foot controls, and adjust water to comfortable temperature.	____	____	____	_____
B. Wet hands and arms under running lukewarm water and lather with detergent to 5 cm above elbows. Keep hands above elbows.	____	____	____	_____
C. Rinse hands and arms thoroughly under running water.	____	____	____	_____
D. Under running water, clean under nails of both hands with nail pick. Discard nail pick after use.	____	____	____	_____
E. Wet clean brush and apply antimicrobial detergent. Scrub the nails of one hand with 15 strokes. Holding brush perpendicular, scrub the palm, each side of the thumb and all fingers, and the posterior side of the hand with 10 strokes each. Scrub each section of the arm 10 times. Continue to scrub for at least 5 to 10 minutes.	____	____	____	_____
F. Discard brush and rinse hands and arms thoroughly. Turn off water with foot or knee controls and back into room entrance with hands elevated in front of and away from the body.	____	____	____	_____
G. Bend slightly forward at the waist, and use a sterile towel to dry one hand thoroughly, moving from fingers to elbow. Dry in a rotating motion.	____	____	____	_____
H. Repeat drying method for other hand, using a different area of the towel or a new sterile towel.	____	____	____	_____
I. Discard towel.	____	____	____	_____

Continued

	S	U	NP	Comments

6. Alternate method of surgical hand hygiene using alcohol-based antiseptic:

A. Wash hands with soap and water for 10 to 15 seconds.

B. Clean nails of both hands under running water with nail pick. Discard nail pick after use and dry hands with a paper towel.

C. Apply enough alcohol-based waterless antiseptic to one palm to cover both hands thoroughly. Spread antiseptic over all hand surfaces. Allow to air dry.

D. Repeat the process and allow hands to air dry before applying sterile gloves.

Continued

378

STUDENT: _____ DATE: _____

INSTRUCTOR: _____ DATE: _____

Procedure Performance Checklist
Skill 33-4 Applying a Sterile Gown and Performing Closed Gloving

	S	U	NP	Comments
1. Apply cap, face mask, eyewear, and foot covers.	___	___	___	_____
2. Perform surgical hand washing and dry hands.	___	___	___	_____
3. Have circulating nurse to open pack containing sterile gown.	___	___	___	_____
4. Have circulating nurse prepare glove package.	___	___	___	_____
5. Reach down to sterile gown package; lift gown directly upward and step back from table.	___	___	___	_____
6. Pick up gown at neckline without touching outside of gown.	___	___	___	_____
7. Hold gown at arm's length; allow it to unfold by itself.	___	___	___	_____
8. Insert each hand through armholes simultaneously. Ask circulating nurse to bring gown over shoulders, leaving sleeves covering hands.	___	___	___	_____
9. Have circulating nurse tie back of gown at neck and waist.	___	___	___	_____
10. Closed gloving procedure:				
A. With hands covered by sleeves, open glove package.	___	___	___	_____
B. With hands covered by sleeves, pick up glove for dominant hand.	___	___	___	_____
C. Place glove palm side down on palm of sleeve-covered hand, with glove fingers pointing toward elbow.	___	___	___	_____
D. Using sleeve-covered nondominant hand, pull glove cuff over dominant hand and gown cuff.	___	___	___	_____
E. Grasping top of glove with nondominant hand, extend fingers of dominant hand.	___	___	___	_____
F. Repeat steps A through E to glove nondominant hand.	___	___	___	_____
G. Adjust fingers until fully extended into both gloves.	___	___	___	_____
11. For wraparound sterile gowns, release front fastener.	___	___	___	_____
12. Handing tie to stationary team member, turn 360 degrees to left and secure tie to gown.	___	___	___	_____

STUDENT: _____ DATE: _____

INSTRUCTOR: _____ DATE: _____

PROCEDURE PERFORMANCE CHECKLIST
Skill 33-5 Open Gloving

	S	U	NP	Comments
1. Perform thorough hand hygiene.	____	____	____	_____
2. Peel apart sides of outer package of glove wrapper.	____	____	____	_____
3. Lay inner package on clean, flat surface just above waist level. Open package, keeping gloves on inside surface of wrapper.	____	____	____	_____
4. If gloves are not prepowdered, apply powder lightly to hands over sink or wastebasket.	____	____	____	_____
5. Identify right and left gloves.	____	____	____	_____
6. Start by applying glove to dominant hand. With thumb and first two fingers of nondominant hand, grasp edge of cuff of glove of dominant hand, touching only inside surface.	____	____	____	_____
7. Carefully pull glove over dominant hand, ensuring cuff does not roll up wrist.	____	____	____	_____
8. With gloved dominant hand, slip fingers underneath second glove's cuff to pick it up.	____	____	____	_____
9. Carefully pull second glove over nondominant hand, and do not allow gloved hand to touch any part of exposed nondominant hand.	____	____	____	_____
10. When both gloves are on, interlock fingers of both hands to secure gloves in position, being careful to touch only sterile sides.	____	____	____	_____
Glove disposal:				
11. Without touching wrist, grasp outside of one cuff with other gloved hand.	____	____	____	_____
12. Pull glove off, turning it inside out. Discard in receptacle.	____	____	____	_____
13. Tuck fingers of bare hand inside remaining glove cuff. Peel glove off, inside out. Discard in receptacle.	____	____	____	_____
14. Perform hand hygiene.	____	____	____	_____

PROCEDURE PERFORMANCE CHECKLIST

Skill 34-1 Administering Oral Medications

	S	U	NP	Comments
1. Assess for any contraindications to client receiving oral medication.	____	____	____	_____
2. Assess client's medical history, history of allergies, medication history, and diet history.	____	____	____	_____
3. Review assessment and laboratory data that may influence drug administration.	____	____	____	_____
4. Assess client's knowledge regarding health and medication usage.	____	____	____	_____
5. Assess client's preferences for fluids.	____	____	____	_____
6. Check accuracy and completeness of each record with prescriber's written medication order.	____	____	____	_____
7. Prepare medications:				
A. Perform hand hygiene.	____	____	____	_____
B. Arrange medication tray and cups in medication preparation area or move medication cart to position outside client's room.	____	____	____	_____
C. Unlock medicine drawer or cart.	____	____	____	_____
D. Prepare medications for one client at a time. Keep all pages of records for one client together.	____	____	____	_____
E. Select correct drug from stock supply or unit-dose drawer.	____	____	____	_____
F. Calculate drug dose as necessary. Double-check calculation.	____	____	____	_____
G. To prepare tablets or capsules from a floor stock bottle, pour required number into bottle cap and transfer medication to medication cup. Do not touch medication with fingers. Extra tablets or capsules may be returned to bottle. Break prescored medications using a gloved hand or a pill-cutting device.	____	____	____	_____
H. To prepare unit-dose tablets or capsules, place packaged tablet or capsule directly into medicine cup. (Do not remove wrapper.)	____	____	____	_____
I. Place tablets or capsules to be given to client at the same time in one medicine cup unless client requires preadministration assessments.	____	____	____	_____

Continued

	S	U	NP	Comments

J. If client has difficulty swallowing and the pill may be crushed, use a pill-crushing device. If a pill-crushing device is not available, place tablet between two medication cups and grind with a blunt instrument. Mix ground tablet in small amount of soft food (e.g., custard or applesauce).

K. Prepare liquids:

   (1) Gently shake container if indicated. Remove bottle cap from container and place cap upside down.

   (2) Hold bottle with label against palm of hand while pouring.

   (3) Hold medication cup at eye level and fill to desired level on scale. Draw up volumes of liquid medication of less than 10 ml in syringe without needle.

   (4) Discard any excess liquid into sink. Wipe lip and neck of bottle with paper towel.

L. When preparing narcotics, check narcotic record for previous drug count and compare with supply available.

M. Check expiration date on all medications.

N. Compare record with prepared drug and container.

O. Return stock containers or unused unit-dose medications to shelf or drawer and read label again.

P. Do not leave drugs unattended.

8. Administering medications:

A. Take medications to client at correct time.

B. Identify client by comparing name on record with name on client's identification bracelet. Ask client to state name.

C. Explain to client the purpose of each medication and its action. Allow client to ask any questions about drugs he or she is receiving.

D. Assist client to sitting position or to side-lying position if sitting is contraindicated.

E. Administer drugs properly:

   (1) Allow client to hold solid medications in hand or cup before placing in mouth.

   (2) Offer water or juice to help client swallow medications. Give client cold carbonated water if available and not contraindicated.

Continued

	S	U	NP	Comments

(3) For drugs administered sublingually, instruct client to place medication under tongue and allow it to dissolve completely. Caution client against swallowing tablet. ____ ____ ____ _____

(4) For drugs administered buccally, instruct client to place medication in mouth against mucous membranes of the cheek until it dissolves. Avoid administering liquids until medication has dissolved. ____ ____ ____ _____

(5) Mix powdered medications with liquids at bedside and give to client to drink. ____ ____ ____ _____

(6) Caution client against chewing or swallowing lozenges. ____ ____ ____ _____

(7) Give effervescent powders and tablets to client immediately after they have dissolved. ____ ____ ____ _____

F. If client is unable to hold medications, place medication cup to client's lips and gently introduce each drug into the mouth, one at a time. ____ ____ ____ _____

G. If tablet or capsule falls to the floor, discard it and repeat preparation. ____ ____ ____ _____

H. Stay in room until client has completely swallowed each medication. Ask client to open mouth if you are uncertain whether medication has been swallowed. ____ ____ ____ _____

I. When administering highly acidic medications, offer client a nonfat snack if not contraindicated. ____ ____ ____ _____

J. Assist client in returning to a comfortable position. ____ ____ ____ _____

K. Dispose of soiled supplies. Perform hand hygiene. ____ ____ ____ _____

9. Return to client's room within 30 minutes to evaluate client's response to medication. ____ ____ ____ _____

10. Ask client or family member to identify drug name and explain purpose, action, dosage schedule, and potential side effects of drug. ____ ____ ____ _____

11. Notify prescriber if the client exhibits a toxic effect or allergic reaction or if there is an onset of side effects. If either of these occurs, withhold further doses of medication. ____ ____ ____ _____

12. Record administration (or withholding) of oral medications. ____ ____ ____ _____

PROCEDURE PERFORMANCE CHECKLIST
Skill 34-2 Administering Nasal Instillations

	S	U	NP	Comments
1. For nasal drops, determine which of client's sinuses is affected.	____	____	____	_____
2. Assess client's history of hypertension, heart disease, diabetes mellitus, and hyperthyroidism.	____	____	____	_____
3. Review prescriber's order.	____	____	____	_____
4. Determine if client has allergies to medication.	____	____	____	_____
5. Identify client.	____	____	____	_____
6. Perform hand hygiene. Inspect condition of client's nose and sinuses. Palpate sinuses for tenderness.	____	____	____	_____
7. Assess client's knowledge regarding use of and technique for instillation and willingness to learn self-administration.	____	____	____	_____
8. Explain procedure to client regarding positioning and sensations to expect.	____	____	____	_____
9. Arrange supplies and medications at bedside. Apply gloves, if indicated.	____	____	____	_____
10. Instruct client to clear or blow nose gently, unless contraindicated.	____	____	____	_____
11. Administer nasal drops:				
A. Assist client to supine position.	____	____	____	_____
B. Position client's head properly:	____	____	____	_____
(1) For access to posterior pharynx, tilt client's head backward.	____	____	____	_____
(2) For access to ethmoid or sphenoid sinus, tilt client's head back over edge of bed or place small pillow under client's shoulder and tilt head back.	____	____	____	_____
(3) For access to frontal and maxillary sinuses, tilt client's head back over edge of bed or pillow with head turned toward side to be treated.	____	____	____	_____
C. Support client's head with nondominant hand.	____	____	____	_____
D. Instruct client to breathe through mouth.	____	____	____	_____
E. Hold dropper 1 cm above client's nares and instill prescribed number of drops toward midline of ethmoid bone.	____	____	____	_____
F. Have client remain in supine position 5 minutes.	____	____	____	_____

Continued

	S	U	NP	Comments

G. Offer facial tissue to client to blot runny nose, but caution client against blowing nose for several minutes.

12. Assist client to a comfortable position after drug is absorbed.

13. Dispose of soiled supplies in proper container and perform hand hygiene.

14. Observe client for onset of side effects for 15 to 30 minutes after administration.

15. Ask if client is able to breathe through nose after decongestant administration.

16. Reinspect condition of nasal passages between instillations.

17. Ask client to review risks of overuse of decongestants and methods for administration.

18. Have client demonstrate self-medication.

19. Record medication administration and client's response.

20. Report any unusual systemic effects.

STUDENT: _____ DATE: _____

INSTRUCTOR: _____ DATE: _____

PROCEDURE PERFORMANCE CHECKLIST
Skill 34-3 Administering Ophthalmic Medications

	S	U	NP	Comments
1. Review prescriber's medication order.	___	___	___	_____
2. Identify client.	___	___	___	_____
3. Assess condition of client's external eye structures.	___	___	___	_____
4. Determine whether client has any known allergies to eye medications. Ask if client is allergic to latex.	___	___	___	_____
5. Determine whether client has any symptoms of visual alterations.	___	___	___	_____
6. Assess client's level of consciousness and ability to follow directions.	___	___	___	_____
7. Assess client's knowledge regarding drug therapy and desire to self-administer medication.	___	___	___	_____
8. Assess client's ability to manipulate and hold eye dropper.	___	___	___	_____
9. Explain procedure to client.	___	___	___	_____
10. Perform hand hygiene. Arrange supplies at client's bedside. Apply clean gloves.	___	___	___	_____
11. Ask client to lie supine or to sit back in chair with head slightly hyperextended.	___	___	___	_____
12. Wash away any crusts or drainage along client's eyelid margins or inner canthus. Soak any crusts that are dried and difficult to remove by applying a damp washcloth or cotton ball over eye for a few minutes.	___	___	___	_____
13. Hold cotton ball or clean tissue in nondominant hand on client's cheekbone just below lower eyelid.	___	___	___	_____
14. With tissue or cotton ball resting below lower lid, gently press downward with thumb or forefinger against bony orbit.	___	___	___	_____
15. Ask client to look at ceiling.	___	___	___	_____
A. Instill eye drops:				
(1) With dominant hand resting on client's forehead, hold filled medication eye dropper or ophthalmic solution approximately 1 to 2 cm above conjunctival sac.	___	___	___	_____
(2) Drop prescribed number of medication drops into conjunctival sac.	___	___	___	_____

Continued

	S	U	NP	Comments

(3) If client blinks or closes eye or if drops land on outer lid margins, repeat procedure.

(4) After instilling drops, ask client to close eye gently.

(5) For drugs that cause systemic effects, with a clean tissue apply gentle pressure with your finger on the client's nasolacrimal duct for 30 to 60 seconds.

B. Instill eye ointment:

   (1) Holding ointment applicator above lower lid margin, apply thin stream of ointment evenly along inner edge of lower eyelid on conjunctiva from inner canthus to outer canthus.

   (2) Have client close eye and rub lid gently in circular motion with cotton ball, if rubbing is not contraindicated.

C. Intraocular disk procedures:

   (1) Application:

      a. Open package containing disk. Gently press fingertip against disk so it adheres to finger. Position convex side of disk on fingertip.

      b. With other hand, gently pull client's lower eyelid away from the eye. Ask client to look up.

      c. Place disk in the conjunctival sac so that it floats on the sclera between the iris and lower eyelid.

      d. Pull client's lower eyelid out and over disk.

   (2) Removal:

      a. Perform hand hygiene and apply gloves.

      b. Explain procedure to client.

      c. Gently pull on client's lower eyelid to expose disk.

      d. Using forefinger and thumb of opposite hand, pinch disk and lift it out of client's eye.

16. If excess medication is on eyelid, gently wipe eyelid from inner to outer canthus.

17. If client has an eye patch, apply clean patch by placing it over affected eye so entire eye is covered. Tape securely without applying pressure to eye.

Continued

	S	U	NP	Comments
18. Remove gloves. Dispose of soiled supplies in proper receptacle and perform hand hygiene.	____	____	____	_____
19. Note client's response to instillation. Ask if any discomfort was felt.	____	____	____	_____
20. Observe client's response to medication by assessing visual changes and noting any side effects.	____	____	____	_____
21. Ask client to discuss drug's purpose, action, side effects, and technique of administration.	____	____	____	_____
22. Have client demonstrate self-administration of next dose.	____	____	____	_____
23. Record drug administration and appearance of client's eye.	____	____	____	_____
24. Record and report any undesirable side effects.	____	____	____	_____

STUDENT: _____ DATE: _____

INSTRUCTOR: _____ DATE: _____

Skill 34-4 Administering Vaginal Medications

	S	U	NP	Comments
1. Check medication order.	____	____	____	_____
2. Review client's history of allergies.	____	____	____	_____
3. Perform hand hygiene.	____	____	____	_____
4. Identify client.	____	____	____	_____
5. Inspect client's external genitalia and vaginal canal.	____	____	____	_____
6. Assess client's ability to manipulate applicator and position herself.	____	____	____	_____
7. Explain procedure to client.	____	____	____	_____
8. Arrange supplies at client's bedside.	____	____	____	_____
9. Provide privacy.	____	____	____	_____
10. Assist client to dorsal recumbent position.	____	____	____	_____
11. Keep client's abdomen and lower extremities draped.	____	____	____	_____
12. Apply clean gloves.	____	____	____	_____
13. Provide adequate lighting.	____	____	____	_____
14. Insert suppository with gloved hand:				
A. Take suppository from wrapper and lubricate smooth or rounded end. Lubricate gloved finger of dominant hand.	____	____	____	_____
B. Retract client's labial folds with nondominant gloved hand.	____	____	____	_____
C. Insert rounded end of suppository 7.5 to 10 cm along posterior wall of vaginal canal.	____	____	____	_____
D. Withdraw finger and wipe away lubricant from client's orifice and labia.	____	____	____	_____
15. Apply cream or foam:				
A. Fill applicator as directed.	____	____	____	_____
B. Retract client's labial folds with nondominant gloved hand.	____	____	____	_____
C. With dominant gloved hand, insert applicator 5 to 7.5 cm; push plunger.	____	____	____	_____
D. Withdraw applicator and place it on paper towel. Wipe away lubricant from client's orifice and labia.	____	____	____	_____
16. Dispose of supplies. Remove and discard gloves. Perform hand hygiene.	____	____	____	_____
17. Instruct client to remain flat on her back for at least 10 minutes.	____	____	____	_____
18. Wash applicator and store for future use, if indicated.	____	____	____	_____
19. Offer client perineal pad.	____	____	____	_____

Continued

	S	U	NP	Comments
20. Inspect condition of client's vaginal canal and external genitalia between applications.	____	____	____	_____
21. Record medication administration and report adverse reactions.	____	____	____	_____

STUDENT: _____ DATE: _____

INSTRUCTOR: _____ DATE: _____

PROCEDURE PERFORMANCE CHECKLIST
Skill 34-5 Administering Rectal Suppositories

	S	U	NP	Comments
1. Check medication order.	____	____	____	_____
2. Review client's medical record for rectal surgery/bleeding.	____	____	____	_____
3. Perform hand hygiene.	____	____	____	_____
4. Apply disposable gloves.	____	____	____	_____
5. Identify client.	____	____	____	_____
6. Explain procedure to client.	____	____	____	_____
7. Arrange supplies at client's bedside.	____	____	____	_____
8. Provide privacy.	____	____	____	_____
9. Position client in Sims' position. Keep client draped, except for anal area.	____	____	____	_____
10. Examine external condition of client's anus. Palpate rectal walls.	____	____	____	_____
11. Dispose of gloves, if soiled, and reapply new gloves.	____	____	____	_____
12. Remove suppository from wrapper and lubricate rounded end. Lubricate gloved finger of dominant hand.	____	____	____	_____
13. Ask client to take slow, deep breaths through mouth and to relax anal sphincter.	____	____	____	_____
14. Retract client's buttocks with nondominant hand. With index finger of dominant hand, gently insert suppository through anus, past the internal sphincter, and place against rectal wall, 10 cm for adults or 5 cm for children and infants.	____	____	____	_____
15. Withdraw finger and wipe client's anal area clean.	____	____	____	_____
16. Remove and dispose of gloves.	____	____	____	_____
17. Keep client flat on back or on side for 5 minutes.	____	____	____	_____
18. If suppository contains a laxative or fecal softener, be sure that client will receive help to reach bedpan or toilet.	____	____	____	_____
19. Perform hand hygiene.	____	____	____	_____
20. Observe client for effects of suppository 30 minutes after administration.	____	____	____	_____
21. Record medication administration or client refusal.	____	____	____	_____

STUDENT: _____ DATE: _____

INSTRUCTOR: _____ DATE: _____

<small>PROCEDURE PERFORMANCE CHECKLIST</small>
Skill 34-6 Using Metered-Dose or Dry Powder Inhalers

	S	U	NP	Comments
1. Review medication order.	___	___	___	_____
2. Identify client.	___	___	___	_____
3. Assess client's ability to hold, manipulate, and depress canister and inhaler.	___	___	___	_____
4. Assess client's readiness and ability to learn.	___	___	___	_____
5. Assess client's knowledge and understanding of his or her disease and purpose of the action of prescribed medications.	___	___	___	_____
6. Assess drug schedule and number of inhalations prescribed for each dose.	___	___	___	_____
7. Assess client's technique for using an inhaler if he or she has been previously instructed in self-medication.	___	___	___	_____
8. Perform instruction in a comfortable environment.	___	___	___	_____
9. Provide adequate time for teaching session.	___	___	___	_____
10. Perform hand hygiene. Arrange necessary equipment.	___	___	___	_____
11. Allow client the opportunity to manipulate inhaler, canister, and spacer device. Explain and demonstrate how canister fits into inhaler.	___	___	___	_____
12. Explain what metered dose is and warn client about overuse of the inhaler, including drug side effects.	___	___	___	_____
13. Explain and demonstrate steps for administering inhaled dose of medication:	___	___	___	_____
A. Insert MDI canister into the holder.	___	___	___	_____
B. Remove mouthpiece cover from inhaler.	___	___	___	_____
C. Shake inhaler well.	___	___	___	_____
D. Have client take a deep breath and exhale.	___	___	___	_____
E. Instruct the client to position the inhaler in one of two ways:	___	___	___	_____
(1) Close mouth around MDI, with opening toward back of throat.	___	___	___	_____
(2) Position the device 2 to 4 cm from the mouth.	___	___	___	_____
F. With the inhaler properly positioned, have client hold it with thumb at the mouthpiece and the index and middle fingers at the top.	___	___	___	_____
G. Instruct client to tilt head back slightly, inhale deeply and slowly through mouth while fully depressing medication canister.	___	___	___	_____

Continued

	S	U	NP	Comments

H. Instruct client to hold breath for approximately 10 seconds. ____ ____ ____ _____

I. Have client exhale through pursed lips. ____ ____ ____ _____

14. Explain and demonstrate steps to administer inhaled dose of medication using a spacer such as an aerochamber:

  A. Remove mouthpiece cover from inhaler and mouthpiece of aerochamber. ____ ____ ____ _____

  B. Insert MDI into end of spacer. ____ ____ ____ _____

  C. Shake inhaler well. ____ ____ ____ _____

  D. Have client profile completely; then place aerochamber mouthpiece in mouth and close lips. Tell client not toinsert mouthpiece beyond raised lip and to avoid covering small exhalation slots with lips. ____ ____ ____ _____

  E. Have client depress medication canister, spraying one puff into aerochamber. ____ ____ ____ _____

  F. Instruct client to breathe slowly and fully for 3 to 5 seconds. ____ ____ ____ _____

  G. Have client hold a full breath for 10 seconds. ____ ____ ____ _____

  H. Remove MDI and spacer before exhaling. ____ ____ ____ _____

15. Explain steps to administer DPI:

  A. Remove cover from mouthpiece. Do not shake. ____ ____ ____ _____

  B. Hold inhaler upright and turn wheel to the right and left until click is heard. ____ ____ ____ _____

  C. Exhale away from inhaler prior to inhalation. ____ ____ ____ _____

  D. Position mouthpiece between the lips. ____ ____ ____ _____

  E. Inhale deeply and forcefully through the mouth. ____ ____ ____ _____

  F. Hold breath for 5 to 10 seconds. ____ ____ ____ _____

16. Instruct client to wait 2 to 5 minutes between inhalations or as ordered by prescriber. ____ ____ ____ _____

17. Instruct client against repeating inhalations before next scheduled dose. ____ ____ ____ _____

18. Explain that client may feel gagging sensation in throat caused by droplets of medication. ____ ____ ____ _____

19. Instruct client in removing medication canister and cleaning inhaler in warm water. ____ ____ ____ _____

20. Ask if client has any questions and answer them. ____ ____ ____ _____

21. Have client explain and demonstrate steps in use of inhaler. ____ ____ ____ _____

22. Ask client to explain drug schedule. ____ ____ ____ _____

23. Ask client to describe side effects of medication and criteria for calling physician. ____ ____ ____ _____

Continued

	S	U	NP	Comments
24. After medication instillation, assess client's respirations and auscultate lungs.	____	____	____	_____
25. Record client education and client's ability to perform self-administration of medication.	____	____	____	_____
26. Record medication administration and any undesirable effects.	____	____	____	_____

PROCEDURE PERFORMANCE CHECKLIST
Skill 34-7 Preparing Injections

	S	U	NP	Comments
1. Check medication order.	____	____	____	_____
2. Review pertinent information related to medication.	____	____	____	_____
3. Assess client's body build, muscle size, and weight.	____	____	____	_____
4. Perform hand hygiene and assemble supplies.	____	____	____	_____
5. Check expiration date of vial or ampule.	____	____	____	_____
6. Prepare medication:				
A. Ampule preparation:	____	____	____	_____
(1) Tap top of ampule lightly and quickly with finger until fluid moves from neck of ampule.	____	____	____	_____
(2) Place small gauze pad around neck of ampule.	____	____	____	_____
(3) Snap neck of ampule quickly and firmly while pointing it away from hands.	____	____	____	_____
(4) Draw up medication quickly using filter needle.	____	____	____	_____
(5) Hold ampule upside down or set it on a flat surface. Insert syringe or filter needle into center of ampule opening. Do not allow needle tip or shaft to touch rim of ampule.	____	____	____	_____
(6) Aspirate medication into syringe by gently pulling back on plunger.	____	____	____	_____
(7) Keep needle tip under surface of liquid. Tip ampule to bring all fluid within reach of needle.	____	____	____	_____
(8) If air bubbles are aspirated, do not expel air into ampule.	____	____	____	_____
(9) To expel excess air bubbles, remove needle from ampule. Hold syringe with needle pointing up. Tap side of syringe to cause bubbles to rise toward needle. Draw back slightly on plunger, then push plunger upward to eject air. Do not eject fluid.	____	____	____	_____

Continued

	S	U	NP	Comments

(10) If syringe contains excess fluid, use sink for disposal. Hold syringe vertically with needle tip up and slanted slightly toward sink. Slowly eject excess fluid into sink. Recheck fluid level in syringe by holding it vertically.

(11) Cover needle with its safety sheath or cap. Change needle on syringe or use filter needle if you suspect medication is on needle shaft.

B. Vial containing a solution:

   (1) Remove cap covering top of unused vial to expose sterile rubber seal, keeping rubber seal sterile. If using a multidose vial that has been used before, firmly and briskly wipe surface of rubber seal with alcohol swab and allow it to dry.

   (2) Pick up syringe and remove needle cap. Pull back on plunger to draw amount of air into syringe equivalent to volume of medication to be aspirated from vial.

   (3) With vial on flat surface, insert tip of needle with beveled tip entering first through center of rubber seal. Apply pressure to tip of needle during insertion.

   (4) Inject air into vial's airspace, holding on to plunger. Hold plunger with firm pressure; plunger may be forced backward by air pressure within the vial.

   (5) Invert vial while keeping firm hold on syringe and plunger. Hold vial between thumb and middle fingers of nondominant hand. Grasp end of syringe barrel and plunger with thumb and forefinger of dominant hand to counteract pressure in vial.

   (6) Keep tip of needle below fluid level.

   (7) Allow air pressure from vial to fill syringe gradually with medication. Pull back slightly on plunger to obtain correct amount of solution.

Continued

	S	U	NP	Comments

(8) When desired volume has been obtained, position needle into vial's airspace. Tap side of syringe barrel carefully to dislodge any air bubbles. Eject any air remaining at top of syringe into vial.

(9) Remove needle from vial by pulling back on barrel of syringe.

(10) Hold syringe at a 90-degree angle at eye level to ensure correct volume and absence of air bubbles. Remove any remaining air by tapping barrel to dislodge any air bubbles. Draw back slightly on plunger, then push plunger upward to eject air. Do not eject fluid.

(11) If medication is to be injected into client's tissue, change needle to appropriate gauge and length according to route of medication.

(12) For multidose vial, make label that includes date of mixing, concentration of drug per milliliter, and nurse's initials.

C. Vial containing a powder (reconstituting medications):

(1) Remove cap covering vial of powdered medication and cap covering vial of proper diluent.

(2) Draw up diluent into syringe by following steps 6B(2) through 6B(10).

(3) Insert tip of needle through center of rubber seal of powdered medication. Inject diluent into vial. Remove needle.

(4) Mix medication thoroughly. Roll vial in palms. Do not shake.

(5) Read label carefully to determine dose after reconstitution.

(6) Prepare medication in syringe.

7. Dispose of soiled supplies. Place broken ampule and/or used vials and used needle in puncture-proof and leak-proof container. Clean work area and perform hand hygiene.

PROCEDURE PERFORMANCE CHECKLIST
Skill 34-8 Administering Injections

	S	U	NP	Comments
1. Review prescriber's medication order.	___	___	___	_____
2. Assess client's history of allergies.	___	___	___	_____
3. Check expiration date of vial or ampule.	___	___	___	_____
4. Observe client's verbal and nonverbal responses to receiving an injection.	___	___	___	_____
5. Assess for contraindications to subcutaneous or intramuscular injections.	___	___	___	_____
6. Perform hand hygiene. Prepare correct medication dose from ampule or vial. Check carefully. Be sure all air is expelled.	___	___	___	_____
7. Perform hand hygiene. Identify client by checking identification armband and asking client's name. Compare with record.	___	___	___	_____
8. Explain steps of procedure to client and tell client injection will cause a slight burning or sting.	___	___	___	_____
9. Provide privacy.				
10. Apply disposable gloves.	___	___	___	_____
11. Keep sheet or gown draped over client's body parts not requiring exposure.	___	___	___	_____
12. Select appropriate injection site. Inspect skin surface of site for bruises, inflammation, or edema:				
A. For subcutaneous (SQ) injections: Palpate sites for masses or tenderness. Avoid these areas. For daily insulin injections, rotate site daily. Check that needle is correct size by grasping skinfold at site with thumb and forefinger. Measure fold from top to bottom.	___	___	___	_____
B. For intramuscular (IM) injections: Note integrity and size of muscle and palpate for tender or hard areas. Avoid these areas. If injections are given frequently, rotate sites.	___	___	___	_____
C. For intradermal (ID) injections: Note lesions or discoloration of forearm. Select site three to four fingerwidths below antecubital space and a handwidth above wrist. Inspect SQ sites, if necessary.	___	___	___	_____
13. Assist client to a comfortable position:				
A. For SQ injections: Have client relax arm, leg, or abdomen, depending on site chosen.	___	___	___	_____
B. For IM injections: Have client lie flat, on side, or prone, depending on site chosen.	___	___	___	_____

Continued

	S	U	NP	Comments

    C. For ID injections: Have client extend elbow and support it and forearm on flat surface. _____ _____ _____ _____

    D. Talk with client about subject of interest. _____ _____ _____ _____

14. Relocate site using anatomical landmarks. _____ _____ _____ _____

15. Cleanse site with an antiseptic swab. Apply swab at center of site and rotate outward in a circular direction for about 5 cm.

16. Hold swab or gauze between third and fourth fingers of nondominant hand. _____ _____ _____ _____

17. Remove needle cap or sheath from needle by pulling it straight off. _____ _____ _____ _____

18. Hold syringe between thumb and forefinger of dominant hand:

    A. For SQ and IM injections: Hold as dart, with palm down. _____ _____ _____ _____

    B. For ID injections: Hold with bevel of needle pointing up. _____ _____ _____ _____

19. Administer injection:

    A. SQ injection:

      (1) For average-size client, spread skin tightly across injection site or pinch skin with nondominant hand. _____ _____ _____ _____

      (2) Inject needle quickly and firmly at a 45- to 90-degree angle, then release skin, if pinched. _____ _____ _____ _____

      (3) For obese client, pinch skin at site and inject needle at 90-degree angle below tissue fold. _____ _____ _____ _____

      (4) Inject medication slowly. _____ _____ _____ _____

    B. IM injection:

      (1) Position nondominant hand at proper anatomical landmarks and pull skin down to administer in a Z-track. _____ _____ _____ _____

      (2) If client's muscle mass is small, grasp body of muscle between thumb and fingers. _____ _____ _____ _____

      (3) Inject needle quickly into muscle at a 90-degree angle. After needle enters site, grasp lower end of syringe barrel with nondominant hand. Move dominant hand to end of plunger. Avoid moving syringe while slowly pulling back on plunger to aspirate drug. If blood appears in syringe, remove needle, discard medication and syringe, and repeat procedure. _____ _____ _____ _____

      (4) Inject medication slowly. _____ _____ _____ _____

Continued

406

	S	U	NP	Comments

(5) Wait 10 seconds, then smoothly and steadily withdraw needle while placing antiseptic swab or dry gauze gently above or over injection site.

C. ID injection:

(1) With nondominant hand, stretch skin across injection site with forefinger or thumb.

(2) Place needle against client's skin and insert it slowly at a 5- to 15-degree angle until resistance is felt. Advance needle through epidermis approximately 3 mm below skin surface so that needle tip can be seen through skin.

(3) Inject medication slowly. Remove needle and begin again if no resistance is felt.

(4) While injecting medication, notice that a small bleb approximately 6 mm in diameter appears on skin's surface.

20. Withdraw needle while applying alcohol swab or gauze gently over site.

21. Apply gentle pressure. Do not massage site. Apply bandage if needed.

22. Assist client to a comfortable position.

23. Discard uncapped needle or needle enclosed in safety shield and attached syringe into puncture- and leak-proof receptacle. If unable to leave client's bedside, use a one-handed technique to recap needle.

24. Remove and dispose of gloves. Perform hand hygiene.

25. Stay with client and observe for any immediate reactions.

26. Return to room in 10 to 30 minutes to evaluate client's response to injection and medication.

27. Inspect injection site and ask about client's sensations.

28. Observe client's response to medication.

29. Ask client to explain purpose and effects of medication.

30. For ID injections, use skin pencil and draw circle around perimeter of injection site. Check site within 48 to 72 hours of injection.

31. Record medication administration.

Continued

	S	U	NP	Comments
32. Record and report client's response to injection and any undesirable effects caused by the medication.	___	___	___	_____

STUDENT: _____ DATE: _____

INSTRUCTOR: _____ DATE: _____

PROCEDURE PERFORMANCE CHECKLIST
Skill 34-9 Adding Medications to Intravenous Fluid Containers

	S	U	NP	Comments
1. Check prescriber's order to determine type of intravenous (IV) solution to use and type of medication and dosage.	____	____	____	_____
2. Collect necessary information for safe administration of the drug.	____	____	____	_____
3. Assess for the compatibility of multiple medications in a single IV solution.	____	____	____	_____
4. Assess client's systemic fluid balance.	____	____	____	_____
5. Assess client's history of allergies.	____	____	____	_____
6. Perform hand hygiene.	____	____	____	_____
7. Assess IV insertion site for signs of infiltration or phlebitis.	____	____	____	_____
8. Assemble supplies in medication room.	____	____	____	_____
9. Prepare prescribed medication from vial or ampule.	____	____	____	_____
10. Identify client.				
11. Assess client's understanding of medication therapy.				
12. Add medication to new container:	____	____	____	_____
A. Solutions in bags: Locate medication injection port on plastic IV solution bag.	____	____	____	_____
B. Solutions in bottles: Locate injection site on IV solution bottle, which is often covered by a metal or plastic cap.	____	____	____	_____
C. Wipe off port or injection site with alcohol or antiseptic swab.	____	____	____	_____
D. Remove needle cap or sheath from syringe and insert needle through center of injection port or site. Inject medication.	____	____	____	_____
E. Withdraw syringe from bag or bottle.	____	____	____	_____
F. Mix medication and IV solution by holding bag or bottle and turning it gently end to end.	____	____	____	_____
G. Complete medication label with name, dose of medication, date, time, and initials. Stick label on bottle or bag.	____	____	____	_____
13. Bring assembled items to client's bedside.	____	____	____	_____
14. Explain procedure to client and alert client to expected sensations.	____	____	____	_____
15. Regulate infusion at ordered rate.	____	____	____	_____
16. Add medication to existing container:				
A. Prepare vented IV bottle or plastic bag:				
(1) Check volume of solution remaining in bottle or bag.	____	____	____	_____
(2) Close off IV infusion clamp.	____	____	____	_____

Continued

	S	U	NP	Comments

(3) Wipe off medication port with an alcohol or antiseptic swab.

(4) Insert syringe needle through injection port and inject medication.

(5) Withdraw syringe.

(6) Lower bag or bottle from IV pole and gently mix. Rehang bag.

B. Complete medication label and stick it to bag or bottle.

C. Regulate infusion to desired rate.

17. Properly dispose of equipment and supplies. Do not cap needle of syringe. Discard sheathed needles as a unit with needle covered.

18. Perform hand hygiene.

19. Observe client for signs and symptoms of drug reaction.

20. Observe client for signs and symptoms of fluid volume excess.

21. Periodically return to client's room to assess IV insertion site and rate of infusion.

22. Observe client for signs or symptoms of IV infiltration.

23. Record solution and medication added to parenteral fluid on appropriate form and report any side effects observed.

STUDENT: _____ DATE: _____

INSTRUCTOR: _____ DATE: _____

	S	U	NP	Comments
1. Check medication order.	____	____	____	_____
2. Perform hand hygiene. Assess IV or heparin (saline) lock site for infiltration or phlebitis. Assess potency of IV line, if in place.	____	____	____	_____
3. Assemble and prepare equipment and supplies.	____	____	____	_____
4. Prepare medication from vial or ampule. Check dilution instructions. Apply a small-gauge needle to syringe.	____	____	____	_____
5. Perform hand hygiene. Apply disposable gloves.	____	____	____	_____
6. Identify client.	____	____	____	_____
7. Administer medication by IV push (existing line):				
A. Select injection port of tubing closest to needle insertion site.	____	____	____	_____
B. Cleanse injection port with antiseptic swab. Allow port to dry.	____	____	____	_____
C. Connect syringe to IV line: Insert small-gauge needle into port or remove cap on port and attach tip of syringe directly to needleless system.	____	____	____	_____
D. Occlude IV line by pinching tubing above port. Aspirate for blood return.	____	____	____	_____
E. Release tubing and inject medication slowly. Time administration of medication.	____	____	____	_____
F. Withdraw syringe and recheck IV rate.	____	____	____	_____
8. Administer medication by IV push (IV lock or needleless system):				
A. Prepare flush solutions per agency policy.	____	____	____	_____
B. Administer medication.	____	____	____	_____
(1) Cleanse lock's injection port with antiseptic swab.	____	____	____	_____
(2) Insert syringe.	____	____	____	_____
(3) Aspirate for blood return.	____	____	____	_____
(4) Flush reservoir with 1 ml saline.	____	____	____	_____
(5) Remove syringe.	____	____	____	_____
(6) Cleanse lock's injection port with antiseptic swab again.	____	____	____	_____
(7) Insert medication syringe into injection port.	____	____	____	_____
(8) Inject prepared medication slowly. Time administration.	____	____	____	_____
(9) Withdraw needle and syringe.	____	____	____	_____
(10) Cleanse injection parts.	____	____	____	_____

Continued

	S	U	NP	Comments
(11) Flush port with 1 ml saline or heparin (or per agency policy).	____	____	____	_____
9. Dispose of all equipment properly.	____	____	____	_____
10. Remove and dispose of gloves. Perform hand hygiene.	____	____	____	_____
11. Observe client closely for adverse reactions during and for several minutes after administration.	____	____	____	_____
12. Record medication administration.	____	____	____	_____

PROCEDURE PERFORMANCE CHECKLIST

Skill 34-11 Administering Intravenous Medications by Piggyback, Intermittent Intravenous Infusion Sets, and Miniinfusion Pumps

	S	U	NP	Comments
1. Check prescriber's order to determine type of IV solution to be used; type of medication; and dose, route, and time of administration.	____	____	____	_____
2. Collect necessary information for safe administration of the drug.	____	____	____	_____
3. Assess compatibility of drug with existing IV solution.	____	____	____	_____
4. Assess patency of client's existing IV infusion line by noting infusion rate of main IV line.	____	____	____	_____
5. Perform hand hygiene. Assess IV insertion site for signs of infiltration or phlebitis.	____	____	____	_____
6. Assess client's history of allergies.	____	____	____	_____
7. Assess client's understanding of the purpose of the drug therapy.	____	____	____	_____
8. Assemble supplies at client's bedside. Prepare client by informing him or her that medication will be given through IV equipment.	____	____	____	_____
9. Perform hand hygiene.	____	____	____	_____
10. Identify client by looking at armband and asking client's name.	____	____	____	_____
11. Explain purpose of medication and side effects to client. Encourage client to report symptoms of discomfort at site.	____	____	____	_____
12. Administer infusion:				
A. Piggyback or tandem infusion:				
(1) Connect infusion tubing to medication bag. Allow solution to fill tubing by opening regulator flow clamp. Close cap and cap end when tubing is full.	____	____	____	_____
(2) Hang piggyback medication bag above level of primary fluid bag. Hang tandem infusion at same level as primary fluid bag.	____	____	____	_____
(3) Connect tubing of piggyback or tandem infusion to appropriate connector on primary infusion line:	____	____	____	_____
(a) Stopcock: Wipe off stopcock port with alcohol swab and connect tubing. Turn stopcock to open position.	____	____	____	_____

Continued

	S	U	NP	Comments

(b) Needleless system: Wipe off needleless port and insert tip of piggyback or tandem infusion tubing. ___ ___ ___ _____

(c) Tubing port: Connect sterile needle to end of piggyback or tandem infusion tubing, remove cap, cleanse injection port on main IV line, and insert needle through center of port. Secure with tape. ___ ___ ___ _____

(4) Regulate flow rate of medication solution by adjusting regulator clamp. ___ ___ ___ _____

(5) After medication has infused, check flow regulator on primary infusion. ___ ___ ___ _____

(6) Regulate main infusion line to desired rate, if necessary. ___ ___ ___ _____

(7) Leave secondary bag and tubing in place for future drug administration or discard in appropriate containers. ___ ___ ___ _____

B. Volume-control administration set:

(1) Assemble supplies in medication room. ___ ___ ___ _____

(2) Prepare medication from vial or ampule. ___ ___ ___ _____

(3) Fill volume-control set with desired amount of fluid (50 to 100 ml) by opening clamp between volume-control set and main IV bag. ___ ___ ___ _____

(4) Close clamp and check to be sure clamp on air vent of volume-control set chamber is open. ___ ___ ___ _____

(5) Clean injection port with antiseptic swab. ___ ___ ___ _____

(6) Remove needle cap or sheath and insert syringe needle through port, then inject medication. Gently rotate volume-control set between hands. ___ ___ ___ _____

(7) Regulate IV infusion rate to allow medication to infuse in recommended time. ___ ___ ___ _____

(8) Label volume-control set with name of drug, dosage, total volume including diluent, and time of administration. ___ ___ ___ _____

(9) Dispose of uncapped needle or needle enclosed in safety shield and syringe in proper container. ___ ___ ___ _____

C. Miniinfusor administration:

(1) Connect prefilled syringe to miniinfusion tubing. ___ ___ ___ _____

Continued

414

	S	U	NP	Comments
(2) Carefully apply pressure to syringe plunger, allowing tubing to fill with medication.	___	___	___	_____
(3) Place syringe into miniinfusor pump. Be sure syringe is secure.	___	___	___	_____
(4) Connect miniinfusion tubing to main IV line.	___	___	___	_____
(5) Explain purpose of medication and side effects to client. Ask client to report symptoms of discomfort at site.	___	___	___	_____
(6) Hang infusion pump with syringe on IV pole alongside main IV bag. Press button on pump to begin infusion.	___	___	___	_____
(7) After medication has infused, check flow regulator on primary infusion. Regulate main infusion line to desired rate as needed. (Note: If stopcock is used, turn off miniinfusion line.)	___	___	___	_____
(8) Perform hand hygiene.	___	___	___	_____
13. Observe client for signs of adverse reactions.	___	___	___	_____
14. During infusion, periodically check infusion rate and condition of IV site.	___	___	___	_____
15. Ask client to explain purpose and side effects of medication.	___	___	___	_____
16. Record medication administration and IV infusion.	___	___	___	_____
17. Report any adverse reactions.	___	___	___	_____

STUDENT: _____ DATE: _____

INSTRUCTOR: _____ DATE: _____

PROCEDURE PERFORMANCE CHECKLIST
Skill 37-1 Applying Restraints

	S	U	NP	Comments
1. Assess client's need for restraint.	___	___	___	_____
2. Assess client's behavior.	___	___	___	_____
3. Review agency policies regarding restraints. Check physician's order for purpose and type of restraint.	___	___	___	_____
4. Review restraint manufacturer's instructions before entering client's room.	___	___	___	_____
5. Perform hand hygiene and gather equipment.	___	___	___	_____
6. Introduce yourself. Explain to client and family the need for restraint. Attempt to obtain consent.	___	___	___	_____
7. Assess the area of the client's body where the restraint is to be placed.	___	___	___	_____
8. Approach client in a calm manner and explain procedure.	___	___	___	_____
9. Adjust bed to proper height and lower side rail on side of client contact.	___	___	___	_____
10. Provide privacy. Place client in proper body alignment.	___	___	___	_____
11. Pad bony prominences before applying restraints.	___	___	___	_____
12. Apply restraint, making sure it is not over an IV line or other device.	___	___	___	_____
13. Attach restraints to bed frame, not side rails.	___	___	___	_____
14. When client is in a chair, secure jacket restraint by placing ties under armrests and securing them at the back of the chair.	___	___	___	_____
15. Secure restraints with a quick-release tie.	___	___	___	_____
16. Make sure two fingers will fit under secured restraint.	___	___	___	_____
17. Assess proper placement of restraint and condition of client's restrained body part at least every 30 minutes or per agency policy.	___	___	___	_____
18. Remove restraints for 30 minutes every 2 hours. Do not leave restrained client unattended. Initiate special precautions for a violent or noncompliant client.	___	___	___	_____
19. Secure call bell or intercom within client's reach.	___	___	___	_____
20. Leave client's bed or chair with wheels locked. Bed should be in lowest position.	___	___	___	_____
21. Perform hand hygiene.	___	___	___	_____
22. Inspect client for any injury.	___	___	___	_____

Continued

	S	U	NP	Comments

23. Observe IV catheters and urinary catheters to determine that they are positioned correctly and that therapy remains uninterrupted. ___ ___ ___ _____

24. Record client behaviors that may place client at risk for injury. ___ ___ ___ _____

25. Provide sensory stimulation and reorient client as needed. ___ ___ ___ _____

26. Document client's response and expected or unexpected outcomes after restraint is applied. ___ ___ ___ _____

PROCEDURE PERFORMANCE CHECKLIST
Skill 37-2 Seizure Precautions

	S	U	NP	Comments
1. Assess client's history and related medical/surgical conditions.	____	____	____	_____
2. Inspect client's environment for safety hazards.	____	____	____	_____
3. Perform hand hygiene and prepare needed equipment and supplies.	____	____	____	_____
4. Have airway, suction equipment, clean gloves, and pillows available in room.	____	____	____	_____
5. Position client safely if seizure begins. Guide the sitting or standing client to the floor. Cradle client's head in lap or place pillow beneath it. Clear area of furniture. Lower bed and raise side rails (padded) for client in bed.	____	____	____	_____
6. Provide privacy.	____	____	____	_____
7. Turn client on side, if possible, with head flexed slightly forward.	____	____	____	_____
8. Do not restrain client. Loosen client's clothing.	____	____	____	_____
9. Do not place anything in client's mouth.	____	____	____	_____
10. Stay with client. Observe sequence and timing of seizure activity. Note aura, level of consciousness, mobility, incontinence, sleep patterns, or confusion afterward.	____	____	____	_____
11. After seizure, explain occurrence, and offer support.	____	____	____	_____
12. Following seizure, perform hand hygiene and assist client to a position of comfort; place bed in a low position with entitled within reach.	____	____	____	_____
13. For status epilepticus:				
A. Apply clean gloves. Insert airway when client's jaw is relaxed between seizure activity.	____	____	____	_____
B. Obtain oxygen and suction equipment. Prepare for IV insertion.	____	____	____	_____
C. Pad side rails and headboard.	____	____	____	_____
14. Record and report seizure activity and interventions.	____	____	____	_____

PROCEDURE PERFORMANCE CHECKLIST
Skill 38-1 Bathing a Client

	S	U	NP	Comments
1. Assess client's tolerance for activity, discomfort level, cognitive ability, and musculoskeletal function.	____	____	____	_____
2. Assess client's bathing preferences.	____	____	____	_____
3. Ask if client has noticed any skin problems or changes.	____	____	____	_____
4. Review orders for specific precautions concerning client's movement or positioning.	____	____	____	_____
5. Explain procedure to client and ask client about bathing preferences.	____	____	____	_____
6. Prepare room for comfort and privacy.	____	____	____	_____
7. Prepare equipment and supplies.	____	____	____	_____
8. Offer client bedpan or urinal. Provide towel and washcloth.	____	____	____	_____
9. Perform hand hygiene. Apply disposable gloves as needed.	____	____	____	_____
10. Bathe client:				
A. Complete or partial bed bath:				
(1) Lower side rail closest to you, and assist client in assuming a comfortable position that maintains body alignment. Bring client toward side of bed closest to you. Place bed in high position.	____	____	____	_____
(2) Loosen top covers at foot of bed. Place bath blanket over top sheet. Fold and remove top sheet from under blanket.	____	____	____	_____
(3) If top sheet is to be reused, fold it for later replacement. If not, place it in laundry bag.	____	____	____	_____
(4) Remove client's gown or pajamas.	____	____	____	_____
(5) Pull side rail up. Fill washbasin two-thirds full with warm water. Have client test temperature. Place plastic container of lotion in bath water to warm, if desired.	____	____	____	_____
(6) Remove pillow if allowed and raise head of bed 30 to 45 degrees. Place bath towel under client's head. Place second bath towel over client's chest.	____	____	____	_____

Continued

	S	U	NP	Comments

(7) Fold washcloth around fingers of your hand to form mitt. Immerse mitt in water and wring thoroughly. ___ ___ ___ _____

(8) Inquire if client is wearing contact lenses. Wash client's eyes with plain warm water. Use different section of mitt for each eye. Move mitt from inner to outer canthus. Soak any crusts on eyelid for 2 to 3 minutes with damp cloth before attempting removal. Dry eye thoroughly but gently. ___ ___ ___ _____

(9) Ask if client prefers to have soap used on face. Wash, rinse, and dry well client's forehead, cheeks, nose, neck, and ears. ___ ___ ___ _____

(10) Remove bath blanket from client's arm that is closest to you. Place bath towel lengthwise under arm. Raise side rail and move to other side to wash arm, if desired. ___ ___ ___ _____

(11) Bathe client's arm with soap and water using long, firm strokes from distal to proximal areas. Raise and support client's arm above head (if possible) while washing axilla. ___ ___ ___ _____

(12) Rinse and dry arm and axilla thoroughly. Apply deodorant or talcum powder, if used. ___ ___ ___ _____

(13) Fold bath towel in half and lay it on bed beside client. Place basin on towel. Immerse client's hand in water. Allow hand to soak for 3 to 5 minutes before washing hand and fingernails. Remove hand from basin and dry well. ___ ___ ___ _____

(14) Raise side rail and move to other side of bed. Lower side rails and repeat steps 11 through 13 for other arm. ___ ___ ___ _____

(15) Check temperature of bath water, and change water if necessary. ___ ___ ___ _____

Continued

	S	U	NP	Comments

(16) Cover client's chest with bath towel, and fold bath blanket down to umbilicus. Lift edge of towel away from client's chest. Bathe client's chest using long, firm strokes with mitted hand. Wash skinfolds under female clients' breasts. Keep client's chest covered between washing and rinsing. Dry well.

(17) Place bath towel(s) lengthwise over client's chest and abdomen. Fold blanket down to just above client's pubic region.

(18) Lift bath towel. Bathe client's abdomen with mitted hand. Stroke from side to side. Keep client's abdomen covered between washing and rinsing. Dry well.

(19) Help client put on clean gown or pajama top.

(20) Cover client's chest and abdomen with top of bath blanket. Expose client's nearer leg by folding blanket toward midline. Drape client's perineum and other leg.

(21) Bend client's leg at knee by positioning your arm under client's leg. Elevate leg from mattress slightly while grasping client's heel, and slide bath towel lengthwise under leg. Ask client to hold foot still. Place bath basin on towel on bed, and secure its position next to the foot to be washed.

(22) Raise the lower leg and place foot in basin. Allow client's feet to soak after the bath, unless contraindicated.

(23) Use long, firm strokes in washing from client's ankle to knee and from knee to thigh, unless contraindicated. Dry well.

(24) Cleanse client's foot, making sure to bathe between toes. Clean and clip nails as needed. Dry well. Apply lotion to dry skin. Do not massage any reddened area on client's skin.

Continued

	S	U	NP	Comments

(25) Raise side rail and move to other side of bed. Lower side rail and repeat steps 21 through 24 for client's other leg and foot.

(26) Cover client with bath blanket, raise side rail for client's safety, and change bath water.

(27) Lower side rail. Assist client in assuming a prone or side-lying position (as applicable). Place towel lengthwise along client's side.

(28) Keep client draped by sliding bath blanket over his or her shoulders and thighs. Wash, rinse, and dry back from neck to buttocks using long, firm strokes. Give client a back rub.

(29) Apply disposable gloves if not done previously.

(30) Assist client in assuming a side-lying or supine position. Cover client's chest and upper extremities with towel and lower extremities with bath blanket. Expose client's genitalia only. Wash, rinse, and dry perineum. Apply water-repellent ointment to area exposed to moisture.

(31) Dispose of gloves in receptacle.

(32) Apply additional body lotion or oil on client as desired.

(33) Assist client in dressing. Comb client's hair.

(34) Make client's bed.

(35) Remove soiled linen and place it in laundry bag. Clean and replace bathing equipment. Replace call light and client's personal possessions. Leave room as clean and comfortable as possible.

(36) Perform hand hygiene.

B. Tub bath or shower:

(1) Consider client's condition, and review orders for precautions.

(2) Check tub or shower for cleanliness. If necessary, use cleaning techniques outlined in agency policy. Place rubber mat on tub or shower bottom. Place disposable bath mat or towel on floor in front of tub or shower.

Continued

	S	U	NP	Comments

(3) Collect all hygienic aids, toiletry items, and linens requested by client. Place within easy reach of tub or shower. ____ ____ ____ _____

(4) Assist client to bathroom if necessary. Have client wear robe and slippers to bathroom. ____ ____ ____ _____

(5) Demonstrate how to use call signal for assistance. ____ ____ ____ _____

(6) Place "Occupied" sign on bathroom door. ____ ____ ____ _____

(7) Fill bathtub halfway with warm water. Ask client to test water, and adjust temperature if needed. Show client which faucet controls hot water. If client is taking a shower, turn shower on and adjust temperature before client enters shower stall. Provide tub chair or shower seat if needed. ____ ____ ____ _____

(8) Instruct client to use safety bars when getting in and out of tub or shower. Caution client against use of bath oil in tub water. ____ ____ ____ _____

(9) Instruct client not to remain in tub longer than 20 minutes. Check on client every 5 minutes. ____ ____ ____ _____

(10) Return to bathroom when client signals, and knock before entering. ____ ____ ____ _____

(11) Drain tub before client attempts to get out of it. Place bath towel over client's shoulders. Assist client as needed. ____ ____ ____ _____

(12) Assist client in donning clothing, if necessary. ____ ____ ____ _____

(13) Assist client to room and to a comfortable position in bed or chair. ____ ____ ____ _____

(14) Clean tub or shower according to agency policy. Remove soiled linen and place it in laundry bag. Discard disposable equipment in proper receptacle. Place "Unoccupied" sign on bathroom door. Return supplies to storage area.

(15) Perform hand hygiene. ____ ____ ____ _____

11. Observe client's skin, paying particular attention to areas that were previously soiled, reddened, or that showed early signs of breakdown. ____ ____ ____ _____

12. Observe client's range of motion during the bath. ____ ____ ____ _____

Continued

	S	U	NP	Comments
13. Ask client to rate level of comfort.	___	___	___	_____
14. Record bath on flow sheet. Note level of assistance required.	___	___	___	_____
15. Record condition of client's skin and any significant findings.	___	___	___	_____
16. Report evidence of alterations in client's skin integrity.	___	___	___	_____

PROCEDURE PERFORMANCE CHECKLIST
Skill 38-2 Perineal Care

	S	U	NP	Comments
1. Assess client's risk for developing infection of genitalia, urinary tract, or reproductive tract.	____	____	____	_____
2. Assess client's cognitive and musculoskeletal function.	____	____	____	_____
3. Perform hand hygiene. Assess client's genitalia for signs of inflammation, skin breakdown, or infection.	____	____	____	_____
4. Assess client's knowledge of the importance of perineal hygiene.	____	____	____	_____
5. Explain procedure and purpose to client.	____	____	____	_____
6. Prepare necessary equipment and supplies.	____	____	____	_____
7. Provide privacy.	____	____	____	_____
8. Raise bed to comfortable working position. Lower side rail, and assist client in assuming a side-lying position. Place towel lengthwise along client's side and keep client covered with bath blanket.	____	____	____	_____
9. Apply disposable gloves.	____	____	____	_____
10. Remove any fecal matter in a fold of underpad or toilet tissue. Cleanse client's buttocks and anus, washing from front to back. Clean, rinse, and dry area thoroughly. Place an absorbent pad under client's buttocks. Remove and discard underpad and replace with clean pad.	____	____	____	_____
11. Change gloves when they are soiled. Perform hand hygiene.	____	____	____	_____
12. Fold top bed linen down toward foot of bed. Raise client's gown so genital area is exposed: A. "Diamond" drape client.	____	____	____	_____
13. Raise side rail. Fill washbasin with warm water.	____	____	____	_____
14. Place washbasin and toilet tissue on overbed table. Place washcloths in basin.	____	____	____	_____
15. Provide perineal care: A. Female perineal care:				
(1) Assist client to dorsal recumbent position.	____	____	____	_____
(2) Lower side rails, and help client flex knees and spread legs. Note limitations in client's positioning.	____	____	____	_____
(3) Fold lower corner of bath blanket up between client's legs onto abdomen. Wash and dry client's upper thighs.	____	____	____	_____

Continued

	S	U	NP	Comments

(4) Wash client's labia majora. Use nondominant hand to gently retract labia from thigh. With dominant hand, carefully wash in skinfolds. Wipe from perineum to rectum. Repeat on opposite side using a different section of the washcloth. Rinse and dry area thoroughly.

(5) Separate labia with nondominant hand to expose urethral meatus and vaginal orifice. Wash downward from pubic area toward rectum in one smooth stroke. Use separate section of cloth for each stroke. Cleanse thoroughly around labia minora, clitoris, and vaginal orifice.

(6) Pour warm water over perineal area if client uses bedpan. Dry perineal area thoroughly, using front-to-back method.

(7) Fold lower corner of bath blanket back between client's legs and over perineum. Ask client to lower legs and assume comfortable position.

B. Male perineal care:

(1) Lower side rails, and assist client to supine position. Note any restriction in client's mobility.

(2) Fold top half of bath blanket below client's penis. Wash and dry client's upper thighs.

(3) Gently raise client's penis and place bath towel underneath it. Gently grasp shaft of penis. Retract foreskin if client is uncircumcised. Defer procedure until later if client has an erection.

(4) Wash tip of client's penis at urethral meatus first. Using circular motion, cleanse from meatus outward. Discard washcloth and repeat with clean cloth until penis is clean. Rinse and dry area gently.

(5) Return foreskin to its natural position.

(6) Wash shaft of penis with gentle but firm downward strokes. Pay special attention to underlying surface. Rinse and dry penis thoroughly. Instruct client to spread legs apart slightly.

Continued

	S	U	NP	Comments

(7) Gently cleanse scrotum. Lift it carefully and wash underlying skin folds. Rinse and dry.   ___ ___ ___ _____

(8) Fold bath blanket back over client's perineum, assist client to a side-lying position, and cleanse client's anal area.   ___ ___ ___ _____

16. Apply thin layer of skin barrier containing petrolatum or zinc oxide over anal and perineal skin of incontinent clients.   ___ ___ ___ _____

17. Remove gloves and dispose of them in proper receptacle. Perform hand hygiene.   ___ ___ ___ _____

18. Assist client in assuming a comfortable position, and cover client with sheet.   ___ ___ ___ _____

19. Remove bath blanket and dispose of all soiled bed linen. Return unused equipment to storage area.   ___ ___ ___ _____

20. Inspect surface of client's external genitalia and surrounding skin after cleansing.   ___ ___ ___ _____

21. Ask if client feels a sense of cleanliness.   ___ ___ ___ _____

22. Observe for abnormal drainage or discharge from client's genitalia.   ___ ___ ___ _____

23. Report and record procedure, appearance of suture line (if present), and the presence of any abnormal findings.   ___ ___ ___ _____

STUDENT: _____ DATE: _____

INSTRUCTOR: _____ DATE: _____

PROCEDURE PERFORMANCE CHECKLIST
Skill 38-3 Performing Nail and Foot Care

	S	U	NP	Comments
1. Inspect all areas of client's fingers, toes, feet, and nails.	____	____	____	_____
2. Assess circulation to client's toes, feet, and fingers.	____	____	____	_____
3. Observe client's walking gait.	____	____	____	_____
4. Ask female clients whether they frequently use nail polish and polish remover.	____	____	____	_____
5. Assess type of footwear worn by client.	____	____	____	_____
6. Assess client's risk for foot or nail problems.	____	____	____	_____
7. Assess types of home remedies client has used for existing foot problems.	____	____	____	_____
8. Assess client's ability to care for nails or feet.	____	____	____	_____
9. Assess client's knowledge of foot and nail care practices.	____	____	____	_____
10. Explain procedure to client.	____	____	____	_____
11. Obtain physician's order for cutting client's nails if agency policy requires it.	____	____	____	_____
12. Perform hand hygiene. Arrange equipment on overbed table.	____	____	____	_____
13. Provide privacy.	____	____	____	_____
14. Assist ambulatory client to sit in bedside chair. Help bed-bound client to supine position with head of bed elevated. Place disposable bath mat on floor under client's feet, or place towel on mattress.	____	____	____	_____
15. Fill washbasin with warm water. Test temperature.	____	____	____	_____
16. Place basin on bath mat or towel, and help client place feet in basin. Place call light within client's reach.	____	____	____	_____
17. Adjust overbed table to low position, and place it over client's lap.	____	____	____	_____
18. Fill emesis basin with warm water, and place basin on paper towels on overbed table.	____	____	____	_____
19. Instruct client to place fingers in emesis basin and to place arms in a comfortable position.	____	____	____	_____
20. Allow client's feet and fingernails to soak for 10 to 20 minutes unless contraindicated. Rewarm water after 10 minutes.	____	____	____	_____

Continued

431

	S	U	NP	Comments
21. Clean gently under client's fingernails with orange stick while fingers are immersed. Remove emesis basin, and dry client's fingers thoroughly.	___	___	___	_____
22. Clip client's fingernails straight across and even with tops of fingers unless contraindicated. Shape nails with emery board or file.	___	___	___	_____
23. Push client's cuticles back gently with orange stick.	___	___	___	_____
24. Move overbed table away from client.	___	___	___	_____
25. Put on disposable gloves. Scrub callused areas of client's feet with washcloth.	___	___	___	_____
26. Clean gently under client's toenails with orange stick. Remove client's feet from basin and dry thoroughly.	___	___	___	_____
27. Clean and trim toenails using the procedures described in steps 22 and 23. Do not file corners of toenails.	___	___	___	_____
28. Apply lotion to client's feet and hands, and assist client back to bed and into a comfortable position.	___	___	___	_____
29. Remove disposable gloves and place in receptacle. Clean and return equipment and supplies to proper place. Dispose of soiled linen in hamper. Perform hand hygiene.	___	___	___	_____
30. Inspect client's nails and surrounding skin surfaces after soaking and nail trimming.	___	___	___	_____
31. Ask client to explain or demonstrate nail care.	___	___	___	_____
32. Observe client's walk after toenail care.	___	___	___	_____
33. Record and report procedure and observations.	___	___	___	_____
34. Report any breaks in skin or ulcerations to charge nurse or physician.	___	___	___	_____

PROCEDURE PERFORMANCE CHECKLIST
Skill 38-4 Providing Oral Hygiene

	S	U	NP	Comments
1. Perform hand hygiene. Apply disposable gloves.	____	____	____	_____
2. Inspect integrity of client's lips, teeth, buccal mucosa, gums, palate, and tongue.	____	____	____	_____
3. Identify presence of common oral problems.	____	____	____	_____
4. Remove gloves and perform hand hygiene.	____	____	____	_____
5. Assess client's risk for oral hygiene problems or aspiration.	____	____	____	_____
6. Determine client's oral hygiene practices.	____	____	____	_____
7. Assess client's ability to grasp and manipulate a toothbrush.	____	____	____	_____
8. Prepare equipment at bedside.	____	____	____	_____
9. Explain procedure to client and discuss preferences regarding use of hygienic aids.	____	____	____	_____
10. Place paper towels on overbed table, and arrange other equipment within easy reach.	____	____	____	_____
11. Raise bed to comfortable working position. Raise head of bed (if allowed) and lower side rail. Move client, or help client move closer. The client can also be in a side-lying position.	____	____	____	_____
12. Place towel over client's chest.	____	____	____	_____
13. Apply gloves.	____	____	____	_____
14. Apply toothpaste to toothbrush while holding brush over emesis basin. Pour small amount of water over toothpaste.	____	____	____	_____
15. Hold toothbrush bristles at a 45-degree angle to client's gumline. Brush inner and outer surfaces of client's upper and lower teeth. Clean biting surfaces of teeth, and brush sides of teeth.	____	____	____	_____
16. Have client hold brush at a 45-degree angle and lightly brush over surface and sides of tongue. Instruct client to avoid initiating gag reflex.	____	____	____	_____
17. Allow client to rinse mouth thoroughly.	____	____	____	_____
18. Allow client to gargle to rinse mouth with mouthwash as desired.	____	____	____	_____
19. Assist in wiping client's mouth.	____	____	____	_____
20. Allow client to floss.	____	____	____	_____
21. Allow client to rinse mouth thoroughly with cool water and spit into emesis basin. Assist in wiping client's mouth.	____	____	____	_____

Continued

	S	U	NP	Comments

22. Assist client to a comfortable position, remove emesis basin and bedside table, raise side rail, and lower bed to original position. ____ ____ ____ _____

23. Wipe off overbed table. Discard soiled linens and paper towels in appropriate containers. Remove and dispose of soiled gloves. Return equipment to proper place. ____ ____ ____ _____

24. Perform hand hygiene. ____ ____ ____ _____

25. Ask client if any area of the oral cavity feels uncomfortable or irritated. ____ ____ ____ _____

26. Apply gloves and inspect condition of client's oral cavity. ____ ____ ____ _____

27. Ask client to describe proper oral hygiene techniques. ____ ____ ____ _____

28. Observe client brushing his or her teeth. ____ ____ ____ _____

29. Record and report procedure and observations. ____ ____ ____ _____

PROCEDURE PERFORMANCE CHECKLIST

Skill 38-5 Performing Mouth Care for an Unconscious or Debilitated Client

	S	U	NP	Comments
1. Perform hand hygiene. Apply disposable gloves.	___	___	___	_____
2. Test client for presence of gag reflex.	___	___	___	_____
3. Inspect condition of client's oral cavity.	___	___	___	_____
4. Remove gloves. Perform hand hygiene.	___	___	___	_____
5. Assess client's risk for oral hygiene problems.	___	___	___	_____
6. Explain procedure to client.	___	___	___	_____
7. Perform hand hygiene. Apply disposable gloves.	___	___	___	_____
8. Place paper towels on overbed table and arrange equipment. If needed, prepare suction.	___	___	___	_____
9. Provide privacy.	___	___	___	_____
10. Raise bed to its highest horizontal level. Lower side rail.	___	___	___	_____
11. Position client on side, close to side of bed. Turn client's head toward mattress. Raise side rail.	___	___	___	_____
12. Place towel under client's head and place emesis basin under client's chin.	___	___	___	_____
13. Separate client's upper and lower teeth with padded tongue blade. Insert blade when client is relaxed, if possible. Do not use force.	___	___	___	_____
14. Clean client's mouth using toothbrush or sponge toothettes moistened with peroxide and water. Clean chewing and inner tooth surfaces first. Clean outer tooth surfaces. Swab roof of mouth, gums, and insides of cheeks. Gently swab or brush tongue, but avoid stimulating the gag reflex. Rinse client's mouth with a clean swab, toothette, or bulb syringe. Repeat rinse several times.	___	___	___	_____
15. Suction secretions as they accumulate, if necessary.	___	___	___	_____
16. Apply thin layer of water-soluble jelly to client's lips.	___	___	___	_____
17. Inform client that procedure is complete.	___	___	___	_____
18. Reposition client comfortably, raise side rail, and return bed to original position.	___	___	___	_____
19. Clean equipment and return it to its proper place. Place soiled linen in proper receptacle.	___	___	___	_____
20. Remove gloves and dispose of them in proper receptacle. Perform hand hygiene.	___	___	___	_____
21. Apply gloves and inspect client's oral cavity.	___	___	___	_____
22. Ask debilitated client if mouth feels clean.	___	___	___	_____

Continued

	S	U	NP	Comments
23. Assess client's respirations on an ongoing basis.	____	____	____	_____
24. Record and report procedure and pertinent observations.	____	____	____	_____

STUDENT: _____   DATE: _____

INSTRUCTOR: _____   DATE: _____

PROCEDURE PERFORMANCE CHECKLIST
Skill 38-6 Making an Occupied Bed

	S	U	NP	Comments
1. Determine if client is incontinent or has excess drainage on bed linen.	____	____	____	_____
2. Check chart for orders or specific precautions for movement and positioning of client.	____	____	____	_____
3. Explain procedure to client.	____	____	____	_____
4. Perform hand hygiene.	____	____	____	_____
5. Assemble and arrange equipment on bedside chair or table.	____	____	____	_____
6. Provide privacy.	____	____	____	_____
7. Adjust bed height to comfortable working position. Lower side rail on near side of bed. Remove call light.	____	____	____	_____
8. Loosen top linen sheet at foot of bed.	____	____	____	_____
9. Remove bedspread and blanket separately by folding them into squares and placing them in linen bag (if not to be reused). Do not allow linen to contact uniform. Do not fan or shake linen.	____	____	____	_____
10. Fold blanket and spread if they will be reused. Fold them into neat squares and place them over back of chair.	____	____	____	_____
11. Cover client with bath blanket in following manner: Unfold bath blanket over top sheet. Ask client to hold top edge of bath blanket, or tuck top of bath blanket under client's shoulder. Grasp top sheet under bath blanket at client's shoulders, and bring sheet down to foot of bed. Remove sheet and discard it in linen bag.	____	____	____	_____
12. With assistance, slide mattress toward head of bed.	____	____	____	_____
13. Position client on his or her side on the far side of the bed, facing away. Adjust pillow under client's head, and raise farthest side rail.	____	____	____	_____
14. Loosen bottom bed linens, moving from head to foot of bed. Fanfold first draw sheet and then bottom sheet toward client. Tuck edges of linen just under client's buttocks, back, and shoulders.	____	____	____	_____
15. Wipe off moisture on mattress with towel and appropriate disinfectant.	____	____	____	_____

Continued

	S	U	NP	Comments

16. Apply clean linen to exposed half of bed:
    A. Place clean mattress pad on bed by folding it lengthwise with center crease in middle of bed. Fanfold top layer over mattress. ____ ____ ____ _____
    B. Unfold bottom sheet lengthwise so center crease is situated lengthwise along center of bed. Fanfold sheet's top layer toward center of bed alongside client. Smooth bottom layer of sheet over mattress, near side. Allow sheet's edge to hang about 25 cm over mattress edge. Lower hem of bottom sheet should lie seam down and even with bottom edge of mattress. ____ ____ ____ _____
17. Miter bottom sheet at head of bed:
    A. Face head of bed diagonally. Place hand away from head of bed under top cover of mattress, near mattress edge, and lift. ____ ____ ____ _____
    B. Tuck top edge of bottom sheet smoothly under mattress. ____ ____ ____ _____
    C. Face side of bed and pick up top edge of sheet at approximately 45 cm down from top of mattress. ____ ____ ____ _____
    D. Lift sheet and lay it on top of mattress to form neat triangular fold, with lower base of triangle even with mattress side edge. ____ ____ ____ _____
    E. Tuck lower edge of sheet, which is hanging free below mattress, under mattress. Tuck with palms down without pulling triangular fold. ____ ____ ____ _____
    F. Hold portion of sheet covering side edge of mattress in place with one hand. Pick up top of triangular linen fold and bring it down over side of mattress. Tuck this portion of sheet under mattress. ____ ____ ____ _____
18. Tuck remaining portion of sheet under mattress, moving toward foot of bed. Keep linen smooth. ____ ____ ____ _____
19. Open draw sheet so it unfolds in half. Lay center fold along middle of bed lengthwise, and position sheet so it will be under client's buttocks and torso. Fanfold top layer toward client with edge alongside client's back. Smooth bottom layer out over mattress and tuck excess edge under mattress. ____ ____ ____ _____
20. Place waterproof pad under draw sheet with center fold against client's side. Fanfold far half toward client. ____ ____ ____ _____
21. Have client roll slowly toward you. Raise side rail on working side of bed and go to other side. ____ ____ ____ _____

Continued

	S	U	NP	Comments

22. Lower side rail. Assist client in positioning on other side, over the folds of linen. Loosen edges of soiled linen from underneath mattress. ____ ____ ____ _____

23. Remove soiled linen by folding it into a bundle or squares, with soiled side turned in. Discard in linen bag. ____ ____ ____ _____

24. Spread clean, fanfolded linen smoothly over edge of mattress from head to foot of bed. ____ ____ ____ _____

25. Assist client in rolling back into supine position. Reposition pillow. ____ ____ ____ _____

26. Miter top corner of bottom sheet (see step 20). When tucking corner, be sure sheet is smooth and wrinkle-free. ____ ____ ____ _____

27. Grasp remaining edge of bottom sheet. Keep back straight and pull as excess linen is tucked under mattress. Proceed from head to foot of bed. ____ ____ ____ _____

28. Smooth fanfolded draw sheet over bottom sheet. Grasp edge of sheet with palms down, lean back, and tuck sheet under mattress. Tuck from middle to top and to bottom. ____ ____ ____ _____

29. Place top sheet over client, with center fold lengthwise down middle of bed. Open sheet from head to foot, and unfold it over client. ____ ____ ____ _____

30. Ask client to hold clean top sheet, or tuck sheet around client's shoulders. Remove bath blanket and discard in linen bag. ____ ____ ____ _____

31. Place blanket on bed, unfolding it so that crease runs lengthwise along middle of bed. Unfold blanket to cover client. Top edge of blanket should be parallel with edge of top sheet and 15 to 20 cm down from top sheet's edge. ____ ____ ____ _____

32. Place spread over bed according to step 31. Be sure top edge of spread extends about 2.5 cm above blanket's edge. Tuck top edge of spread over and under top edge of blanket. ____ ____ ____ _____

33. Make cuff by turning edge of top sheet down over edge of blanket and spread. ____ ____ ____ _____

34. Lift mattress corner slightly with one hand and tuck top linens under mattress. Top sheet and blanket are tucked under together. Allow for movement of client's feet. ____ ____ ____ _____

35. Make modified mitered corner with top sheet, blanket, and spread:
    A. Pick up side edge of top sheet, blanket, and spread approximately 45 cm up from foot of mattress. Lift linens to form triangular fold, and lay it on bed. ____ ____ ____ _____

Continued

	S	U	NP	Comments

B. Tuck lower edge of sheet, which is hanging free below mattress, under mattress. Do not pull triangular fold.

C. Pick up triangular fold and bring it down over mattress while holding linen in place along side of mattress. Do not tuck tip of triangle.

36. Raise side rail. Make other side of bed. Spread sheet, blanket, and bedspread out evenly. Fold top edge of spread over blanket, and make cuff with top sheet (see step 37). Make modified corner at foot of bed (see step 39).

37. Change pillowcase:

A. Have client raise head. Remove pillow while supporting client's neck.

B. Remove soiled pillowcase and discard in linen bag.

C. Grasp clean pillowcase at center of closed end. Gather case, turning it inside out over hand holding it. Pick up middle of one end of pillow. Pull pillowcase down over pillow with other hand.

D. Fit pillow corners evenly in corners of pillowcase.

38. Support client's head under neck and place pillow under head.

39. Place call light within client's reach. Return bed to comfortable position.

40. Open room curtains. Rearrange furniture. Place personal items easily within client's reach on overbed table or bedside stand. Return bed to comfortable height. Discard dirty linen in linen hamper or chute.

41. Perform hand hygiene.

42. Ask if client feels comfortable.

43. Inspect skin for irritation.

44. Observe for signs of discomfort.

PROCEDURE PERFORMANCE CHECKLIST
Skill 39-1 Suctioning

	S	U	NP	Comments
1. Assess client for signs and symptoms of airway obstruction.	___	___	___	_____
2. Assess signs and symptoms associated with hypoxia and hypercapnia.	___	___	___	_____
3. Determine factors that influence upper or lower airway functioning.	___	___	___	_____
4. Assess client's understanding of procedure.	___	___	___	_____
5. Obtain prescriber's order (if indicated).	___	___	___	_____
6. Explain purpose of procedure, expected sensations, and importance of coughing.	___	___	___	_____
7. Perform hand hygiene. Assist client to a comfortable position.	___	___	___	_____
8. Place pulse oximeter on client's finger, take reading, and leave in place.	___	___	___	_____
9. Place towel across client's chest.	___	___	___	_____
10. Apply face shield if splashing is likely.	___	___	___	_____
11. Connect one end of connecting tubing to suction machine, and place other end in convenient location near client. Turn suction device on, and set vacuum regulator to appropriate negative pressure.	___	___	___	_____
12. Increase supplemental oxygen therapy to 100% as indicated or ordered. Encourage client to breathe deeply.	___	___	___	_____
13. Prepare suction catheter with following sterile technique:				
A. Open suction kit or catheter with use of aseptic technique. Place sterile drape (if available) across client's chest or on overbed table.	___	___	___	_____
B. Unwrap or open sterile basin and place on bedside table. Fill with about 100 ml of sterile normal saline solution or water.	___	___	___	_____
C. Open lubricant. Squeeze small amount onto open sterile catheter package.	___	___	___	_____
14. Apply sterile glove to each hand, or apply nonsterile glove to nondominant hand and sterile glove to dominant hand.	___	___	___	_____
15. Pick up suction catheter with dominant hand without touching nonsterile surfaces. Pick up connecting tubing with nondominant hand. Secure catheter to tubing.	___	___	___	_____
16. Suction small amount of normal saline solution from basin.	___	___	___	_____

Continued

	S	U	NP	Comments

17. Coat distal 6 to 8 cm of catheter with water-soluble lubricant. Do not lubricate for oral suction.   ____ ____ ____ _____

18. Suction airway:

  A. Insert catheter appropriate distance for child or adult.   ____ ____ ____ _____

  B. Nasopharyngeal and nasotracheal:

    (1) Remove client's oxygen delivery device, if applicable. Gently but quickly insert catheter into client's naris during inhalation. Insert it at a slight downward slant or through mouth, without applying suction. Do not force catheter through naris. Position client's head to right or left. Pull catheter back 1 cm if resistance is felt.   ____ ____ ____ _____

    (2) Apply intermittent suction for 10 to 15 seconds, withdrawing catheter while rotating it back and forth between dominant thumb and forefinger. Encourage client to cough. Replace oxygen device, if applicable.   ____ ____ ____ _____

    (3) Rinse catheter and connecting tubing with normal saline or water until cleared.   ____ ____ ____ _____

    (4) Assess for need to repeat suctioning procedure. Allow adequate time between suction passes. Ask client to breathe deeply and cough.   ____ ____ ____ _____

    (5) Perform oropharyngeal suctioning when secretions have been cleared. Do not suction nose again after suctioning mouth.   ____ ____ ____ _____

  C. Oropharyngeal:

    (1) Insert catheter into client's mouth along gumline to pharynx. Move catheter around mouth until secretions are cleared. Encourage client to cough. Replace oxygen mask. Do not dislodge any oral tubing.   ____ ____ ____ _____

    (2) Rinse catheter with water in cup or basin until connecting tubing is cleared of secretions. Turn off suction. Wash face if secretions are present on client's skin.   ____ ____ ____ _____

  D. Endotracheal or tracheal tube:

    (1) Hyperinflate and/or hyperoxygenate client before suctioning.   ____ ____ ____ _____

Continued

	S	U	NP	Comments

(2) Open swivel adapter or remove oxygen or humidity delivery device with nondominant hand.

(3) Insert catheter (without applying suction) into artificial airway with thumb and forefinger of dominant hand until resistance is met or client coughs; then pull catheter back 1 cm.

(4) Apply intermittent suction, and slowly withdraw catheter while rotating it back and forth between dominant thumb and forefinger. Encourage client to cough. Watch for respiratory distress.

(5) Close swivel adapter or replace oxygen delivery device. Encourage client to breathe deeply if able.

(6) Rinse catheter and connecting tubing with normal saline until clear. Use continuous suction.

(7) Assess client's cardiopulmonary status.

(8) Repeat steps 18D(1) through 18D(7) once or twice more to clear secretions. Allow adequate time between suction passes.

(9) Perform nasopharyngeal and oropharyngeal suctioning. Do not reinsert catheter into endotracheal or tracheostomy tube.

19. Disconnect catheter. Roll catheter around fingers of dominant hand. Pull glove off inside out so that catheter remains coiled in glove. Pull off other glove over first glove. Discard in appropriate receptacle. Turn off suction device.

20. Remove towel, place in laundry or appropriate receptacle, and reposition client.

21. Readjust oxygen to original level, if indicated.

22. Reposition client as indicated by condition. Reapply clean gloves for client's personal care.

23. Discard remainder of normal saline into appropriate receptacle. Discard or clean and replace basin.

24. Remove and discard face shield.

25. Perform hand hygiene.

26. Place unopened suction kit on suction machine or at head of bed according to institution preference.

Continued

	S	U	NP	Comments
27. Compare client's respiratory assessments and vital signs before and after suctioning.	____	____	____	_____
28. Ask client if breathing is easier and if congestion is decreased.	____	____	____	_____
29. Observe airway secretions.	____	____	____	_____
30. Record and report the amount and characteristics of secretions, respiratory status, and client's response to procedure.	____	____	____	_____

PROCEDURE PERFORMANCE CHECKLIST
Skill 39-2 Care of an Artificial Airway

	S	U	NP	Comments
1. Perform cardiopulmonary assessment.	___	___	___	_____
2. Explain procedure to client.	___	___	___	_____
3. Position client.	___	___	___	_____
4. Place towel across client's chest.	___	___	___	_____
5. Perform hand hygiene.	___	___	___	_____
6. Perform airway care:	___	___	___	_____
A. Endotracheal tube (ET) care:				
(1) Assess client for signs and symptoms indicating the need to perform care of the artificial airway.	___	___	___	_____
(2) Identify factors that increase risk of complications from artificial airways.	___	___	___	_____
(3) Suction endotracheal tube:				
(a) Instruct client not to bite or move ET tube.	___	___	___	_____
(b) Leave Yankauer suction catheter connected to suction source.	___	___	___	_____
(4) Prepare tape. Cut piece of tape long enough to go completely around client's head from naris to naris plus 15 cm (6 inches)—about 30 to 60 cm (1 to 2 feet). Lay adhesive side up on bedside table. Cut and lay 8 to 16 cm (3 to 6 inches) of tape, adhesive side down, in center of long strip to prevent tape from sticking to hair.	___	___	___	_____
(5) Apply gloves. Have an assistant also apply a pair of gloves and hold ET tube firmly so that tube does not move.	___	___	___	_____
(a) Carefully remove tape from ET tube and client's face. If tape is difficult to remove, moisten with water or adhesive tape remover. Discard tape in appropriate receptacle if nearby. If not, place soiled tape on bedside table or on distant end of towel.	___	___	___	_____
(b) Use adhesive remover swab to remove excess adhesive left on face after tape removal.	___	___	___	_____
(c) Remove oral airway or bite block if present.	___	___	___	_____

Continued

	S	U	NP	Comments

(d) Clean mouth, gums, and teeth opposite ET tube with mouthwash solution and 4 × 4 gauze, sponge-tipped applicators, or saline swabs. Brush teeth as indicated. If necessary, administer oropharyngeal suctioning with Yankauer catheter. _____ _____ _____ _____

(e) Oral ET tube only: Note "cm" ET tube marking at lips or gums. With help of assistant, move ET tube to opposite side or center of mouth. Do not change tube depth. _____ _____ _____ _____

(f) Repeat oral cleaning on opposite side of mouth. _____ _____ _____ _____

(g) Clean face and neck with soapy washcloth; rinse and dry. Shave male client as necessary. _____ _____ _____ _____

(h) Pour small amount of tincture of benzoin on clean 2 × 2 gauze and dot on upper lip (oral ET tube) or across nose (nasal ET tube) and cheeks to ear. Allow to dry completely. _____ _____ _____ _____

(i) Slip tape under client's head and neck, adhesive side down. Take care not to twist tape or catch hair. Do not allow tape to stick to itself. It helps to stick tape gently to tongue blade, which serves as a guide. Then slide tongue blade under client's neck. Center tape so that double-faced tape extends around back of neck from ear to ear. _____ _____ _____ _____

(j) On one side of face, secure tape from ear to naris (nasal ET tube) or edge of mouth (oral ET tube). Tear remaining tape in half lengthwise, forming two pieces that are 1/2 to 3/4 inch wide. Secure bottom half of tape across upper lip (oral ET tube) or across top of nose (nasal ET tube). Wrap top half of tape around tube. _____ _____ _____ _____

Continued

	S	U	NP	Comments

(k) Gently pull other side of tape firmly to pick up slack and secure to remaining side of face. Assistant can release hold when tube is secure. Nurse may want assistant to help reinsert oral airway. ____ ____ ____ _____

(l) Clean oral airway in warm soapy water and rinse well. Hydrogen peroxide can aid in removal of crusted secretions. Shake excess water from oral airway. ____ ____ ____ _____

(m) Reinsert oral airway without pushing tongue into oropharynx. ____ ____ ____ _____

B. Tracheostomy care:

(1) Observe for signs and symptoms of need to perform tracheostomy care. ____ ____ ____ _____

(2) Suction tracheostomy. Before removing gloves, remove soiled tracheostomy dressing and discard in glove with coiled catheter. ____ ____ ____ _____

(3) While client is replenishing oxygen stores, prepare equipment on bedside table. Open sterile tracheostomy kit. Open three 4 × 4 gauze packages using aseptic technique and pour normal saline (NS) on one package and hydrogen peroxide on another. Leave third package dry. ____ ____ ____ _____

(a) Open two cotton-tipped swabbed packages and pour NS on one package and hydrogen peroxide on the other. ____ ____ ____ _____

(b) Open sterile tracheostomy package. ____ ____ ____ _____

(c) Unwrap sterile basin and pour about 2 cm (3/4 inch) hydrogen peroxide into it.

(d) Open small sterile brush package and place aseptically into sterile basin.

(e) If using large roll of twill tape, cut appropriate length of tape and lay aside in dry area. Do not recap hydrogen peroxide and NS. ____ ____ ____ _____

(4) Apply gloves. Keep dominate hand sterile throughout procedure. ____ ____ ____ _____

(5) Remove oxygen source. ____ ____ ____ _____

Continued

	S	U	NP	Comments

(6) If a nondisposable inner cannula is used:

   (a) Remove with nondominant hand. Drop inner cannula into hydrogen peroxide basin. ____ ____ ____ _____

   (b) Place tracheostomy collar or T tube and ventilator oxygen source over or near outer cannula. ____ ____ ____ _____

   (c) To prevent oxygen desaturation in affected clients, quickly pick up inner cannula and use small brush to remove secretions from inside and outside. ____ ____ ____ _____

   (d) Hold inner cannula over basin and rinse with NS, using nondominant hand to pour. ____ ____ ____ _____

   (e) Replace inner cannula and secure "locking" mechanism. Reapply ventilator or oxygen sources. ____ ____ ____ _____

(7) If a disposable inner cannula is used:

   (a) Remove cannula from manufacturer's packaging. ____ ____ ____ _____

   (b) Withdraw inner cannula and replace with new cannula. Lock into position. ____ ____ ____ _____

   (c) Dispose of contaminated cannula in appropriate receptacle. ____ ____ ____ _____

(8) Using hydrogen peroxide-prepared cotton-tipped swabs and 4 × 4 gauze, clean exposed outer cannula surfaces and stoma under faceplate, extending 5 to 10 cm (2 to 4 inches) in all directions from stoma. Clean in circular motion from stoma site outward, using dominant hand to handle sterile supplies. ____ ____ ____ _____

(9) Using NS-prepared cotton-tipped swabs and 4 × 4 gauze, rinse hydrogen peroxide from tracheostomy tube and skin surfaces. ____ ____ ____ _____

(10) Using dry 4 × 4 gauze, pat lightly at skin and exposed outer cannula surfaces. ____ ____ ____ _____

(11) Instruct assistant, if available, to hold tracheostomy tube securely in place while ties are cut. ____ ____ ____ _____

Continued

	S	U	NP	Comments
(a) Cut length of twill tape long enough to go around client's neck two times, about 60 to 75 cm (24 to 30 inches) for an adult. Cut ends on a diagonal.	___	___	___	_____
(b) Insert one end of tie through faceplate eyelet and pull ends even.	___	___	___	_____
(c) Slide both ends of tie behind head and around neck to other eyelet, and insert one tie through second eyelet.	___	___	___	_____
(d) Pull snugly.	___	___	___	_____
(e) Tie ends securely in double square knot, allowing space for only one finger in tie.	___	___	___	_____
(f) Insert fresh tracheostomy dressing under clean ties and faceplate.	___	___	___	_____
(g) Position client comfortably and assess respiratory status.	___	___	___	_____
7. Replace any oxygen delivery devices.	___	___	___	_____
8. Remove and discard gloves. Perform hand hygiene.	___	___	___	_____
9. Compare respiratory assessments made before and after artificial airway care. Observe for tissue breakdown or persistent dried secretions.	___	___	___	_____
10. Observe depth and position of tubes.	___	___	___	_____
11. Assess security of tape and tubes.	___	___	___	_____
12. Assess skin around mouth and oral mucosa and tracheostomy stoma.	___	___	___	_____
13. Identify unexpected outcomes and intervene as necessary.	___	___	___	_____
14. Record and report intervention and client's response.	___	___	___	_____

STUDENT: _____ DATE: _____

INSTRUCTOR: _____ DATE: _____

PROCEDURE PERFORMANCE CHECKLIST
Skill 39-3 Care of Clients with Chest Tubes

	S	U	NP	Comments
1. Assess client for respiratory distress and chest pain, breath sounds over affected lung area, and vital signs.	____	____	____	_____
2. Observe the following:				
A. Chest tube dressing	____	____	____	_____
B. Tubing, for kinks, dependent loops, or clots	____	____	____	_____
C. Chest drainage system	____	____	____	_____
3. Provide two shodded hemostats for each chest tube, and attach them to top of client's bed with adhesive tape.	____	____	____	_____
4. Position client in one of the following ways:				
A. Semi-Fowler's position to evacuate air (pneumothorax)	____	____	____	_____
B. High-Fowler's position to drain fluid (hemothorax)	____	____	____	_____
5. Maintain tube connection between chest and drainage tubes. Make sure it is intact and taped.	____	____	____	_____
6. Coil excess tubing on mattress next to client. Lift coiled tubing q15 minutes to promote drainage. Secure with rubber band and safety pin or system's clamp.	____	____	____	_____
7. Adjust tubing to hang in straight line from top of mattress to drainage chamber. Indicate time that drainage began.	____	____	____	_____
8. Strip or milk chest tube only if indicated.	____	____	____	_____
9. Perform hand hygiene.	____	____	____	_____
10. Observe the following:				
A. Chest tube dressing, tubing, and drainage system	____	____	____	_____
B. Water seal for fluctuations with client's inspiration and expiration	____	____	____	_____
C. Bubbling in water-seal bottle or chamber	____	____	____	_____
D. Type and amount of fluid drainage	____	____	____	_____
E. Client vital signs and skin color	____	____	____	_____
F. Bubbling in the suction-control chamber	____	____	____	_____
G. Client's pain level	____	____	____	_____
11. Record and report status of chest tubes, dressing, and client's responses.	____	____	____	_____

STUDENT: _____ DATE: _____

INSTRUCTOR: _____ DATE: _____

Skill 39-4 Applying a Nasal Cannula or Oxygen Mask

	S	U	NP	Comments
1. Assess client's respiratory status.	___	___	___	_____
2. Explain procedure and purpose to client and family.	___	___	___	_____
3. Prepare needed equipment and supplies. Perform hand hygiene.	___	___	___	_____
4. Attach nasal cannula to humidified oxygen source. Adjust oxygen flow to prescribed rate.	___	___	___	_____
5. Place tips of cannula into nares. Adjust band until cannula fits snugly and comfortably.	___	___	___	_____
6. Secure oxygen tubing to clothes, maintaining sufficient slack.	___	___	___	_____
7. Check cannula every 8 hours. Keep humidification jar filled at all times.	___	___	___	_____
8. Assess nares and external nose for skin breakdown.	___	___	___	_____
9. Check oxygen flow rate and physician's orders every 8 hours.	___	___	___	_____
10. Perform hand hygiene.	___	___	___	_____
11. Inspect client for relief of symptoms.	___	___	___	_____
12. Record procedure and observations. Report on therapy and client's response.	___	___	___	_____

PROCEDURE PERFORMANCE CHECKLIST
Skill 39-5 Using Home Liquid Oxygen Equipment

	S	U	NP	Comments
1. Assess client's need for and client's/family's ability to use equipment and observe for hypoxia.	____	____	____	_____
2. Explain procedure to client and family.	____	____	____	_____
3. Perform hand hygiene.	____	____	____	_____
4. Demonstrate steps for oxygen therapy.	____	____	____	_____
5. Prepare primary and portable oxygen. Perform hand hygiene.	____	____	____	_____
6. Have client or family perform each step with guidance.	____	____	____	_____
7. Discuss signs and symptoms of respiratory tract infection and hypoxia.	____	____	____	_____
8. Instruct client and family to notify physician if signs or symptoms of hypoxia or respiration infection occur.	____	____	____	_____
9. Perform hand hygiene.	____	____	____	_____
10. Record teaching, information provided, and client's/family's understanding.	____	____	____	_____

STUDENT: _____ DATE: _____

INSTRUCTOR: _____ DATE: _____

Skill 40-1 Initiating a Peripheral Intravenous Infusion

	S	U	NP	Comments
1. Review client's medical record for order. Follow "six rights" for administration of medications.	____	____	____	_____
2. Observe client for signs and symptoms indicating fluid or electrolyte imbalances.	____	____	____	_____
3. Assess client's prior experience with intravenous (IV) therapy.	____	____	____	_____
4. Determine if client is to have surgery or blood transfusion.	____	____	____	_____
5. Assess laboratory data and client's allergies.	____	____	____	_____
6. Assess client for risk factors.	____	____	____	_____
7. Explain procedure to client.	____	____	____	_____
8. Perform hand hygiene.	____	____	____	_____
9. Assist client to a comfortable sitting or lying position.	____	____	____	_____
10. Organize equipment on bedside stand or overbed table.	____	____	____	_____
11. Change client's gown to a more easily removable gown with snaps at shoulder, if available.	____	____	____	_____
12. Open sterile packages and maintain a sterile technique throughout.	____	____	____	_____
13. Check IV solution. Make sure prescribed additives (e.g., potassium, vitamins) have been added. Check solution for color, clarity, and expiration date. Check bag for leaks.	____	____	____	_____
14. Open infusion set.	____	____	____	_____
15. Place roller clamp about 2 to 5 cm below drip chamber and move roller clamp to "off" position.	____	____	____	_____
16. Remove protective sheath over IV tubing port.	____	____	____	_____
17. Insert infusion set into fluid bag or bottle. Remove protector cap from tubing insertion spike and insert spike into opening of IV bag. Cleanse rubber stopper on bottled solutions with antiseptic, and insert spike into black rubber stopper of IV bottle. Hang solution container on IV pole at minimum height of 35 inches (90 cm) above insertion site.	____	____	____	_____
18. Prime infusion tubing by filling with IV solution. Compress drip chamber and release, allowing it to fill one-third to one-half full.	____	____	____	_____

Continued

	S	U	NP	Comments

19. Remove tubing protector cap and slowly release roller clamp to allow fluid to travel from drip chamber through tubing to needle adapter. Return roller clamp to "off" position after tubing is primed.

20. Clear tubing of air bubbles. Firmly tap IV tubing where air bubbles are located. Check entire length of tubing to ensure that all air bubbles are removed.

21. Replace tubing cap protector on end of tubing.

22. Optional: Prepare heparin or normal saline lock for infusion. Use a sterile technique to connect the IV plug to the loop or short extension tubing. Inject 1 to 3 ml normal saline through the plug and through the loop or short extension tubing.

23. Apply disposable gloves. Eye protection and mask applied, if indicated.

24. Identify site for IV replacement. Place tourniquet 10 to 15 cm above insertion site. Check presence of distal pulse.

25. Select well-dilated vein. Foster vein dilation with the following techniques:
    A. Stroke the extremity from distal to proximal sites below the proposed venipuncture site.
    B. Tell client to open and close the fist of the arm where the site has been selected.
    C. Lower the extremity on which the site has been selected.

26. Release tourniquet temporarily. Clip excess hair at site, if necessary.

27. Cleanse insertion site using firm, circular motion and antiseptic solution. Refrain from touching cleansed site. Allow the site to dry for at least 2 minutes.

28. Reapply tourniquet or BP cuff.

29. Perform venipuncture. Anchor vein by placing thumb over vein and stretching skin against the direction of insertion 5 to 7.5 cm distal to the site.
    A. Butterfly needle: Hold needle at 20- to 30-degree angle with bevel up slightly distal to actual site of venipuncture.
    B. Over-the-needle catheter: Insert over-the-needle catheter with bevel up at 20- to 30-degree angle slightly distal to actual site and in the direction of the vein.

Continued

458

	S	U	NP	Comments

C. Needleless IV catheter safety device: Insert using same technique as for over-the-needle catheter.

30. Look for blood return through tubing of butterfly needle or flashback chamber of over-the-needle catheter. Lower needle until almost flush with skin. Advance butterfly needle until hub rests at venipuncture site. Advance over-the-needle catheter 1/4 inch into vein and then loosen stylet. Advance catheter into vein until hub rests at venipuncture site. Do not reinsert the stylet once it is loosened.

31. Stabilize the catheter with dominant hand. Apply gentle pressure 1 1/4 inches (3 cm) above insertion site. Release tourniquet and remove stylet from over-the-needle catheter. Do not recap the stylet. Slide the catheter off the stylet while gliding the protective guard over the stylet.

32. Connect needle adapter of administration set or heparin lock to hub of over-the-needle catheter or butterfly tubing. Do not touch point of entry of needle adapter.

33. Release roller clamp slowly to begin infusion at a rate to maintain patency of IV line.

34. Secure IV catheter or needle:
   A. Place narrow piece of tape under catheter hub with adhesive side up and cross tape over catheter.
   B. Place second piece of narrow tape directly across hub of catheter.

35. Apply sterile dressing over site.
   A. Transparent dressing:
      (1) Remove adherent backing. Apply dressing to site. Smooth dressing over site, leaving end of catheter hub uncovered.
      (2) Take 1-inch piece of tape and place from end of catheter hub to insertion site over dressing.
      (3) Apply chevron and place only over tape, not dressing.
   B. Sterile gauze dressing:
      (1) Fold 2 × 2 gauze in half and cover with 1-inch tape. Place under tubing/catheter hub junction.
      (2) Place a 2 × 2 gauze pad over venipuncture site. Secure edges with tape.

Continued

	S	U	NP	Comments
(3) Curl loop of tubing alongside arm and secure with tape.	___	___	___	_____
36. For IV fluid administration, adjust flow rate to correct drops per minute:				
A. For heparin lock, flush with 1 to 3 ml of heparin (10 to 100 U/ml).	___	___	___	_____
B. For saline lock, flush with 1 to 3 ml of sterile normal saline.	___	___	___	_____
37. Write date and time, gauge size and size of catheter, and placement of IV line and dressing.	___	___	___	_____
38. Dispose of used needles in appropriate sharps container. Discard supplies. Remove gloves and perform hand hygiene.	___	___	___	_____
39. Observe client every hour to determine if fluid is infusing correctly.	___	___	___	_____
40. Observe client every hour to determine response to therapy.	___	___	___	_____
41. Record peripheral IV insertion.	___	___	___	_____
42. Record and report client's response to IV fluid, amount infused, and integrity and patency of system.	___	___	___	_____

STUDENT: _____ DATE: _____

INSTRUCTOR: _____ DATE: _____

PROCEDURE PERFORMANCE CHECKLIST
Skill 40-2 Regulating Intravenous Flow Rate

	S	U	NP	Comments
1. Check client's medical record for correct solution, additives, and time of infusion.	____	____	____	_____
2. Perform hand hygiene. Observe for patency of intravenous (IV) lineand needle or catheter.	____	____	____	_____
3. Check client's knowledge of how positioning of IV site affects flow rate.	____	____	____	_____
4. Verify with client how venipuncture site feels.	____	____	____	_____
5. Calculate flow rate.	____	____	____	_____
6. Check calibration (drop factor) in drops per milliliter (gtt/ml) of infusion set.	____	____	____	_____
7. Select formula to calculate flow rate after determining ml/hr.	____	____	____	_____
8. Read prescriber's orders and follow "six rights" for correct solution and proper additives.	____	____	____	_____
9. Calculate appropriate flow rate.	____	____	____	_____
10. Place adhesive or fluid indicator tape on IV bottle or bag next to volume markings.	____	____	____	_____
11. Time flow rate by counting drops in drip chamber for 1 minute, then adjust roller clamp to increase or decrease rate of infusion.	____	____	____	_____
12. Follow this procedure for infusion controller or pump:				
A. Place electronic eye on drip chamber below origin of drop and above fluid level in chamber or consult manufacturer's directions for setup of the infusion. If controller is used, ensure that IV bag is 1 m above the IV site.	____	____	____	_____
B. Place IV infusion tubing within ridges of control box in direction of flow or consult manufacturer's directions for use of pump. Select drops per minute or volume per hour. Close door to control chamber. Turn on power and press start button.	____	____	____	_____
C. Monitor infusion rates and IV site for infiltration according to agency policy.	____	____	____	_____
D. Assess patency and integrity of system when alarm sounds.	____	____	____	_____
13. Follow this procedure for volume control device:				
A. Place volume control device between IV bag and insertion spike of infusion set.	____	____	____	_____

Continued

	S	U	NP	Comments

B. Place 2 hours' allotment of fluid into device. ____ ____ ____ _____

C. Assess system at least hourly. Add fluid to volume control device as needed. Regulate flow rate. ____ ____ ____ _____

14. Observe client for signs of overhydration or dehydration. ____ ____ ____ _____

15. Evaluate client for signs of infiltration: inflammation at site, clot in catheter, kink or knot in infusion tubing. ____ ____ ____ _____

16. Record and report solutions, infusion rates, use of electronic infusion device, and client's responses. ____ ____ ____ _____

PROCEDURE PERFORMANCE CHECKLIST
Skill 40-3 Maintenance of IV System

	S	U	NP	Comments
Changing intravenous (IV) solution:				
1. Check prescriber's orders. Clarify rate, if necessary.	___	___	___	_____
2. Note date and time solution was last changed.	___	___	___	_____
3. Determine compatibility of IV fluids and additives.	___	___	___	_____
4. Determine client's understanding of need for continued IV therapy.	___	___	___	_____
5. Assess patency of current IV access site.	___	___	___	_____
6. Prepare next solution at least 1 hour before needed. Check that solution is correct and properly labeled. Check solution expiration date.	___	___	___	_____
7. Prepare to change solution when less than 50 ml of fluid remains in bottle or bag.	___	___	___	_____
8. Explain procedure to client.	___	___	___	_____
9. Keep drip chamber at least half full.	___	___	___	_____
10. Perform hand hygiene.	___	___	___	_____
11. Prepare new solution for changing. Remove protective cover from IV tubing port.	___	___	___	_____
12. Move roller clamp to stop flow rate.	___	___	___	_____
13. Remove old IV fluid container from IV pole.	___	___	___	_____
14. Remove spike from old solution bag or bottle and, without touching tip, insert spike into new bag or bottle.	___	___	___	_____
15. Hang new bag or bottle of solution.	___	___	___	_____
16. Check for air in tubing. Remove bubbles in tubing: Insert a needle and syringe into a port below the air and aspirate into the syringe. Swab port with alcohol and allow to dry before inserting needle into port.	___	___	___	_____
17. Keep drip chamber one-third to one-half full. If the drip chamber is too full, pinch off tubing below the drip chamber, invert the container, squeeze the drip chamber, hang up the bottle, and release the tubing.	___	___	___	_____
18. Regulate flow to prescribed rate.	___	___	___	_____
19. Label time tape and place on bag.	___	___	___	_____
20. Observe client for signs of overhydration or dehydration.	___	___	___	_____
21. Observe IV system for patency and development of complications.	___	___	___	_____

Continued

	S	U	NP	Comments

Changing infusion tubing:

22. Determine when new infusion set is needed. Observe for occlusions in tubing. ____ ____ ____ _____

23. Explain procedure to client. ____ ____ ____ _____

24. Perform hand hygiene. ____ ____ ____ _____

25. Open new infusion set, keeping protective coverings over infusion spike and connector site for butterfly needle or IV catheter. ____ ____ ____ _____

26. Apply nonsterile disposable gloves. ____ ____ ____ _____

27. Remove IV dressing. Do not remove tape securing needle or catheter to skin. Anchor catheter during disconnection. ____ ____ ____ _____

28. For IV infusion:
    A. Move roller clamp on new IV tubing to "off" position. ____ ____ ____ _____
    B. Slow rate of infusion by regulating drip rate on old tubing. Maintain keep vein open (KVO) rate. ____ ____ ____ _____
    C. Compress and fill drip chamber. ____ ____ ____ _____
    D. Remove old tubing from solution and hang or tape drip chamber on IV pole 1 m above IV site. ____ ____ ____ _____
    E. Place insertion spike of new tubing into old solution bag opening and hang solution bag on IV pole. ____ ____ ____ _____
    F. Compress and release drip chamber on new tubing. Slowly fill drip chamber one-third to one-half full. ____ ____ ____ _____
    G. Slowly open roller clamp, remove protective cap from needle adapter, and flush tubing with solution. Replace cap. ____ ____ ____ _____
    H. Turn roller clamp on old tubing to "off" position. ____ ____ ____ _____

29. For heparin lock:
    A. Use sterile technique to connect the new injection cap to the loop or tubing. ____ ____ ____ _____
    B. Swab injection cap with antiseptic. Insert syringe with 1 to 3 ml saline and inject through the injection cap into the loop or short extension tubing. ____ ____ ____ _____

30. Stabilize hub of catheter or needle and apply pressure over vein just above insertion site. Gently disconnect old tubing. Maintain stability of hub and quickly insert needle adapter of new tubing or heparin lock into hub. ____ ____ ____ _____

31. Open roller clamp on new tubing. Allow solution to run rapidly for 30 to 60 seconds. ____ ____ ____ _____

Continued

	S	U	NP	Comments
32. Regulate IV drip according to orders and monitor rate hourly.	____	____	____	_____
33. Apply new dressing if necessary.	____	____	____	_____
34. Discard old tubing in proper container.	____	____	____	_____
35. Remove and dispose of gloves.	____	____	____	_____
36. Perform hand hygiene. Evaluate flow rate and observe connection site for leakage.	____	____	____	_____
37. Record changing of tubing and solution.	____	____	____	_____
38. Place a piece of tape or preprinted label with the date and time of tubing change and attach to tubing below level of drip chamber.	____	____	____	_____

Discontinuing peripheral IV access:

	S	U	NP	Comments
39. Check physicians order for discontinuing IV.	____	____	____	_____
40. Explain procedure to client.	____	____	____	_____
41. Perform hand hygiene and apply disposable gloves.	____	____	____	_____
42. Turn IV tubing roller clamp to "off" position.	____	____	____	_____
43. Remove tape securing tubing. Remove IV site dressing and tape while stabilizing catheter.	____	____	____	_____
44. With dry gauze or alcohol swab held over site, apply light pressure and withdraw the catheter, using a slow steady movement, keeping the hub parallel to the skin.	____	____	____	_____
45. Apply pressure to the site for 2 or 3 minutes, using the dry, sterile gauze pad. Secure with tape.	____	____	____	_____
46. Inspect the catheter for intactness, noting tip integrity and length.	____	____	____	_____
47. Discard used supplies.	____	____	____	_____
48. Remove and discard gloves, and perform hand hygiene.	____	____	____	_____
49. Instruct client to report any redness, pain, drainage, or swelling that may occur after catheter removal.	____	____	____	_____
50. Record discontinuation of IV.	____	____	____	_____

STUDENT: _____ DATE: _____

INSTRUCTOR: _____ DATE: _____

Skill 40-4 Changing a Peripheral Intravenous Dressing

	S	U	NP	Comments
1. Determine when dressing was last changed.	____	____	____	_____
2. Perform hand hygiene. Observe present dressing for moisture and intactness.	____	____	____	_____
3. Observe intravenous (IV) system for proper functioning. Palpate the catheter site through the intact dressing for inflammation or discomfort.	____	____	____	_____
4. Inspect exposed catheter site for swelling or infiltration.	____	____	____	_____
5. Assess client's understanding of need for continued IV infusion.	____	____	____	_____
6. Explain procedure to client and family.	____	____	____	_____
7. Perform hand hygiene. Apply disposable gloves.	____	____	____	_____
8. Remove tape, gauze, and/or transparent dressing from old dressing one layer at a time, leaving tape that secures the IV needle in place or holding that needle in place.	____	____	____	_____
9. Observe insertion site for signs and/or symptoms of infection.	____	____	____	_____
10. Discontinue infusion if necessary.	____	____	____	_____
11. Remove tape securing needle or catheter. Stabilize needle or catheter with one finger. Use adhesive remover to cleanse skin and remove adhesive residue, if needed.	____	____	____	_____
12. Keep one finger over catheter at all times until tape or dressing is replaced.	____	____	____	_____
13. Cleanse peripheral IV insertion site with alcohol and then with povidone-iodine solution starting at insertion site and working outward, creating concentric circles. Allow each solution to dry for 2 minutes.	____	____	____	_____
14. Apply new transparent or gauze dressing.	____	____	____	_____
15. Remove and discard gloves.	____	____	____	_____
16. Anchor IV tubing with additional pieces of tape. Minimize tape placed over polyurethane dressing.	____	____	____	_____
17. Write date and time of dressing change and size and gauge of catheter directly on dressing.	____	____	____	_____
18. Discard equipment and perform hand hygiene.	____	____	____	_____
19. Observe functioning and patency of IV system in response to changing dressing.	____	____	____	_____
20. Monitor client's body temperature.	____	____	____	_____
21. Record appearance of IV site, dressing, and status of IV.	____	____	____	_____

PROCEDURE PERFORMANCE CHECKLIST

Skill 43-1 Inserting a Small-Bore Nasoenteric Tube for Enteral Feedings

	S	U	NP	Comments
1. Assess client for the need for enteral tube feeding.	____	____	____	_____
2. Review client's medical history for nasal problems and risk of aspiration.	____	____	____	_____
3. Review prescriber's order for type of tube and enteral feeding schedule.	____	____	____	_____
4. Perform hand hygiene.	____	____	____	_____
5. Assess patency of nares. Close each of client's nostrils alternately, and ask client to breathe.	____	____	____	_____
6. Assess for gag reflex.	____	____	____	_____
7. Auscultate for bowel sounds.	____	____	____	_____
8. Explain procedure to client.	____	____	____	_____
9. Stand on same side of bed as nares for insertion. Assist client to high-Fowler's position unless contraindicated. Place pillow behind client's head and shoulders.	____	____	____	_____
10. Place bath towel over client's chest. Keep facial tissues within reach.	____	____	____	_____
11. Determine length of tube to be inserted and mark with tape: Measure distance from tip of client's nose to earlobe to xiphoid process of sternum.	____	____	____	_____
12. Prepare nasogastric or nasointestinal tube for intubation:				
A. Do not ice plastic tubes.	____	____	____	_____
B. Inject 10 ml of water from 30 ml or larger Luer-Lok or catheter-tip syringe into the tube.	____	____	____	_____
C. Make certain that guidewire is securely positioned against weighted tip and that both Luer-Lok connections are snugly fitted together.	____	____	____	_____
13. Cut tape 10 cm long or prepare tube fixation device.	____	____	____	_____
14. Apply disposable gloves.	____	____	____	_____
15. Dip tube with surface lubricant into glass of water.	____	____	____	_____
16. Insert tube through client's nostril to back of throat. Aim back and down toward ear.	____	____	____	_____
17. Have client flex head toward chest after tube has passed through nasopharynx.	____	____	____	_____
18. Emphasize client's need to breathe through mouth and swallow during procedure.	____	____	____	_____

Continued

	S	U	NP	Comments

19. When tip of tube reaches carina (about 10 inches (25 cm), stop, hold end of twice near ear and listen for air exchange. ____ ____ ____ _____

20. Advance tube each time client swallows until desired length has been passed. Do not force tube. If resistance is met or client starts to cough, choke, or become cyanotic, stop advancing the tube and pull it back. ____ ____ ____ _____

21. Check for position of tube in back of throat with penlight and tongue blade. ____ ____ ____ _____

22. Perform measures to verify placement of tube: ____ ____ ____ _____

23. Anchor tube to nose, avoiding pressure on nares. Mark exit site with indelible ink. ____ ____ ____ _____
   A. Apply tape.
     (1) Apply tincture of benzoin or other skin adhesive on tip of client's nose and tube. Allow to become "tacky." ____ ____ ____ _____
     (2) Remove gloves and split one end of tape lengthwise 5 cm. ____ ____ ____ _____
     (3) Place the intact end of tape over bridge of client's nose. Wrap each of the 5 cm strips around tube as it exits client's nose. ____ ____ ____ _____
   B. Apply tube fixation device.
     (1) Apply wide end of adhesive patch to nose. ____ ____ ____ _____
     (2) Slip connector around tube as it exits nose. ____ ____ ____ _____

24. Fasten end of nasogastric tube to client's gown by looping rubber band around tube in slip knot. Pin rubber band to gown. ____ ____ ____ _____

25. For intestinal placement, position client on right side if possible until confirmation of placement. Otherwise, assist client to a comfortable position. ____ ____ ____ _____

26. Remove gloves. Dispose of equipment and perform hand hygiene. ____ ____ ____ _____

27. Obtain x-ray film of client's abdomen. ____ ____ ____ _____

28. Apply gloves and administer oral hygiene. Cleanse tubing at nostril. ____ ____ ____ _____

29. Inspect client's nares and oropharynx for any irritation after insertion. ____ ____ ____ _____

30. Ask if client feels comfortable. ____ ____ ____ _____

31. Observe client for gagging or any difficulty breathing. Auscultate lung sounds. ____ ____ ____ _____

32. Record and report type and size of tube insertion and position and client's tolerance of procedure. ____ ____ ____ _____

Continued

PROCEDURE PERFORMANCE CHECKLIST
Skill 43-2 Administering Enteral Tube Feedings via Nasoenteric Tubes

	S	U	NP	Comments
1. Assess client's need for enteral tube feedings.	____	____	____	_____
2. Obtain client's baseline weight and laboratory values. Assess client for fluid volume excess or deficit and electrolyte and metabolic abnormalities.	____	____	____	_____
3. Verify prescriber's order for formula, rate, route, and frequency of feeding.	____	____	____	_____
4. Explain procedure to client.	____	____	____	_____
5. Perform hand hygiene.	____	____	____	_____
6. Auscultate client for bowel sounds before feeding.	____	____	____	_____
7. Prepare feeding container to administer formula:				
A. Check expiration date of formula.	____	____	____	_____
B. Have formula at room temperature.	____	____	____	_____
C. Connect tubing to container as needed or prepare ready-to-hang container.	____	____	____	_____
D. Shake formula container well and fill container and tubing with formula.	____	____	____	_____
8. Have syringe and formula ready for intermittent feeding.	____	____	____	_____
9. Place client in high-Fowler's position or elevate head of bed 30 degrees.	____	____	____	_____
10. Determine tube placement.	____	____	____	_____
11. Check for gastric residual.	____	____	____	_____
12. Flush tubing with 30 ml water.	____	____	____	_____
13. Initiate feeding:				
A. Syringe or intermittent feeding:				
(1) Pinch proximal end of feeding tube.	____	____	____	_____
(2) Remove plunger from syringe and attach barrel of syringe to end of tube.	____	____	____	_____
(3) Fill syringe with measured amount of formula. Release tube and hold syringe high enough to allow it to be emptied gradually by gravity. Refill. Repeat until prescribed amount has been delivered to the client.	____	____	____	_____
(4) If feeding bag is used, hang feeding bag on IV pole. Fill bag with prescribed amount of formula and allow bag to empty gradually over at least 30 minutes.	____	____	____	_____

Continued

	S	U	NP	Comments

B. Continuous-drip method:
   (1) Hang feeding bag and tubing on IV pole. _____ _____ _____ _____
   (2) Connect distal end of tubing to the proximal end of the feeding tube. _____ _____ _____ _____
   (3) Connect tubing through infusion pump and set rate. _____ _____ _____ _____

14. Advance tube feeding gradually per guidelines. _____ _____ _____ _____

15. Flush tubing with water after completion of bolus or intermittent feeding unless contraindicated. _____ _____ _____ _____

16. When tube feedings are not being administered, cap or clamp the proximal end of the feeding tube. _____ _____ _____ _____

17. Rinse bag and tubing with warm water whenever feedings are interrupted. _____ _____ _____ _____

18. Change bag and tubing every 24 hours. _____ _____ _____ _____

19. Measure amount of aspirate every 4 hours. _____ _____ _____ _____

20. Monitor client's finger-stick blood glucose every 6 hours until maximum administration is reached and maintained for 24 hours. _____ _____ _____ _____

21. Monitor client's intake and output every 24 hours. _____ _____ _____ _____

22. Weigh client daily until maximum administration rate is reached and maintained for 24 hours, then weigh client three times per week. _____ _____ _____ _____

23. Observe return of normal laboratory values. _____ _____ _____ _____

24. Record and report type of feeding, status of feeding tube, client's tolerance, and adverse effects. _____ _____ _____ _____

PROCEDURE PERFORMANCE CHECKLIST

Skill 43-3 Administering Enteral Feedings via Gastrostomy or Jejunostomy Tube

	S	U	NP	Comments
1. Assess client's need for enteral tube feedings.	___	___	___	_____
2. Verify order for formula, rate, route, and frequency.	___	___	___	_____
3. Assess gastrostomy/jejunostomy site for integrity.	___	___	___	_____
4. Explain procedure to client.	___	___	___	_____
5. Auscultate client for bowel sounds before feeding. Consult physician if bowel sounds are absent.	___	___	___	_____
6. Obtain client's baseline weight and laboratory values.	___	___	___	_____
7. Perform hand hygiene.	___	___	___	_____
8. Prepare feeding container to administer formula:				
A. Have formula at room temperature.	___	___	___	_____
B. Connect tubing to container as needed or prepare ready-to-hang bag.	___	___	___	_____
C. Shake formula well. Fill container and tubing with formula.	___	___	___	_____
9. Have syringe and formula ready for intermittent feeding.	___	___	___	_____
10. Elevate head of bed 30 to 45 degrees.	___	___	___	_____
11. Apply clean gloves. Verify tube placement:				
A. Gastrostomy tube: Aspirate client's gastric secretions and check appearance and pH. Return aspirated contents unless the volume exceeds 100 ml.	___	___	___	_____
B. Jejunostomy tube: Aspirate client's intestinal secretions and check appearance and pH.	___	___	___	_____
12. Flush tube with 30 ml of water.	___	___	___	_____
13. Initiate feedings:				
A. Syringe feedings:				
(1) Pinch proximal end of gastrostomy/jejunostomy tube.	___	___	___	_____
(2) Remove plunger and attach barrel of syringe to end of tube, then fill syringe with formula.	___	___	___	_____
(3) Release tube and elevate syringe. Allow syringe to empty gradually by gravity. Refill until prescribed amount of formula has been delivered to client.	___	___	___	_____

Continued

	S	U	NP	Comments

B. Continuous-drip feedings:
   (1) Fill feeding container with enough formula for length of feeding. _____ _____ _____ _____
   (2) Hang container into IV pole and clear tubing of air. _____ _____ _____ _____
   (3) Thread tubing into pump according to manufacturer's directions. _____ _____ _____ _____
   (4) Connect tubing to end of feeding tube. _____ _____ _____ _____
   (5) Begin infusion at prescribed rate. _____ _____ _____ _____

14. Administer water via tube as ordered. _____ _____ _____ _____

15. Flush tube with 30 ml water every 4 to 6 hours and before and after medication administration. _____ _____ _____ _____

16. Cap or clamp proximal end of tube between feedings. _____ _____ _____ _____

17. Rinse container and tubing after intermittent feedings. _____ _____ _____ _____

18. Assess client's skin around tube exit site. Cleanse skin daily with warm water and mild soap. Dressings around the exit site are not recommended.

19. Dispose of supplies and perform hand hygiene. _____ _____ _____ _____

20. Measure the amount of aspirate every 4 hours. _____ _____ _____ _____

21. Evaluate client's tolerance to feeding. Monitor client's finger-stick blood glucose every 6 hours until maximum administration rate is reached and maintained for 24 hours. _____ _____ _____ _____

22. Monitor intake and output every 24 hours. _____ _____ _____ _____

23. Weigh client daily until maximum administration rate is reached and maintained for 24 hours, then weigh client three times per week. _____ _____ _____ _____

24. Observe return of normal laboratory values. _____ _____ _____ _____

25. Inspect stoma site for integrity. _____ _____ _____ _____

26. Record and report amount and type of feeding, status of tube, client's tolerance, and any adverse effects. _____ _____ _____ _____

STUDENT: _____ DATE: _____

INSTRUCTOR: _____ DATE: _____

Skill 44-1 Collecting a Midstream (Clean-Voided) Urine Specimen

	S	U	NP	Comments
1. Assess client's voiding status.	___	___	___	_____
2. Assess client's understanding of procedure.	___	___	___	_____
3. Explain procedure to client.	___	___	___	_____
4. Provide fluids a half-hour before collecting specimen, unless contraindicated.	___	___	___	_____
5. Provide privacy.	___	___	___	_____
6. Have client cleanse perineal area, or assist client with this process.	___	___	___	_____
7. Perform hand hygiene and apply nonsterile gloves. Assist female client onto bedpan if nonambulatory.	___	___	___	_____
8. Change gloves if necessary.	___	___	___	_____
9. Open sterile kit and prepare appropriately. Open specimen container. Place cap with inside surface facing up. Apply sterile gloves.	___	___	___	_____
10. Pour antiseptic over cotton balls or gauze.	___	___	___	_____
11. Assist or allow client to cleanse perineal area and collect specimen:	___	___	___	_____
A. Female client:				
(1) Cleanse client's perineal area. Rinse and dry per agency policy.	___	___	___	_____
(2) After client begins urinating, pass container into stream and collect 30 to 60 ml of urine.	___	___	___	_____
B. Male client:				
(1) Cleanse client's penis. Rinse and dry per agency policy.	___	___	___	_____
(2) After client begins urinating, pass container into stream and collect 30 to 60 ml of urine.	___	___	___	_____
12. Remove container before urine flow stops.	___	___	___	_____
13. Place cap on container.	___	___	___	_____
14. Cleanse urine from outside of container. Place container in plastic specimen bag.	___	___	___	_____
15. Remove bedpan (if applicable) and assist client to a comfortable position.	___	___	___	_____
16. Label specimen and attach laboratory requisition slip.	___	___	___	_____
17. Remove and dispose of gloves and perform hand hygiene.	___	___	___	_____
18. Take specimen to laboratory within 15 minutes or refrigerate.	___	___	___	_____
19. Record date and time specimen was obtained.	___	___	___	_____

Continued

STUDENT: _____ DATE: _____

INSTRUCTOR: _____ DATE: _____

Skill 44-2 Inserting a Straight or an Indwelling Catheter

	S	U	NP	Comments
1. Assess client's urinary status.	____	____	____	_____
2. Review client's medical record.	____	____	____	_____
3. Assess client's knowledge of the purpose of catheterization.	____	____	____	_____
4. Explain procedure to client.	____	____	____	_____
5. Arrange for assistance if necessary.	____	____	____	_____
6. Perform hand hygiene.	____	____	____	_____
7. Provide privacy.	____	____	____	_____
8. Raise bed to appropriate working height.	____	____	____	_____
9. Stand on left side of bed if right-handed (or vice versa). Clear bedside table and arrange equipment.	____	____	____	_____
10. Raise side rail on opposite side of bed, and put side rail down on working side.	____	____	____	_____
11. Place waterproof pad under client.	____	____	____	_____
12. Position client:	____	____	____	_____
A. Female client:				
(1) Assist client to dorsal recumbent position. Ask client to relax thighs so hip joints can be externally rotated.	____	____	____	_____
(2) Position client in side-lying position with upper leg flexed at knee and hip if client cannot be in dorsal recumbent position.	____	____	____	_____
B. Male client: Assist client to supine position with thighs slightly abducted.	____	____	____	_____
13. Drape client:				
A. Female client: Diamond-drape client.	____	____	____	_____
B. Male client: Drape client's upper trunk with bath blanket and cover lower extremities with bed sheets so only genitalia are exposed.	____	____	____	_____
14. Apply disposable gloves. Wash client's perineal area with soap and water as needed. Dry area thoroughly. Remove gloves and discard. Perform hand hygiene.	____	____	____	_____
15. Position light to illuminate perineal area.	____	____	____	_____
16. Open package containing drainage system. Place drainage bag over edge of bottom of bed frame, and bring drainage tube up between side rail and mattress (indwelling catheter only).	____	____	____	_____
17. Open catheterization kit according to directions, keeping bottom container sterile.	____	____	____	_____
18. Place plastic bag that contained kit to use for waste disposal.	____	____	____	_____

Continued

	S	U	NP	Comments

19. Apply sterile gloves.

20. Organize supplies on sterile field. Open inner sterile package containing catheter. Pour sterile antiseptic solution into correct compartment containing sterile cotton balls. Open packet containing lubricant. Remove specimen container (lid should be loosely placed on top) and prefilled syringe from collection compartment of tray, and set them aside on sterile field.

21. Test balloon by injecting fluid from prefilled syringe into balloon port.

22. Lubricate 2.5 to 5 cm (1-2 inches) of catheter for female clients and 12.5 to 17.5 cm (5-7 inches) for male clients.

23. Apply sterile drape:

   A. Female client:

     (1) Allow top edges of drape to form cuff over both gloved hands. Place drape down on bed between client's thighs. Slip cuffed edge just under client's buttocks.

     (2) Pick up fenestrated sterile drape and allow it to unfold without touching an unsterile object. Apply drape over client's perineum, exposing labia.

   B. Male client:

     (1) First method: Apply drape over client's thighs and under penis without completely opening fenestrated drape.

     (2) Second method: Apply drape over client's thighs just below penis. Pick up fenestrated sterile drape, allow it to unfold, and drape it over penis with fenestrated slit resting over penis.

24. Place sterile tray and contents on sterile drape between client's thighs. Open specimen container.

25. Cleanse urethral meatus:

   A. Female client:

     (1) Retract client's labia with nondominant hand to fully expose urethral meatus. Maintain position of nondominant hand throughout procedure.

     (2) With forceps, pick up cotton ball saturated with antiseptic solution and clean perineal area, wiping front to back from clitoris toward anus. Wipe along the far labial fold, near labial fold, and directly over center of urethral meatus.

Continued

478

	S	U	NP	Comments

B. Male client:

(1) Retract foreskin of client's penis with nondominant hand. Grasp penis at shaft just below glans. Retract urethral meatus between thumb and forefinger. Maintain nondominant hand in this position throughout procedure.   ____ ____ ____ _____

(2) With forceps, pick up cotton ball saturated with antiseptic solution and clean penis. Move cotton ball in circular motion from urethral meatus down to base of glans. Repeat cleansing three more times, using clean cotton ball each time.   ____ ____ ____ _____

26. Pick up catheter with gloved dominant hand 7.5 to 10 cm (3-4 inches) from catheter tip. Hold end of catheter loosely coiled in palm of dominant hand.   ____ ____ ____ _____

27. Insert catheter: ____ ____ ____ _____

A. Female client: ____ ____ ____ _____

(1) Ask client to bear down gently as if to void urine, and slowly insert catheter through urethral meatus.   ____ ____ ____ _____

(2) Advance catheter a total of 5 to 7.5 cm (2-3 inches) in adult or until urine flows out catheter's end. Advance catheter another 2.5 to 5 cm (1-2 inches) when urine appears. Do not force. Place end of catheter in urine tray receptacle.   ____ ____ ____ _____

(3) Release labia and hold catheter securely with nondominant hand. Inflate balloon of retention catheter.   ____ ____ ____ _____

B. Male client:

(1) Lift client's penis to position perpendicular to client's body and apply light traction.   ____ ____ ____ _____

(2) Ask client to bear down as if to void urine, and slowly insert catheter through urethral meatus.   ____ ____ ____ _____

(3) Advance catheter 17 to 22.5 cm (7-9 inches) in adult or until urine flows out catheter's end. Withdraw catheter if resistance is felt. Advance catheter another 2.5 to 5 cm when urine appears. Do not force to insert catheter.   ____ ____ ____ _____

(4) Lower client's penis and hold catheter securely in nondominant hand. Place end of catheter in urine tray   ____ ____ ____ _____

Continued

	S	U	NP	Comments

receptacle. Inflate balloon of
retention catheter.

28. Collect urine specimen as needed. Fill
specimen cup or jar to desired level by
holding end of catheter in dominant hand
over cup.

29. Allow client's bladder to empty fully if
institution policy permits.

30. Remove straight, single-use catheter:
Withdraw catheter slowly but smoothly
until removed.

31. Indwelling catheter:
   A. Slowly inflate balloon with fluid from
      prefilled syringe.
   B. Release catheter with nondominant hand
      and pull gently to feel resistance.

32. Attach end of retention catheter to collecting
tube of drainage system. Keep drainage bag
below level of bladder. Do not place bag on
side rails of bed.

33. Anchor catheter, allowing sufficient slack for
client movement.
   A. Female client: Secure catheter tubing to
      client's inner thigh with strip of
      nonallergenic tape or tube holder.
   B. Male client: Secure catheter tubing to
      top of thigh or lower abdomen.

34. Assist client to a comfortable position.
Wash and dry client's perineal area as needed.

35. Dispose of equipment, drapes, and urine in
proper receptacles.

36. Remove and dispose of gloves.

37. Perform hand hygiene.

38. Palpate client's bladder.

39. Ask if client is comfortable.

40. Observe character and amount of urine in
drainage system.

41. Determine that no urine is leaking from
catheter or tubing connections.

42. Record and report catheterization,
characteristics and amount of urine, specimen
collection (if performed), and client's
response to procedure and teaching concepts.

43. Initiate intake and output records.

44. Report absence of urine immediately.

STUDENT: _____ DATE: _____

INSTRUCTOR: _____ DATE: _____

PROCEDURE PERFORMANCE CHECKLIST
Skill 44-3 Indwelling Catheter Care

	S	U	NP	Comments
1. Assess client for bowel incontinence or discomfort at catheter insertion site.	____	____	____	_____
2. Prepare equipment and supplies.	____	____	____	_____
3. Explain procedure to client.	____	____	____	_____
4. Provide privacy.	____	____	____	_____
5. Perform hand hygiene.	____	____	____	_____
6. Position client properly.	____	____	____	_____
7. Place waterproof pad under client.	____	____	____	_____
8. Drape client.	____	____	____	_____
9. Apply disposable gloves.	____	____	____	_____
10. Undo anchor tapes to free catheter tubing.	____	____	____	_____
11. Expose and assess client's urethral meatus.	____	____	____	_____
12. Cleanse client's perineal tissues with soap and water.				
A. Female client: Cleanse urinary meatus and labia. Clean toward anus. Move down catheter.	____	____	____	_____
B. Male client: Cleanse around catheter, then around meatus and glans in circular motion.	____	____	____	_____
13. Reassess client's meatus for discharge.	____	____	____	_____
14. With soap and water, wipe in a circular motion approximately 10 cm (4 inches) down the length of the catheter.	____	____	____	_____
15. Apply antibiotic ointment (if ordered) at meatus and along catheter. Reposition the foreskin for the uncircumsized male.	____	____	____	_____
16. Assist client to a comfortable position.	____	____	____	_____
17. Dispose of supplies and gloves.	____	____	____	_____
18. Perform hand hygiene.	____	____	____	_____
19. Record and report client's status.	____	____	____	_____

PROCEDURE PERFORMANCE CHECKLIST
Skill 44-4 Closed and Open Catheter Irrigation

	S	U	NP	Comments
1. Verify prescriber's order.	____	____	____	_____
2. Assess appearance and amount of client's urine.	____	____	____	_____
3. Determine type of catheter used.	____	____	____	_____
4. Determine patency of catheter.	____	____	____	_____
5. Measure urine in drainage bag.	____	____	____	_____
6. Explain procedure to client.	____	____	____	_____
7. Perform hand hygiene. Apply disposable gloves for closed method.	____	____	____	_____
8. Provide privacy.	____	____	____	_____
9. Assess client for bladder distention.	____	____	____	_____
10. Position client properly.	____	____	____	_____
11. Closed intermittent irrigation:				
A. Prepare solution and draw into syringe.	____	____	____	_____
B. Clamp indwelling catheter below injection port.	____	____	____	_____
C. Cleanse port with swab.	____	____	____	_____
D. Insert syringe at 30-degree angle.	____	____	____	_____
E. Slowly inject fluid into catheter and bladder.	____	____	____	_____
F. Withdraw syringe, remove clamp, and allow solution to drain into bag.	____	____	____	_____
12. Closed continuous irrigation:				
A. Using aseptic technique, insert tip of irrigation tubing into bag containing solution.	____	____	____	_____
B. Close clamp on tubing and hang solution on IV pole.	____	____	____	_____
C. Open clamp, allow solution to flow through tubing, and close clamp.	____	____	____	_____
D. Wipe off irrigation part of triple lumen catheter or attach sterile Y connector to double lumen catheter and then attach to irrigation tubing.	____	____	____	_____
E. Connect to irrigation tubing using a triple lumen catheter or Y connector to double lumen catheter. Connect tubing securely.	____	____	____	_____
F. For intermittent flow, clamp tubing on drainage, open irrigation tubing, allow prescribed amount to enter bladder, close irrigation clamp, and open drainage clamp.	____	____	____	_____

Continued

	S	U	NP	Comments
G. For continuous irrigation, calculate drip rate, adjust clamp on tubing, and establish security and patency of system.	___	___	___	_____
13. Open irrigation:				
A. Prepare sterile supplies.	___	___	___	_____
B. Apply sterile gloves.	___	___	___	_____
C. Position waterproof drape.	___	___	___	_____
D. Aspirate 30 ml of solution into sterile irrigating syringe.	___	___	___	_____
E. Move sterile collection close to client's thighs. Disconnect catheter from drainage tubing, allow urine to flow into basin, and cover open end of tubing with sterile cap.	___	___	___	_____
F. Insert syringe, gently instill solution, and withdraw syringe.	___	___	___	_____
G. Allow solution to drain into basin; repeat until drainage is clear.	___	___	___	_____
H. When irrigation is completed, reestablish closed drainage system.	___	___	___	_____
I. If solution does not return, have client change position, or gently aspirate solution.	___	___	___	_____
14. Reanchor catheter to client.	___	___	___	_____
15. Assist client to a comfortable position.	___	___	___	_____
16. Lower bed and raise side rails, if indicated.	___	___	___	_____
17. Dispose of supplies. Remove and dispose of gloves.	___	___	___	_____
18. Perform hand hygiene.	___	___	___	_____
19. Calculate irrigation fluid used and subtract from total drainage.	___	___	___	_____
20. Record and report type and amount of irrigation, character of drainage, and any unexpected findings.	___	___	___	_____

PROCEDURE PERFORMANCE CHECKLIST

Skill 45-1 Administering a Cleansing Enema

	S	U	NP	Comments
1. Assess status of client.	____	____	____	_____
2. Assess client for presence of increased intracranial pressure, glaucoma, or recent rectal or prostate surgery.	____	____	____	_____
3. Check client's medical record.	____	____	____	_____
4. Review prescriber's order for enema.	____	____	____	_____
5. Determine client's understanding of purpose of enema.	____	____	____	_____
6. Collect appropriate equipment.	____	____	____	_____
7. Identify client and explain procedure.	____	____	____	_____
8. Assemble enema bag with appropriate solution and rectal tube.	____	____	____	_____
9. Perform hand hygiene and apply gloves.	____	____	____	_____
10. Provide privacy.	____	____	____	_____
11. Raise bed to appropriate working height and raise side rail on client's left side.	____	____	____	_____
12. Assist client to left side-lying position with right knee flexed.	____	____	____	_____
13. Place waterproof pad under client's hips and buttocks.	____	____	____	_____
14. Cover client with bath blanket so that only rectal area is exposed and anus is clearly visible.	____	____	____	_____
15. Place bedpan or commode in easily accessible position.	____	____	____	_____
16. Administer enema:				
A. Enema bag:				
(1) Add warmed solution to enema bag. Warm tap water as it flows from faucet, place saline container in basin of hot water before adding saline to enema bag, and check temperature of solution.	____	____	____	_____
(2) Raise container, release clamp, and allow solution to flow long enough to fill tubing.	____	____	____	_____
(3) Reclamp tubing.	____	____	____	_____
(4) Lubricate 6 to 8 cm (2½ to 3 inches) of tip of rectal tube with lubricating jelly.	____	____	____	_____
(5) Gently separate client's buttocks and locate anus. Instruct client to relax by breathing out slowly through mouth.	____	____	____	_____

Continued

	S	U	NP	Comments

(6) Insert tip of rectal tube slowly by pointing tip in direction of client's umbilicus.

(7) Hold tubing in client's rectum constantly until end of fluid instillation.

(8) Open regulating clamp, and allow solution to enter slowly, with container at client's hip level.

(9) Raise enema container slowly to appropriate level above client's anus.

(10) Lower container or clamp tubing if client complains of cramping or if fluid escapes around rectal tube.

(11) Clamp tubing after all solution is instilled.

B. Prepackaged disposable container:

(1) Remove plastic cap from rectal tip.

(2) Gently separate client's buttocks and locate rectum. Instruct client to relax by breathing out slowly through mouth.

(3) Insert tip of bottle gently into rectum (7.5 to 10 cm in adult, 5 to 7.5 cm in child, 2.5 to 3.75 cm in infant).

(4) Squeeze bottle until all of solution has entered client's rectum and colon. Instruct client to retain solution until the urge to defecate occurs.

17. Place layers of toilet tissue around tube at anus and gently withdraw rectal tube.

18. Explain to client that feeling of distention is normal. Ask client to retain solution as long as possible while lying quietly in bed. If client is an infant or young child, gently hold client's buttocks together for a few minutes.

19. Discard enema container and tubing in receptacle, or rinse container thoroughly with soap and warm water if it is to be reused.

20. Assist client to bathroom or help position client on bedpan.

21. Observe character of client's feces and solution (caution client against flushing toilet before inspection).

22. Assist client as needed in washing anal area with warm soap and water.

23. Remove and discard gloves. Perform hand hygiene.

24. Inspect color, consistency, and amount of stool and fluid passed.

Continued

	S	U	NP	Comments
25. Assess condition of client's abdomen.	___	___	___	_____
26. Record type and volume of enema given and characteristics of results.	___	___	___	_____
27. Report to physician if client fails to defecate.	___	___	___	_____

STUDENT: _____ DATE: _____

INSTRUCTOR: _____ DATE: _____

PROCEDURE PERFORMANCE CHECKLIST
Skill 45-2 Inserting and Maintaining a Nasogastric Tube

	S	U	NP	Comments
1. Perform hand hygiene. Inspect condition of client's nasal and oral cavities.	____	____	____	_____
2. Ask if client has history of nasal surgery and note if deviated nasal septum is present.	____	____	____	_____
3. Palpate client's abdomen for distention, pain, and rigidity. Auscultate for bowel sounds.	____	____	____	_____
4. Assess client's level of consciousness and ability to follow instructions.	____	____	____	_____
5. Check medical record for prescriber's order, type of nasogastric (NG) tube to be placed, and whether tube is to be attached to suction or drainage bag.	____	____	____	_____
6. Prepare equipment at bedside.	____	____	____	_____
7. Explain procedure to client.	____	____	____	_____
8. Perform hand hygiene and apply disposable gloves.	____	____	____	_____
9. Position client in high-Fowler's position with pillow behind client's head and shoulders. Raise bed to a comfortable working level.	____	____	____	_____
10. Place bath towel over client's chest. Give facial tissues to client.	____	____	____	_____
11. Provide privacy.	____	____	____	_____
12. Stand on client's right side if you are right-handed and on left side if left-handed.	____	____	____	_____
13. Instruct client to relax and breathe normally while occluding one naris. Repeat this action for other naris. Select nostril with greater air flow.	____	____	____	_____
14. Measure distance to insert tube using traditional Hanson method.	____	____	____	_____
15. Mark length of tube to be inserted with small piece of tape placed so it can easily be removed.	____	____	____	_____
16. Curve 10 to 15 cm (5-6 inches) of end of tube tightly around index finger, then release.	____	____	____	_____
17. Lubricate 7.5 to 10 cm (3-4 inches) of end of tube with water-soluble lubricating jelly.	____	____	____	_____
18. Alert client that procedure is to begin.	____	____	____	_____
19. Instruct client to extend neck back against pillow. Insert tube slowly through naris, with curved end pointing downward.	____	____	____	_____

Continued

	S	U	NP	Comments

20. Continue to pass tube along floor of nasal passage, aiming down toward ear. When resistance is felt, apply gentle downward pressure to advance tube (do not force past resistance).

21. If resistance is met, try to rotate the tube and see if it advances. If there is still resistance, withdraw tube, allow client to rest, relubricate tube, and insert into client's other naris.

22. Continue insertion of tube until just past client's nasopharynx by gently rotating tube toward client's opposite naris.

   A. Stop tube advancement, allow client to relax, and provide tissues.

   B. Explain to client that next step requires that client swallow. Give client glass of water, unless contraindicated.

23. With tube just above client's oropharynx, instruct client to flex head forward, take a small sip of water, and swallow. Advance tube 2.5 to 5 cm with each swallow of water. If client is not allowed fluids, instruct client to dry swallow or suck air through straw.

24. If client begins to cough, gag, or choke, withdraw tube slightly and stop advancement. Instruct client to breathe easily and take sips of water. Pull tube back slightly if client continues to cough.

25. If client continues to gag, check back of pharynx using flashlight and tongue blade.

26. Continue to advance tube to the desired distance. Once tube is correctly advanced, remove tape used to mark length of tube and place the prepared split tape with nonsplit side on client's nose. Anchor tape with one of split ends while checking tube placement.

27. Check tube placement:

   A. Ask client to talk.

   B. Inspect posterior pharynx for presence of coiled tube.

   C. Aspirate gently back on syringe to obtain gastric contents. Observe color.

   D. Measure pH of aspirate with color-coded pH paper that has range of whole numbers from 1 to 11.

   E. If tube is not in client's stomach, advance it another 2.5 to 5 cm and repeat steps 27B through 27C.

Continued

	S	U	NP	Comments

28. Anchor the tube:
   A. Clamp end of tube or connect it to drainage bag or suction machine after insertion. ____ ____ ____ _____

   B. Tape tube to client's nose; avoid putting pressure on nares:
     (1) Apply small amount of tincture of benzoin to lower end of client's nose and allow to dry. Secure tape over client's nose. ____ ____ ____ _____

     (2) Carefully wrap two split ends of tape around tube. ____ ____ ____ _____

     (3) Alternatively, apply tube fixation device using shaped adhesive patch. ____ ____ ____ _____

   C. Fasten end of NG tube to client's gown by looping rubber band around tube in slip knot. Pin rubber band to gown. ____ ____ ____ _____

   D. Elevate head of bed 30 degrees, unless contraindicated. ____ ____ ____ _____

   E. Explain to client that sensation of tube should decrease somewhat with time. ____ ____ ____ _____

   F. Remove and dispose of gloves and perform hand hygiene. ____ ____ ____ _____

29. Identify tube placement in nose with mark or tape or measure length from nares to connector. ____ ____ ____ _____

30. Irrigate tube:
   A. Wash hands and apply disposable gloves. ____ ____ ____ _____

   B. Check for tube placement. Reconnect NG tube to connecting tube. ____ ____ ____ _____

   C. Draw up 30 ml of normal saline into regular or catheter-tipped syringe. ____ ____ ____ _____

   D. Clamp NG tube. Disconnect it from connection tubing and lay end of connection tubing on towel. ____ ____ ____ _____

   E. Insert tip of irrigating syringe into end of NG tube. Remove clamp. Hold syringe with tip pointed at floor and inject saline slowly and evenly. Do not force solution. ____ ____ ____ _____

   F. If resistance occurs, check for kinks in tubing. Turn client onto left side. ____ ____ ____ _____

   G. After instilling saline, immediately aspirate or pull back slowly on syringe to withdraw fluid. ____ ____ ____ _____

   H. Reconnect NG tube to drainage or suction. (If solution does not return, repeat irrigation). ____ ____ ____ _____

   I. Remove and dispose of gloves and perform hand hygiene. ____ ____ ____ _____

Continued

	S	U	NP	Comments

31. Discontinue NG tube:
    A. Verify order to discontinue NG tube. ____ ____ ____ _____
    B. Explain procedure to client and reassure
       client that removal is less distressing
       than insertion. ____ ____ ____ _____
    C. Perform hand hygiene and apply
       disposable gloves. ____ ____ ____ _____
    D. Turn off suction and disconnect NG tube
       from drainage bag or suction. Remove
       tape from bridge of client's nose and
       unpin tube from client's gown. ____ ____ ____ _____
    E. Stand on client's right side if you are
       right-handed and left side if you are
       left-handed. ____ ____ ____ _____
    F. Hand the client facial tissue. Place clean
       towel across client's chest. Instruct client
       to take and hold a deep breath. ____ ____ ____ _____
    G. Clamp or kink tubing securely and then
       pull tube out steadily and smoothly into
       towel held in other hand while client
       holds breath. ____ ____ ____ _____
    H. Measure amount of drainage and note
       character of content. Dispose of tube and
       drainage equipment. ____ ____ ____ _____
    I. Clean client's nares and provide mouth care. ____ ____ ____ _____
    J. Assist client to a comfortable position
       and explain procedure for drinking fluids,
       if not contraindicated. ____ ____ ____ _____
32. Clean equipment and return to proper place.
    Place soiled linen in proper receptacle. ____ ____ ____ _____
33. Remove and dispose of gloves and
    perform hand hygiene. ____ ____ ____ _____
34. Observe amount and character of contents
    draining from NG tube. Ask if client feels
    nauseated. ____ ____ ____ _____
35. Palpate client's abdomen periodically for
    distention, pain, and rigidity, and
    auscultate for the presence of bowel
    sounds. Turn off suction while auscultating. ____ ____ ____ _____
36. Inspect condition of client's nares and nose. ____ ____ ____ _____
37. Observe position of tubing. ____ ____ ____ _____
38. Ask if client's throat feels sore of if there
    is irritation in the pharynx. ____ ____ ____ _____
39. Record time and type of NG tube inserted,
    client's tolerance of procedure, confirmation
    of placement, character of client's gastric
    contents, pH value of contents, and
    whether tube is clamped or connected to
    drainage device. ____ ____ ____ _____

PROCEDURE PERFORMANCE CHECKLIST
Skill 45-3 Pouching an Ostomy

	S	U	NP	Comments
1. Auscultate client for bowel sounds.	___	___	___	_____
2. Perform hand hygiene. Observe client's skin barrier and pouch for leakage and length of time in place.	___	___	___	_____
3. Observe stoma for color, swelling, trauma, and healing.	___	___	___	_____
4. Measure the stoma with each pouching change.	___	___	___	_____
5. Observe client's abdominal incision (if present).	___	___	___	_____
6. Observe effluent from stoma and keep a record of intake and output. Ask client about skin tenderness.	___	___	___	_____
7. When assessing client's skin for irritation, check that the pouching system is not leaking.	___	___	___	_____
8. Avoid unnecessary changing of entire pouching system.	___	___	___	_____
9. Assess client's abdomen for best type of pouching system to use.	___	___	___	_____
10. Assess client's self-care ability.	___	___	___	_____
11. After skin barrier and pouch removal, assess client's skin around stoma.	___	___	___	_____
12. Determine client's emotional response and knowledge and understanding of an ostomy and its care.	___	___	___	_____
13. Explain procedure to client. Encourage client's interaction and questions.	___	___	___	_____
14. Assemble equipment. Provide privacy.	___	___	___	_____
15. Position client either standing, supine, or seated and drape client.	___	___	___	_____
16. Perform hand hygiene. Apply disposable gloves.	___	___	___	_____
17. Place towel or disposable waterproof barrier under client.	___	___	___	_____
18. Remove used pouch and skin barrier gently by pushing the skin away from the barrier.	___	___	___	_____
19. Cleanse client's peristomal skin gently with warm tap water using gauze pads or clean washcloth. Do not scrub the skin. Dry area completely by patting the skin with gauze or towel.	___	___	___	_____
20. Measure the stoma for correct size of pouching system needed.	___	___	___	_____

Continued

	S	U	NP	Comments

21. Select appropriate pouch for client based on assessment. With a custom cut-to-fit pouch, use an ostomy guide to cut opening 1/16 to 1/8 of an inch larger than stoma before removing backing. Prepare pouch by removing backing from barrier and adhesive. With ileostomy, apply thin circle of barrier paste around opening in pouch. Allow to dry.

22. Apply skin barrier and pouch. If creases occur next to stoma, use barrier paste to fill in; let dry 1 to 2 minutes.
   A. For one-piece pouching system:
      (1) Use skin sealant wipes on skin directly under adhesive skin barrier or pouch; allow to dry. Press the adhesive backing of the pouch and/or skin barrier smoothly against the skin, starting from the bottom and working up and around the sides.
      (2) Hold pouch by barrier, center over stoma, and press down gently on barrier. Bottom of pouch should point toward client's knees.
      (3) Maintain gentle finger pressure around barrier for 1 to 2 minutes.
   B. For two-piece pouching system: Apply flange as in steps above for one-piece system, then snap on pouch and maintain finger pressure.

23. Apply nonallergenic paper tape around pectin skin barrier using "picture frame" method. A belt may be attached for extra security, rather than tape.

24. A small amount of ostomy deodorant may be put in pouch.

25. Fold bottom of drainable open-ended pouches up once and close with closure device.

26. Properly dispose of old pouch and soiled equipment. Spray room deodorant if necessary.

27. Remove gloves and perform hand hygiene.

28. Change pouch every 3 to 7 days unless leaking.

29. Ask if client feels discomfort around stoma.

30. Note appearance of stoma skin and incision (if present).

Continued

	S	U	NP	Comments

31. Auscultate client for bowel sounds and observe characteristics of stool. ____ ____ ____ _____

32. Observe client's nonverbal behaviors as pouch is applied. Ask if client has any questions about pouching. ____ ____ ____ _____

33. Record type of pouch used and skin barrier applied. ____ ____ ____ _____

34. Record amount and appearance of client's stool and texture and condition of peristomal skin and sutures. ____ ____ ____ _____

35. Record and report abdominal distention and excessive tenderness, nature of client's bowel sounds, and any unexpected findings. ____ ____ ____ _____

36. Record client's level of participation and need for teaching. ____ ____ ____ _____

PROCEDURE PERFORMANCE CHECKLIST

Skill 46-1 Moving and Positioning Clients in Bed

	S	U	NP	Comments
1. Assess client's body alignment and comfort level while client is lying down.	____	____	____	_____
2. Assess client for risk factors that may contribute to complications of immobility.	____	____	____	_____
3. Assess client's physical ability to help with moving and positioning. Get extra help if needed.	____	____	____	_____
4. Check prescriber's order.	____	____	____	_____
5. Perform hand hygiene.	____	____	____	_____
6. Assess for presence of tubes, incisions, and equipment.	____	____	____	_____
7. Assess motivation of client and family.	____	____	____	_____
8. Raise bed to comfortable working height.	____	____	____	_____
9. Perform hand hygiene.	____	____	____	_____
10. Explain procedure to client.	____	____	____	_____
11. Position client flat, if tolerated.	____	____	____	_____
12. Position client in bed:				
A. Move immobile client up in bed (one nurse):	____	____	____	_____
(1) Place client on back with head of bed flat. Stand on one side of bed.	____	____	____	_____
(2) Remove pillow from under client's head and shoulders and place pillow at head of bed.	____	____	____	_____
(3) Begin at client's feet. Face foot of bed at 45-degree angle. Place feet apart with foot nearest head of bed behind other foot. Flex knees and hips as needed to bring arms level with client's legs. Shift weight from front to back leg, and slide client's legs diagonally toward head of bed.	____	____	____	_____
(4) Move parallel to client's hips. Flex knees and hips as needed to bring arms level with client's hips.	____	____	____	_____
(5) Slide client's hips diagonally toward head of bed.	____	____	____	_____
(6) Move parallel to client's head and shoulders. Flex knees and hips as needed to bring arms level with client's body.	____	____	____	_____
(7) Slide arm closest to head of bed under client's neck, and reach hand	____	____	____	_____

Continued

	S	U	NP	Comments

under client to support client's
shoulder.

    (8) Place other arm under client's
upper back. ___ ___ ___ _____

    (9) Slide client's trunk, shoulders, head,
and neck diagonally toward
head of bed. ___ ___ ___ _____

   (10) Elevate side rail. Move to other side
of bed and lower side rail. ___ ___ ___ _____

   (11) Repeat procedure, alternating sides
until client reaches desired position
in bed. ___ ___ ___ _____

   (12) Center client in middle of bed by
moving body in same three sections
as just described. ___ ___ ___ _____

B. Assist client to move up in bed (one or
two nurses):

    (1) Remove pillow from under client's
head and shoulders and place
pillow at head of bed. ___ ___ ___ _____

    (2) Face head of bed. ___ ___ ___ _____

       (a) Place one arm under client's
shoulders and one arm under
client's thighs. ___ ___ ___ _____

       (b) Alternative position: Position
one nurse at client's upper body.
That nurse will place arm nearest
head of bed under client's head
and opposite shoulder and other
arm under client's closest arm
and shoulder. Position other nurse
at client's lower torso. That nurse
will place arms under client's
lower back and torso. ___ ___ ___ _____

    (3) Place feet apart, with foot nearest
head of bed behind other foot. ___ ___ ___ _____

    (4) Flex knees and hips. Shift weight
from front to back leg, and move
client and draw sheet or pull sheet
to desired position in bed. ___ ___ ___ _____

    (5) Have client assist by pushing with
heels and elevating trunk, as able. ___ ___ ___ _____

C. Move immobile client up in bed with
drawsheet or pull sheet (two nurses):

    (1) Place drawsheet or pull sheet under
client by turning client side to side.
Drawsheet extends from shoulders
to thighs. Return to supine position. ___ ___ ___ _____

    (2) Position one nurse at each side of client. ___ ___ ___ _____

Continued

	S	U	NP	Comments
(3) Grasp drawsheet or pull sheet firmly near the client.	___	___	___	_____
(4) Place feet apart with forward-backward stance. Flex knees and hips. Shift weight from front to back leg, and move client and drawsheet or pull sheet to desired position in bed.	___	___	___	_____
(5) Realign client in correct body alignment.	___	___	___	_____

D. Position client in supported Fowler's position:

	S	U	NP	Comments
(1) Elevate head of bed 45 to 60 degrees.	___	___	___	_____
(2) Rest client's head against mattress or on small pillow.	___	___	___	_____
(3) Use pillows to support client's arms and hands if client does not have control of use of them.	___	___	___	_____
(4) Position pillow at client's lower back.	___	___	___	_____
(5) Place small pillow or roll under client's thigh.	___	___	___	_____
(6) Place small pillow or roll under client's ankles.	___	___	___	_____

E. Position hemiplegic client in supported Fowler's position:

	S	U	NP	Comments
(1) Elevate head of bed 45 to 60 degrees.	___	___	___	_____
(2) Position client in sitting position as straight as possible and support client's affected shoulder.	___	___	___	_____
(3) Position client's head on small pillow with chin slightly forward. Hyperextension of the neck must be avoided.	___	___	___	_____
(4) Provide support for client's involved arm and hand on overbed table in front of client. Place arm away from client's side and support elbow with pillow.	___	___	___	_____
(a) Position flaccid hand in normal resting position with wrist slightly extended, arches of hand maintained, and fingers partially flexed. Clasp client's hands together.	___	___	___	_____
(b) Position spastic hand with wrist in neutral position or slightly extended and fingers extended with palm down or left in relaxed position with palm up.	___	___	___	_____
(5) Flex client's knees and hips by placing pillow or folded blanket under client's knees.	___	___	___	_____

Continued

	S	U	NP	Comments

(6) Support client's feet in dorsiflexion with firm pillow, foot board, or high-top sneakers.

F. Position client in supine position:

(1) Place client on back, with head of bed flat.

(2) Place small rolled towel under lumbar area of client's back.

(3) Place pillow under client's upper shoulders, neck, or head.

(4) Place trochanter rolls or sandbags parallel to lateral surface of client's thighs.

(5) Place small pillow or roll under client's ankles to elevate heels.

(6) Place foot board or firm pillows against bottom of client's feet.

(7) Place high-top sneakers or foot splints on client's feet.

(8) Place pillows under client's pronated forearms, and keep client's upper arms parallel to client's body.

(9) Place hand rolls in client's hands.

G. Position hemiplegic client in supine position:

(1) Place client on back, with head of bed flat.

(2) Place folded towel or small pillow under client's shoulder or affected side.

(3) Keep affected arm away from client's body, with elbow extended and palm up.

(4) Place folded towel under client's hip on involved side.

(5) Flex client's affected knee 30 degrees by supporting it on a pillow or folded blanket.

(6) Support client's feet with soft pillows at right angle to leg.

H. Position client in prone position:

(1) With client supine, roll client over arm with arm positioned close to client's body, elbow straight, and hand under hip. Position client on abdomen in center of bed.

(2) Turn client's head to one side and support head with small pillow.

(3) Place small pillow under client's abdomen, below level of diaphragm.

Continued

	S	U	NP	Comments

(4) Support client's arms in flexed position level at shoulders.

(5) Support client's lower legs, and use pillow to elevate toes.

I. Position hemiplegic client in prone position:
   (1) Move client toward unaffected side.
   (2) Roll client onto side.
   (3) Place pillow on client's abdomen.
   (4) Roll client onto abdomen by positioning involved arm close to client's body with elbow straight and hand under hip. Roll client carefully over arm.
   (5) Turn client's head toward involved side.
   (6) Position client's involved arm out to side with elbow bent, hand toward head of bed, and fingers extended (if possible).
   (7) Flex client's knees slightly by placing pillow under client's legs from knees to ankles.
   (8) Keep client's feet at right angles to legs by using pillow high enough to keep toes off mattress.

J. Position client in lateral position:
   (1) Lower head of bed completely or as low as client can tolerate.
   (2) Position client to side of bed.
   (3) Turn client onto side.
   (4) Roll client onto side, toward you.
   (5) Place pillow under client's head and neck.
   (6) Bring client's shoulder blade forward.
   (7) Position both arms in slightly flexed position, with upper arm supported by pillow level and other arm by mattress.
   (8) Place tuck-back pillow behind client's back.
   (9) Place pillow under semiflexed upper leg for support.
   (10) Place sandbag parallel to plantar surface of client's dependent foot.

K. Position client in Sims' position:
   (1) Lower head of bed completely.
   (2) Place client in supine position.
   (3) Position client in lateral position, lying partially on abdomen.

Continued

	S	U	NP	Comments

(4) Carefully lift client's dependent shoulder and bring arm back behind client.

(5) Place small pillow under client's head.

(6) Place pillow under client's flexed upper arm to support arm on level with shoulder.

(7) Place pillow under client's flexed upper legs to support leg on level with hip.

(8) Place sandbags parallel to plantar surface of client's feet.

L. Logrolling the client (three nurses):

(1) Place pillow between client's knees.

(2) Cross client's arms over chest.

(3) Position two nurses on side of bed to which the client will be turned. Position third nurse on the other side of bed.

(4) Fanfold or roll the draw sheet.

(5) Move the client as one unit in a smooth, continuous motion on the count of three.

(6) Nurse on the opposite side of the bed places pillows along the length of the client.

(7) Gently lean the client as a unit back toward the pillows.

13. Perform hand hygiene.

14. Evaluate client's comfort level and ability to assist in position change.

15. Evaluate client's body alignment and presence of any pressure areas.

16. Record each position change and include amount of assistance needed and client's response and tolerance.

17. Record and report any signs of redness (e.g., in areas over bony prominences).

PROCEDURE PERFORMANCE CHECKLIST

Skill 46-2 Using Safe and Effective Transfer Techniques

	S	U	NP	Comments
1. Assess client's neuromuscular and sensory status.	___	___	___	_____
2. Assess previous mode of transfer.	___	___	___	_____
3. Determine special transfer equipment needed for home.	___	___	___	_____
4. Assess client's level of motivation.	___	___	___	_____
5. Identify client's risks for problems with transferring.	___	___	___	_____
6. Perform hand hygiene.	___	___	___	_____
7. Explain procedure to client.	___	___	___	_____
8. Provide privacy.	___	___	___	_____
9. Transfer client:				
A. Assist client to sitting position (bed at waist level):				
(1) Place client in supine position.	___	___	___	_____
(2) Face head of bed and remove pillows.	___	___	___	_____
(3) Place feet apart, with foot nearer bed behind other foot.	___	___	___	_____
(4) Place hand farther from client under client's shoulders and support client's head and cervical vertebrae.	___	___	___	_____
(5) Place other hand on bed surface.	___	___	___	_____
(6) Raise client to sitting position by shifting weight from front to back leg.	___	___	___	_____
(7) Push against bed using arm that is placed on bed surface.	___	___	___	_____
B. Assist client to sitting position on side of bed with bed in low position:				
(1) Turn client to side, facing you, on side of bed on which client will be sitting.	___	___	___	_____
(2) Raise head of bed 30 degrees.	___	___	___	_____
(3) Stand opposite client's hips. Turn diagonally so you face client and far corner of foot of bed.	___	___	___	_____
(4) Place feet apart, with foot closer to head of bed in front of other foot.	___	___	___	_____
(5) Place arm nearer head of bed under client's shoulder to support client's head and neck.	___	___	___	_____
(6) Place other arm over client's thighs.	___	___	___	_____
(7) Move client's lower legs and feet over side of bed. Pivot toward rear leg, allowing client's upper legs to swing downward.	___	___	___	_____

Continued

	S	U	NP	Comments
(8) Shift weight to rear leg and elevate client at the same time.	___	___	___	_____
(9) Remain in front of client until client regains balance.	___	___	___	_____
C. Transfer client from bed to chair with bed in low position:				
(1) Assist client to sitting position on side of bed. Position chair at 45-degree angle to bed.	___	___	___	_____
(2) Apply transfer belt of other transfer aids to client, if needed.	___	___	___	_____
(3) Ensure that client has stable, nonskid shoes. Place strong leg forward and weak leg back.	___	___	___	_____
(4) Spread feet apart.	___	___	___	_____
(5) Flex hips and knees, and align knees with client's knees.	___	___	___	_____
(6) Grasp transfer belt from underneath, if used, or reach through client's axillae and place hands on client's scapulas.	___	___	___	_____
(7) Rock client up to standing position on count of three while straightening hips and legs and keeping knees slightly flexed. Instruct client to use hands to push up, if able.	___	___	___	_____
(8) Maintain stability of client's weak or paralyzed leg with knee.	___	___	___	_____
(9) Pivot on foot farther from chair.	___	___	___	_____
(10) Instruct client to use armrests on chair for support, and ease client into chair.	___	___	___	_____
(11) Flex hips and knees while lowering client into chair.	___	___	___	_____
(12) Assess client for proper alignment for sitting position. Provide support for paralyzed extremities. Use lap board or sling to support flaccid arm. Stabilize legs with bath blanket or pillow.	___	___	___	_____
(13) Praise client's progress, effort, and performance.	___	___	___	_____
D. Perform three-person carry from bed to stretcher (bed at stretcher level):				
(1) Stand side by side with two other nurses, facing side of client's bed.	___	___	___	_____
(2) Assume responsibility for one of three areas: head and shoulders, hips, or thighs and ankles.	___	___	___	_____
(3) Assume wide base of support.	___	___	___	_____

Continued

	S	U	NP	Comments

(4) Lifters will place arms under client's head and shoulders, hips, and thighs and ankles, with fingers securely around other side of client's body.   ____ ____ ____ _____

(5) Lifters will roll client toward them. On count of three, lift client and hold against chest.   ____ ____ ____ _____

(6) On second count of three, all lifters step back and pivot toward stretcher, moving forward if needed.   ____ ____ ____ _____

(7) Lifters will lower client onto center of stretcher by flexing knees and hips until elbows are level with edge of stretcher.   ____ ____ ____ _____

(8) Assess client's body alignment, place safety straps across client's body, and raise side rails of bed.   ____ ____ ____ _____

E. Use mechanical/hydraulic lift to transfer client from bed to chair:

(1) Bring lift to bedside.   ____ ____ ____ _____

(2) Position chair near bed and allow adequate space to maneuver lift.   ____ ____ ____ _____

(3) Raise bed to high position, with mattress flat. Lower side rail.   ____ ____ ____ _____

(4) Keep bed side rail up on side opposite nurse.   ____ ____ ____ _____

(5) Roll client away from you.   ____ ____ ____ _____

(6) Place hammock or canvas strips under client to form sling; fit lower edge under client's knees and upper edge around client's shoulders.   ____ ____ ____ _____

(7) Raise side rail of bed.   ____ ____ ____ _____

(8) Go to opposite side of bed and lower side rail.   ____ ____ ____ _____

(9) Roll client to opposite side and pull hammock or canvas strips through.   ____ ____ ____ _____

(10) Roll client supine onto canvas seat.   ____ ____ ____ _____

(11) Remove client's glasses, if appropriate. Assess that any tubes remain intact and untangled.   ____ ____ ____ _____

(12) Place lift's horseshoe bar under side of bed (on side with chair).   ____ ____ ____ _____

(13) Lower horizontal bar to sling level by releasing hydraulic valve. Lock valve.   ____ ____ ____ _____

(14) Attach hooks on strap (chain) to holes in sling. Hook short chains or straps to top holes of sling, and hook longer chains to bottom of sling.   ____ ____ ____ _____

(15) Elevate head of bed.   ____ ____ ____ _____

Continued

	S	U	NP	Comments
(16) Fold client's arms over chest.	____	____	____	_____
(17) Pump hydraulic handle using long, slow, even strokes until client is raised off bed.	____	____	____	_____
(18) Use steering handle to pull lift from bed and maneuver to chair.	____	____	____	_____
(19) Roll base around chair.	____	____	____	_____
(20) Release check valve slowly and lower client into chair.	____	____	____	_____
(21) Close check valve as soon as client is down and straps can be released.	____	____	____	_____
(22) Remove straps and mechanical/ hydraulic lift.	____	____	____	_____
(23) Check client's sitting alignment.	____	____	____	_____
10. Perform hand hygiene.	____	____	____	_____
11. Assess client's tolerance and alignment with each transfer.	____	____	____	_____
12. Record each transfer and position change and client's response and tolerance.	____	____	____	_____
13. Record and report any signs of redness (e.g., over bony prominences).	____	____	____	_____

STUDENT: _____ DATE: _____

INSTRUCTOR: _____ DATE: _____

Skill 47-1 Assessment for Risk of Pressure Ulcer Development

	S	U	NP	Comments
1. Identify client's general risk for pressure ulcer formation.	____	____	____	_____
2. Determine client's ability to communicate discomfort.	____	____	____	_____
3. Assess extent that skin is exposed to moisture.	____	____	____	_____
4. Observe client's mobility and ability to initiate and assist with position changes.	____	____	____	_____
5. Assess food intake pattern.	____	____	____	_____
6. Evaluate presence of friction and/or shear.	____	____	____	_____
7. Document the risk assessment.	____	____	____	_____
8. Assess client's and family's understanding of risks for pressure ulcers.	____	____	____	_____
9. a. Observe client's skin for areas at risk for change in color or texture.	____	____	____	_____
b. Observe tolerance of client for position change.	____	____	____	_____
c. Monitor success of toileting program.	____	____	____	_____
d. Evaluate nutritional status and laboratory values.	____	____	____	_____
10. Compare client's subsequent risk assessment scores.	____	____	____	_____
11. Record and report client's risk assessment and any preventive measures used.	____	____	____	_____

PROCEDURE PERFORMANCE CHECKLIST
Skill 47-2 Treating Pressure Ulcers

	S	U	NP	Comments
1. Assess client's level of comfort and need for pain medication.	___	___	___	_____
2. Determine if client has allergies to topical agents.	___	___	___	_____
3. Review prescriber's order for topical agent or dressing.	___	___	___	_____
4. Provide privacy.	___	___	___	_____
5. Perform hand hygiene. Apply disposable gloves. Position client to allow dressing removal.	___	___	___	_____
6. Assess pressure ulcer and surrounding skin to determine ulcer stage:	___	___	___	_____
A. Note color, moisture, and appearance of skin around ulcer and of ulcer itself.	___	___	___	_____
B. Measure two maximum perpendicular diameters.	___	___	___	_____
C. Measure depth of pressure ulcer using sterile cotton-tipped applicator or other device.	___	___	___	_____
D. Measure depth of skin undermined by lateral tissue necrosis. Use a cotton-tipped applicator and gently probe under skin edges.	___	___	___	_____
7. Assess the periwound skin.	___	___	___	_____
8. Change to sterile gloves (check agency policy).	___	___	___	_____
9. Cleanse ulcer thoroughly with normal saline or cleansing agent: Use irrigating syringe for deep ulcers.	___	___	___	_____
10. Apply topical agents as prescribed:				
A. Enzymes:				
(1) Apply thin, even later of ointment over necrotic areas of ulcer only.	___	___	___	_____
(2) Apply gauze dressing directly over ulcer.	___	___	___	_____
(3) Tape dressing securely in place.	___	___	___	_____
B. Hydrogel:				
(1) Cover surface of ulcer with hydrogel using applicator or gloved hand.	___	___	___	_____
(2) Apply dry fluffy gauze or hydrocolloid or transparent dressing over hydrogel to completely cover ulcer.	___	___	___	_____
C. Calcium alginate:				
(1) Pack wound with alginate using applicator or gloved hand.	___	___	___	_____

Continued

	S	U	NP	Comments
(2) Apply dry gauze, foam, or hydrocolloid over alginate.	___	___	___	_____
11. Reposition client comfortably, off of pressure ulcer.	___	___	___	_____
12. Remove and dispose of gloves. Discard soiled supplies. Perform hand hygiene.	___	___	___	_____
13. Complete assessment for ulcer healing scale.	___	___	___	_____
14. Compare subsequent ulcer measurements.	___	___	___	_____
15. Do not use the pressure ulcer staging system to measure pressure ulcer healing.	___	___	___	_____
16. Record and report ulcer appearance and treatment.	___	___	___	_____

PROCEDURE PERFORMANCE CHECKLIST

Skill 47-3 Applying Dry and Wet-to-Dry Moist Dressings

	S	U	NP	Comments
1. Determine size and location of wound to be dressed.	____	____	____	_____
2. Assess client's level of comfort. Apply prescribed analgesic, if needed.	____	____	____	_____
3. Review orders for dressing change procedure.	____	____	____	_____
4. Explain procedure to client and instruct client not to touch wound area or sterile supplies.	____	____	____	_____
5. Provide privacy.	____	____	____	_____
6. Assist client to a comfortable position. Drape client with bath blanket to expose only wound site.	____	____	____	_____
7. Place disposable bag within reach of work area. Fold top of bag to make cuff.	____	____	____	_____
8. Apply face mask and protective eyewear, if required. Perform hand hygiene.	____	____	____	_____
9. Apply disposable gloves and remove tape, bandage, or ties from wound site.	____	____	____	_____
10. Remove tape: Pull parallel to skin, toward dressing, and remove remaining adhesive from client's skin.	____	____	____	_____
11. With gloved hand, carefully remove gauze dressings one layer at a time, taking care not to dislodge drains or tubes. Keep soiled undersurface away from client's sight. If dressing sticks on a wet-to-dry dressing, alert client of potential discomfort and gently free dressing.	____	____	____	_____
12. Observe character and amount of drainage on dressing and appearance of wound.	____	____	____	_____
13. Dispose of soiled dressings in disposable bag. Remove and dispose of gloves. Perform hand hygiene.	____	____	____	_____
14. Open sterile dressing tray or individually wrapped sterile supplies. Place on bedside table.	____	____	____	_____
15. Cleanse wound:				
A. Open bottle of cleansing solution (if ordered) and pour into sterile basin.	____	____	____	_____
B. Apply sterile gloves.	____	____	____	_____
C. Use syringe and allow solution to flow gently over wound. Continue until irrigation flow is clear.	____	____	____	_____
D. Dry surrounding skin.	____	____	____	_____

Continued

	S	U	NP	Comments

16. Apply sterile dressings:
   A. Dry dressing:
      (1) Apply sterile gloves.
      (2) Inspect wound.
      (3) Cleanse wound.
      (4) Dry area.
      (5) Apply sterile dressing.
      (6) Apply topper dressing, if needed.
   B. Wet-to-dry dressing:
      (1) Pour prescribed solution into sterile basin and add fine-mesh gauze.
      (2) Apply sterile gloves.
      (3) Inspect wound for color, character of drainage, type of sutures, and drains.
      (4) Cleanse wound with prescribed antiseptic solution or normal saline.
      (5) Apply moist fine-mesh gauze as a single layer directly onto wound surface. If wound is deep, gently pack gauze into wound with forceps.
      (6) Apply dry, sterile 4 x 4 gauze over wet gauze.
      (7) Cover with large dressing pads or gauze.

17. Apply tape over dressing, gauze roll, or dressing stabilizing or securing ties. For application of dressing stabilizing or securing ties:
   A. Expose adhesive surface of tape on end of each tie.
   B. Place ties on opposite sides of dressing.
   C. Place adhesive directly on skin or use skin barrier.
   D. Secure dressing by lacing ties across it.

18. Remove and dispose of gloves. Remove mask and eyewear.

19. Dispose of supplies and perform hand hygiene.

20. Assist client to a comfortable position.

21. Report brisk, bright-red bleeding or evidence of wound dehiscence or evisceration to physician immediately.

22. Record and report wound appearance, client's response, and characteristics of drainage at shift change.

PROCEDURE PERFORMANCE CHECKLIST

Skill 47-4 Implementation of Vacuum Assisted Closure

	S	U	NP	Comments
1. Position client comfortably. Drape to expose only wound site. Instruct client not to touch wound or sterile supplies.	___	___	___	_____
2. Perform hand hygiene. Place disposable waterproof bag within reach of work area with top folded to make a cuff.	___	___	___	_____
3. Push therapy "on/off" button.	___	___	___	_____
A. Apply gloves. Keeping tube connectors with VAC unit, disconnect tubes from each other to drain fluids into canister.	___	___	___	_____
B. Prior to lowering, tighten clamp on canister tube.	___	___	___	_____
4. With dressing tube unclamped, introduce 10 to 30 ml of normal saline, if ordered, into tubing to soak underneath foam.	___	___	___	_____
5. Gently stretch transparent film horizontally and slowly pull up from the skin.	___	___	___	_____
6. Remove old VAC dressing, observing appearance and drainage. Avoid tension on any drains that are present. Discard dressing and remove gloves.	___	___	___	_____
7. Apply sterile or clean gloves. Irrigate the wound with normal saline or other solution as ordered. Gently blot to dry.	___	___	___	_____
8. Measure wound as ordered. Remove and discard gloves.	___	___	___	_____
9. Apply new sterile or clean gloves.	___	___	___	_____
10. Prepare VAC foam:				
A. Select appropriate foam.	___	___	___	_____
B. Using sterile scissors, cut foam to wound size.	___	___	___	_____
11. Gently place foam in wound, being sure that foam is in contact with entire wound base, margins, and undermined areas.	___	___	___	_____
12. Apply transparent dressing over to foam and secure tubing to the unit.	___	___	___	_____
13. Apply skin protectant around the wound.	___	___	___	_____
14. Cover the VAC foam, 3 to 5 cm of surrounding tissue, and tubing with wrinkle-free transparent film to ensure an occlusive seal. Do not apply tension to drape and tubing.	___	___	___	_____
15. Secure tubing several centimeters away from the dressing.	___	___	___	_____

Continued

	S	U	NP	Comments

16. Connect the tubing from the dressing to the tubing from the canister and VAC unit:
    A. Remove canister from sterile packaging and push into VAC unit until a click is heard. An alarm will sound if the canister is not properly engaged. _____ _____ _____ _____
    B. Connect the dressing tubing to the canister tubing. Make sure both clamps are open. _____ _____ _____ _____
    C. Place VAC unit on a level surface or hand from the foot of the bed. The unit will alarm and deactivate therapy if the unit is tilted beyond 45 degrees. _____ _____ _____ _____
    D. Press in green-lit power button and set pressure as ordered. _____ _____ _____ _____
17. Discard old dressing materials, remove gloves, and perform hand hygiene. _____ _____ _____ _____
18. Inspect wound VAC system to verify that negative pressure is achieved: _____ _____ _____ _____
    A. Verify that display screen reads THERAPY ON. _____ _____ _____ _____
    B. Be sure that clamps are open and tubing is patent. _____ _____ _____ _____
    C. Identify air leaks by listening with stethoscope or by moving hand around edges of wound while applying light pressure. _____ _____ _____ _____
    D. Use strips of transparent film to patch areas where there are leaks. _____ _____ _____ _____
19. Compare appearance of wound with prior assessment. _____ _____ _____ _____
20. Verify airtight dressing seal and proper negative pressure. _____ _____ _____ _____
21. Identify unexpected outcomes and intervene as necessary. _____ _____ _____ _____
22. Record and report intervention and client's response. _____ _____ _____ _____

514

PROCEDURE PERFORMANCE CHECKLIST
Skill 47-5 Performing Wound Irrigation

	S	U	NP	Comments
1. Assess client's level of pain. Administer prescribed analgesic 30 to 45 minutes before starting wound irrigation procedure.	___	___	___	_____
2. Review client's record for prescription for irrigation of open wound.	___	___	___	_____
3. Assess signs and symptoms related to client's open wound.	___	___	___	_____
4. Explain procedure to client.	___	___	___	_____
5. Assist client to a comfortable position that will permit gravitational flow of irrigating solution through wound and into collection receptacle.	___	___	___	_____
6. Warm irrigation solution to approximate body temperature.	___	___	___	_____
7. Perform hand hygiene.	___	___	___	_____
8. Form cuff on waterproof bag and place it near bed.	___	___	___	_____
9. Provide privacy.	___	___	___	_____
10. Apply gown and goggles, if needed.	___	___	___	_____
11. Apply disposable gloves. Remove soiled dressing and discard in waterproof bag. Remove and dispose of gloves.	___	___	___	_____
12. Prepare equipment and open sterile supplies.	___	___	___	_____
13. Apply sterile gloves.	___	___	___	_____
14. Irrigate wound with wide opening:				
A. Fill 35 ml syringe with irrigation solution.	___	___	___	_____
B. Attach 19-gauge needle or angiocatheter.	___	___	___	_____
C. Hold syringe tip 2.5 cm (1 inch) above upper end of wound and over area being cleansed.	___	___	___	_____
D. Flush wound with continuous pressure.	___	___	___	_____
E. Repeat steps 17A(1) through 17A(4) until solution draining into basin is clear.	___	___	___	_____
15. Irrigate deep wound with very small opening:				
A. Attach soft angiocatheter to filled irrigating syringe.	___	___	___	_____

Continued

	S	U	NP	Comments

B. Lubricate tip of catheter with irrigating solution, then gently insert tip of catheter and pull out about 1 cm (1/2 inch).

C. Flush wound with slow continuous pressure.

D. Pinch off catheter just below syringe while keeping catheter in place.

E. Remove and refill syringe. Reconnect to catheter and repeat until solution draining into basin is clear.

16. Cleanse wound with hand-held shower:
   A. With client seated comfortably in shower chair, adjust spray to gentle flow; warm water temperature.
   B. Cover shower head with clean washcloth, if needed.
   C. Cleanse wound for 5 to 10 minutes with shower head 30 cm (12 inches) from wound.

17. Obtain cultures, if needed, after cleansing wound with nonbacteriostatic saline.

18. Dry wound edges with gauze; dry client if shower or whirlpool is used.

19. Apply appropriate dressing.

20. Remove gloves and, if worn, mask, goggles, and gown.

21. Assist client to a comfortable position.

22. Dispose of equipment and soiled supplies. Perform hand hygiene.

23. Assess type of tissue in wound bed.

24. Inspect dressing periodically.

25. Evaluate skin integrity.

26. Observe client for signs of discomfort.

27. Record wound irrigation and client response on progress notes.

28. Immediately report any evidence of fresh bleeding, sharp increase in pain, retention of irrigant, or signs of shock to attending physician.

29. Record and report expected and unexpected outcomes.

PROCEDURE PERFORMANCE CHECKLIST
Skill 47-6 Applying an Abdominal or Breast Binder

	S	U	NP	Comments
1. Observe client with need for support of thorax or abdomen. Observe client's ability to breathe deeply and cough effectively.	___	___	___	_____
2. Review client's medical record if particular binder is prescribed.	___	___	___	_____
3. Inspect client's skin for actual or potential alterations in integrity.	___	___	___	_____
4. Inspect client's surgical dressings, if any.	___	___	___	_____
5. Assess client's comfort level.	___	___	___	_____
6. Gather necessary data regarding size of client and appropriate binder.	___	___	___	_____
7. Explain procedure to client.	___	___	___	_____
8. Teach procedure to client or caregiver.	___	___	___	_____
9. Perform hand hygiene. Apply disposable gloves.	___	___	___	_____
10. Provide privacy.	___	___	___	_____
11. Apply binder:				
A. Abdominal binder:				
(1) Position client in supine position with head slightly elevated and knees slightly flexed.	___	___	___	_____
(2) Fanfold far side of binder toward midline of binder.	___	___	___	_____
(3) Assist client in rolling away from you and toward raised side rail while firmly supporting abdominal incision and dressing with hands.	___	___	___	_____
(4) Place fanfolded ends of binder under client.	___	___	___	_____
(5) Assist client in rolling over onto folded ends.	___	___	___	_____
(6) Unfold and stretch ends out smoothly on far side of bed.	___	___	___	_____
(7) Instruct client to roll back into supine position.	___	___	___	_____
(8) Adjust binder so that supine client is centered over binder using symphysis pubis and costal margins as lower and upper landmarks.	___	___	___	_____

Continued

	S	U	NP	Comments

(9) Close binder. Pull one end over center of client's abdomen. While maintaining tension on that end of binder, pull opposite end over center and secure with Velcro closure tabs, metal fasteners, or horizontally placed safety pins.

12. Assess client's comfort level.

13. Adjust binder as necessary.

    B. Breast binder:

    (1) Assist client in placing arms through binder's armholes.

    (2) Assist client to supine position in bed.

    (3) Pad area under client's breasts, if necessary.

    (4) Using Velcro closure tabs or horizontally placed safety pins, secure binder at nipple level first. Continue closure process above and then below nipple line until entire binder is closed.

    (5) Make appropriate adjustments, including individualizing fit of shoulder straps and pinning waistline darts to reduce binder size.

    (6) Instruct and observe client's skill development in self-care related to reapplying breast binder.

14. Remove and dispose of gloves. Perform hand hygiene.

15. Observe wound site for skin integrity, circulation, and characteristics.

16. Assess comfort level of client using analog scale of 0 to 10 and noting any objective signs and symptoms.

17. Assess client's ability to ventilate properly.

18. Identify client's need for assistance with daily activities.

19. Record and report application of binder, condition of client's skin, circulation, integrity of dressing, and client's comfort level.

20. Report ineffective lung expansion to physician immediately.

PROCEDURE PERFORMANCE CHECKLIST
Skill 47-7 Applying an Elastic Bandage

	S	U	NP	Comments
1. Perform hand hygiene and apply gloves, if necessary. Inspect client's skin for alterations in integrity.	____	____	____	_____
2. Inspect client's surgical dressing. Remove gloves and perform hand hygiene.	____	____	____	_____
3. Observe adequacy of client's circulation distal to bandage.	____	____	____	_____
4. Review client's medical record for specific orders related to application of elastic bandage.	____	____	____	_____
5. Identify client's and primary caregiver's present knowledge level and skill if bandaging will be continued when the client goes home.	____	____	____	_____
6. Explain procedure to client.	____	____	____	_____
7. Teach bandaging skill to client or caregiver.	____	____	____	_____
8. Perform hand hygiene. Apply disposable gloves if drainage is present.	____	____	____	_____
9. Provide privacy.	____	____	____	_____
10. Assist client to a comfortable position.	____	____	____	_____
11. Hold roll of elastic bandage in dominant hand and use other hand to lightly hold beginning of bandage at distal body part. Continue transferring roll to dominant hand as bandage is wrapped.	____	____	____	_____
12. Apply bandage from distal point toward proximal boundary using a variety of turns to cover various shapes of body parts.	____	____	____	_____
13. Unroll and very slightly stretch bandage.	____	____	____	_____
14. Overlap turns by one-half to two-thirds width of bandage roll.	____	____	____	_____
15. Secure first bandage with clip or tape before applying additional rolls. Apply additional rolls without leaving any uncovered skin surface. Secure final bandage applied.	____	____	____	_____
16. Remove and dispose of gloves and perform hand hygiene.	____	____	____	_____
17. Assess client's distal circulation when bandage application is complete and at least twice during each 8-hour period.	____	____	____	_____
18. Have client or caregiver demonstrate bandage application.	____	____	____	_____

Continued

19. Record and report condition of client's wound, integrity of dressing, application of bandage, client's circulation, and client's comfort level.

S   U   NP   Comments
___   ___   ___   _____

PROCEDURE PERFORMANCE CHECKLIST

Skill 47-8 Applying a Warm, Moist Compress to an Open Wound

	S	U	NP	Comments
1. Refer to client's record for compress order.	___	___	___	_____
2. Refer to client's medical record to identify any systemic contraindications to heat application.	___	___	___	_____
3. Perform hand hygiene.	___	___	___	_____
4. Inspect condition of client's exposed skin and wound on which compress is to be applied.	___	___	___	_____
5. Assess client's extremities for sensitivity to temperature and pain.	___	___	___	_____
6. Prepare equipment and supplies.	___	___	___	_____
7. Explain procedure and purpose to client. Describe sensations that will be felt, such as increasing warmth and wetness. Explain precautions to prevent burning.	___	___	___	_____
8. Provide privacy.	___	___	___	_____
9. Assist client to a comfortable position in proper body alignment. Place waterproof pad under part of client's body that will be treated.	___	___	___	_____
10. Expose client's body part that will be covered with the compress, and drape rest of client with bath blanket.	___	___	___	_____
11. Prepare compress:				
A. Pour solution into sterile container.	___	___	___	_____
B. If using portable heating source, warm solution. Open sterile packages and drop gauze into container to become immersed in solution.	___	___	___	_____
C. Adjust temperature of aquathermia pad.	___	___	___	_____
12. Apply disposable gloves. Remove any existing dressing covering wound. Dispose of gloves and dressings in proper receptacle.	___	___	___	_____
13. Assess condition of wound and surrounding skin.	___	___	___	_____
14. Apply sterile gloves.	___	___	___	_____
15. Pick up one layer of immersed gauze, wring out any excess solution, and apply gauze lightly to open wound.	___	___	___	_____
16. After a few seconds, lift edge of gauze to assess for redness.	___	___	___	_____
17. If client tolerates compress, pack gauze snugly against the wound. Cover all wound surfaces with hot compress.	___	___	___	_____

Continued

	S	U	NP	Comments

18. Cover moist compress with dry sterile dressing and bath towel. If necessary, pin or tie in place. Remove sterile gloves.

19. Apply aquathermia or waterproof heating pad over towel (optional). Keep in place for desired duration of application.

20. If an aquathermia pad is not used to maintain temperature of application, change hot compress using sterile technique every 5 minutes or as ordered during duration of therapy.

21. After prescribed time, apply disposable gloves and remove pad, towel, and compress. Reassess wound and condition of skin, and replace dry sterile dressing as ordered.

22. Assist client to preferred comfortable position.

23. Dispose of equipment and soiled compress. Perform hand hygiene.

24. Inspect area covered by compress and heating pad every 5 to 10 minutes.

25. Ask every 5 to 10 minutes if client notices an unusual burning sensation not felt before application of compress.

26. Have client explain and demonstrate application of compress.

27. Record type, location, and duration of application of compress. Note solution and temperature.

28. Record and report condition of wound and skin, treatment, instructions provided, and client's response to compress.

PROCEDURE PERFORMANCE CHECKLIST

Skill 49-1 Demonstrating Postoperative Exercises

	S	U	NP	Comments
1. Assess client for risk of postoperative respiratory complications.	____	____	____	_____
2. Assess client's ability to cough and deep breathe.	____	____	____	_____
3. Assess risk for postoperative thrombus formation.	____	____	____	_____
4. Assess client's ability to move independently while in bed.	____	____	____	_____
5. Explain purpose and importance of exercises.	____	____	____	_____
6. Demonstrate exercises:	____	____	____	_____
A. Diaphragmatic breathing				
(1) Assist client to comfortable sitting position on side of bed or in chair or standing position.	____	____	____	_____
(2) Stand or sit facing client.	____	____	____	_____
(3) Instruct client to place palms of hands across from each other, down and along lower borders of anterior rib cage. Place tips of third fingers lightly together. Demonstrate for client.	____	____	____	_____
(4) Have client take slow, deep breaths, inhaling through nose and push abdomen against hands. Tell client to feel middle fingers separate during inhalation. Demonstrate.	____	____	____	_____
(5) Explain that client will feel normal downward movement of diaphragm during inspiration. Explain that abdominal organs descend and chest wall expands.	____	____	____	_____
(6) Avoid using chest and shoulders while inhaling and instruct client in same manner.	____	____	____	_____
(7) Have client hold slow, deep breath for count of three and then slowly exhale through mouth as if blowing out a candle (pursed lips). Tell client middle fingertips will touch as chest wall contracts.	____	____	____	_____
(8) Repeat breathing exercise 3 to 5 times.	____	____	____	_____
(9) Have client practice exercise. Instruct client to take 10 slow, deep breaths every hour while awake during postoperative period until mobile.	____	____	____	_____

Continued

	S	U	NP	Comments

B. Incentive spirometry:
(1) Perform hand hygiene.
(2) Position client in semi- or high-Fowler's position.
(3) Set the spirometer to the volume level to be attained.
(4) Demonstrate correct use of spirometer mouthpiece.
(5) Instruct client to inhale slowly and maintain constant flow through unit, attempting to reach goal volume. When maximal inspiration is reached, client should hold breath for 2 to 3 seconds and then exhale slowly. Number of breaths should not exceed 10 to 12/min each session.
(6) Instruct client to breathe normally for short period.
(7) Instruct client to repeat maneuver until goals are achieved.
(8) Perform hand hygiene.

C. Positive expiratory pressure therapy and "huff" coughing:
(1) Perform hand hygiene.
(2) Set positive expiratory pressure device for the positive pressure setting ordered.
(3) Instruct client to assume semi-Fowler's or high-Fowler's position and place nose clip on client's nose.
(4) Ask client to place lips around mouthpiece of device. Client should take a full breath and then exhale two to three times longer than inhalation.
(5) Remove device from client's mouth and have client take a slow, deep breath and hold for 3 seconds.
(6) Instruct client to exhale in quick, short, forced inhalations.

D. Controlled coughing:
(1) Assist client to an upright position. Explain importance of positioning.
(2) Demonstrate coughing: Take two slow diaphragmatic breaths, inhaling through mouth, exhaling through nose.
(3) Instruct client to then inhale a third breath deeply, hold breath to count of three, and then cough fully two or three times without inhaling.

Continued

524

	S	U	NP	Comments

(4) Caution client against merely clearing throat. ___ ___ ___ _____

(5) If surgical incision is in client's chest or abdominal area, show client how to splint cough with both hands over incision or with pillow. Have client practice technique. ___ ___ ___ _____

(6) Explain how often the patient should cough and splint. ___ ___ ___ _____

(7) Instruct client to examine sputum. ___ ___ ___ _____

E. Turning:

(1) Assist client to supine position on right side of bed (as permitted by surgery). Put side rails up. ___ ___ ___ _____

(2) Ask client to place left hand over incisional area for splinting. ___ ___ ___ _____

(3) Instruct client to keep left leg straight and flex right knee up and over left leg. ___ ___ ___ _____

(4) Ask client to grasp side rail on left side of bed with right hand, pull toward left, and roll onto left side. ___ ___ ___ _____

(5) Teach client when to perform maneuver. ___ ___ ___ _____

F. Leg exercises:

(1) Assist client to supine position. Explain and demonstrate exercises by using passive range-of-motion exercises. ___ ___ ___ _____ / ___ ___ ___ _____

(2) Rotate each of client's ankles in complete circle. Have client draw imaginary circles with big toe and repeat five times. ___ ___ ___ _____

(3) Alternate dorsiflexion and plantar flexion of client's feet. ___ ___ ___ _____

(4) Continue exercises by alternately flexing and extending client's knees; repeat five times. ___ ___ ___ _____

(5) Have client keep knees straight and alternately raise each leg straight up from bed surface; repeat five times. ___ ___ ___ _____

(6) Have client tighten thighs and bring knees down toward mattress, then relax. ___ ___ ___ _____

(7) Instruct client when and how often to perform exercises and to coordinate turning and leg exercises with breathing and coughing exercises. ___ ___ ___ _____

7. Have client practice exercises every 2 hours while awake ___ ___ ___ _____

8. Observe client's ability to perform all exercises. ___ ___ ___ _____

9. Record procedures performed and observations. ___ ___ ___ _____

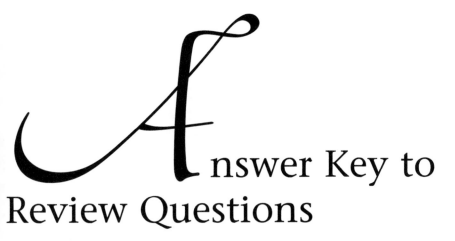

Answer Key to Review Questions

CHAPTER 1	**CHAPTER 5**	**CHAPTER 9**	**CHAPTER 13**
1. c	1. b	1. a	1. b
2. d	2. d	2. c	2. a
3. d	3. c	3. c	3. b
4. a	4. b	4. c	4. c
5. a	5. c	5. a	5. b

CHAPTER 2	**CHAPTER 6**	**CHAPTER 10**	**CHAPTER 14**
1. a	1. c	1. b	1. b
2. d	2. b	2. b	2. c
3. a	3. b	3. a	3. a
4. d	4. d	4. c	4. c
5. c	5. d	5. d	

CHAPTER 15

1. c
2. a
3. a
4. a
5. d

CHAPTER 3	**CHAPTER 7**	**CHAPTER 11**
1. b	1. c	1. c
2. a	2. c	2. d
3. a	3. d	3. d
4. d	4. a	4. a
5. c	5. a	5. c
		6. d

CHAPTER 16

1. a
2. a
3. b
4. a
5. d

CHAPTER 4	**CHAPTER 8**
1. b	1. a
2. d	2. b
3. a	3. b
4. b	4. b
5. a	5. a

CHAPTER 12

1. b
2. a
3. b
4. c
5. b

CHAPTER 17

1. d
2. b
3. d
4. d
5. a

CHAPTER 18

1. b
2. d
3. a
4. a
5. c

CHAPTER 19

1. c
2. c
3. b
4. b
5. a

CHAPTER 20

1. a
2. c
3. c
4. d
5. a

CHAPTER 21

1. d
2. d
3. a
4. b
5. c

CHAPTER 22

1. a
2. c
3. d
4. b
5. d

CHAPTER 23

1. b
2. b
3. b
4. a
5. b

CHAPTER 24

1. b
2. c
3. d
4. c
5. b

CHAPTER 25

1. b
2. c
3. c
4. c
5. d

CHAPTER 26

1. c
2. c
3. b
4. c
5. d

CHAPTER 27

1. b
2. d
3. c
4. a
5. d

CHAPTER 28

1. a
2. a
3. a
4. a
5. c

CHAPTER 29

1. c
2. c
3. b
4. c
5. d

CHAPTER 30

1. d
2. a
3. a
4. d
5. c
6. d

CHAPTER 31

1. d
2. d
3. b
4. c
5. c

CHAPTER 32

1. d
2. a
3. c
4. c
5. c
6. d

CHAPTER 33

1. d
2. b
3. d
4. a
5. b
6. a

CHAPTER 34

1. b
2. a
3. a
4. a
5. b
6. a

CHAPTER 35

1. c
2. c
3. d
4. a

CHAPTER 36

1. c
2. b
3. a
4. b
5. d

CHAPTER 37

1. d
2. d
3. c
4. d
5. a

CHAPTER 38

1. b
2. a
3. c
4. b
5. c

CHAPTER 39

1. a
2. c
3. b
4. b
5. d
6. b

CHAPTER 40

1. b
2. c
3. a
4. c
5. b
6. d

CHAPTER 41

1. a
2. a
3. c
4. d
5. b

CHAPTER 42

1. b
2. d
3. a
4. b
5. c

CHAPTER 43

1. c
2. d
3. c
4. c
5. b
6. a

CHAPTER 44

1. a
2. b
3. b
4. a
5. d

CHAPTER 45

1. b
2. a
3. c
4. b
5. c

CHAPTER 46

1. a
2. d
3. d
4. a
5. d

CHAPTER 47

1. b
2. b
3. a
4. c
5. b
6. d

CHAPTER 48

1. c
2. a
3. b
4. c
5. a

CHAPTER 49

1. d
2. c
3. c
4. a
5. b

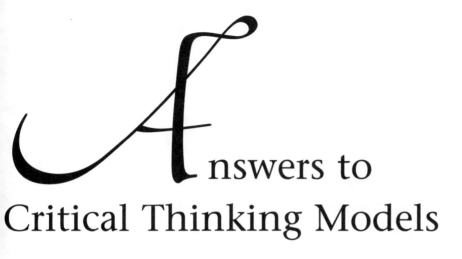

Critical Thinking Models

KNOWLEDGE

- Components of self-concept (identity, body image, self-esteem, role performance)
- Self-concept stressors related to identity, body image, self-esteem, role
- Therapeutic communication principles, nonverbal indicators of distress
  Cultural factors that influence self-concept
  Growth and development (middle-age adult)
- Pharmacologic effects of medicine (pain medication)

EXPERIENCE

- Caring for a client who had an alteration in body image, self-esteem, role, or identity
- Jan's own personal experience of threat to self-concept

Assessment

- Observe Mrs. Johnson's behaviors that suggest an alteration in self-concept
- Assess the Mrs. Johnson's cultural background
- Assess the Mrs. Johnson's coping skills and resources
- Converse with Mrs. Johnson to determine her feelings, perceptions about changes in body image, self-esteem, or role
- Assess the quality of Mrs. Johnson's relationships

STANDARDS

- Support Mrs. Johnson's autonomy to make choices and express values that support positive self-concept.
- Apply intellectual standards of relevance and plausibility for care to be acceptable to Mrs. Johnson
- Jan needs to safeguard Mrs. Johnson's right to privacy by judiciously protecting information of a confidential nature

ATTITUDES

- Display curiosity in considering why Mrs. Johnson might be behaving or responding in this manner
- Jan needs to display integrity when her beliefs and values differ from Mrs. Johnson's; admit to any inconsistencies between her values and his
- Risk taking may be necessary in developing a trusting relationship with Mrs. Johnson

CHAPTER *26* *Critical Thinking Model for Nursing Care Plan for* Alterations in Self-Concept (page 132).

KNOWLEDGE

- A basic understanding of sexual development, sexual orientation, sociocultural dimensions, the impact of self-concept, STDs, safe sex practices.
- Ways to phrase questions regarding sexuality and functioning
- Disease conditions that affect sexual functioning
- How interpersonal relationship factors may affect sexual functioning

EXPERIENCE

- Jack needs to explore his discomfort with discussing topics related to sexuality and develop a plan for addressing these discomforts
- Jack needs to reflect on his personal sexual experiences and how he has responded

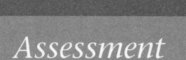

Assessment

- Assess Mr. Clement's developmental stage in regard to sexuality
- Consider self-concept as a factor that will influence sexual satisfaction and functioning
- Physical assessment of urogenital area
- Determine Mr. Clement's sexual concerns
- Assess safe sex practices and the use of contraception
- Assess the medical conditions and medications which may be affecting his sexual functioning
- Assess the impact of high-risk behaviors on sexual health

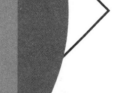

STANDARDS

- Jack needs to apply intellectual standards of relevance and plausibility for care to be acceptable to Mr. Clement
- Jack needs to safeguard Mr. Clement's right to privacy by judiciously protecting information of a confidential nature
- Jack needs to apply the principles of ethic of care

ATTITUDES

- Jack needs to display curiosity, consider why Mr. Clement might behave or respond in a particular manner
- Jack needs to display integrity; his beliefs and values may differ from Mr. Clement's
- Jack needs to admit to any inconsistencies in his and Mr. Clement's values
- Risk taking: Jack needs to be willing to explore both personal and Mr. Clement's sexual issues and concerns

CHAPTER 27 *Critical Thinking Model for Nursing Care Plan for* Sexual Dysfunction (page 139).

KNOWLEDGE

- The concepts of faith, hope, spiritual well-being and religion
- Caring practices in the individual approach to a client
- Available services in the community (health care providers and agencies)

EXPERIENCE

- Leah's past experience in selecting interventions that support client's spiritual well-being

Planning

- Leah needs to collaborate with James and his family on choice of interventions
- Consult with pastoral care or other clergy, holy leaders as appropriate
- Continue appropriate religious rituals specific to James
- Ask if the client's expectations have been met.

STANDARDS

- Standards of autonomy and self determination to support James decisions about the plan

ATTITUDES

- Leah will exhibit confidence in her skills and know to develop a trusting relationship with James
- Be open to any possible CONFLICT between the client's opinion and Leah's; decide how to reach mutually beneficial outcomes

CHAPTER *28* *Critical Thinking Model for Nursing Care Plan for* Spiritual Well-Being (page 145).

534   Answers to Critical Thinking Models

KNOWLEDGE

- Characteristics of a resolution of grief
- Clinical symptoms of an improved level of comfort (applicable for the terminally ill)
- Principles of pallative care

EXPERIENCE

- Previous client responses to planned nursing interventions for management or the loss of a significant other

Evaluation

- Evaluate signs and symptoms of Mr. Miller's grief and his wife's
- Evaluate his wife's ability to provide supportive care
- Evaluate Mr. Miller's level of comfort and symptom relief
- Ask if the client/family's expectations are being met

STANDARDS

- Use established expected outcomes to evaluate Mr. Miller's plan of care (participation in life review)
- Evaluate Mr. Miller's role in end-of-life decisions and (or the grieving) process

ATTITUDES

- Persevere in seeking successful comfort measures for Mr. Miller

CHAPTER *29* *Critical Thinking Model for Nursing Care Plan for* Grief and Loss (page 151).

KNOWLEDGE

- Characteristics of adaptive behaviors
- Characteristics of continuing stress response
- Differentiation of stress and trauma

EXPERIENCE

- Previous client responses to planned nursing interventions

Evaluation

- Reassess Carl for the presence of new or recurring stress related problems or symptoms (fatigue, changes in energy level, weight, or eating habits)
- Determine if change in care promoted Carl's adaptation to stress
- Evaluate if Carl's expectations have been achieved

STANDARDS

- Use of established expected outcomes to evaluate Carl's plan of care (rest and relaxation, stable weight, positive feelings about wife and their relationship)
- Apply the intellectual standard of relevance; be sure that Carl achieves goals relevant to his needs

ATTITUDES

- Janet needs to demonstrate perseverance in redesigning interventions to promote Carl's adaptation to stress
- Janet needs to display integrity in accurately evaluating nursing interventions

CHAPTER *30*   *Critical Thinking Model for Nursing Care Plan for* Care Giver Role Strain (page 157).

KNOWLEDGE

- The role of physical therapist and exercise trainers in improving Mrs. Swain's activity and exercise program
- Determine Mrs. Swain's ability to increase her level of activity
- Impact of medication on Mrs. Swain's activity tolerance

EXPERIENCE

- Mary needs to consider previous client and personal experiences to therapies designed to improve exercise and activity tolerance
- Mary's personal experience with exercise regimens

Planning

- Mary needs to consult and collaborate with members of the health team to increase Mrs. Swain's activity
- Involve Mrs. Swain and her family in designing her activity and exercise plan
- Mary needs to consider Mrs. Swain's ability to increase her activity level and follow a exercise program

STANDARDS

- Therapies need to be individualized to Mrs. Swain's activity tolerance
- Mary needs to apply the goals of the American College of Sports Medicine in the application

ATTITUDES

- Mary needs to be responsible and creative in designing interventions to improve Mrs. Swain's activity tolerance

CHAPTER *36* *Critical Thinking Model for Nursing Care Plan for* Activity Intolerance (page 220).

KNOWLEDGE

- Basic human needs
- The potential risks to a client's safety from physical and environmental hazards
- The influence of developmental stage on safety needs (older adult)
- The influence of illness and medications on Ms. Cohen's safety (immobilization and visual impairment)

EXPERIENCE

- Past experiences of Mr. Key in caring for clients with mobility or sensory impairments that threaten safety
- Personal experiences in caring for the older adult

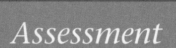

Assessment

- Identification of actual and potential threats to Ms. Cohen's safety
- Determine the impact of Ms. Cohen's underlying disease on her safety
- The presence of risks for Ms. Cohen's developmental stage

STANDARDS

- Mr. Key needs to apply intellectual standards of accuracy, significance, completeness, and fairness when assessing for threats to Ms. Cohen's safety
- ANA standards of nursing practice
- Fall prevention protocols (Practice Standards)

ATTITUDES

- Perseverance is needed when identifying all threats to Ms. Cohen's safety
- Responsibility for collecting unbiased accurate data regarding Ms. Cohen's threat to safety
- Fairness is appropriate to objectively evaluate the risk to Ms. Cohen's safety within the home and the community

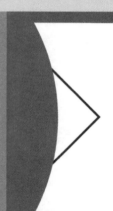

CHAPTER *37*   *Critical Thinking Model for Nursing Care Plan for* Risk for Injury (page 227).

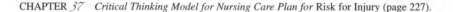

KNOWLEDGE

- Principles of comfort and safety
- Adult learning principles to apply when educating the client and family
- Services available through community agencies

EXPERIENCE

- Care of previous clients that required adaptation of hygiene approaches

Planning

- Involve Mrs. Wyatt and her family in planning and adapting approaches as well as in hygience instruction
- Know community resources applicable to Mrs. Wyatt's needs
- Consider the timing of other care activities when choosing the best time for hygienic care

STANDARDS

- Individualize the hygiene care to meet Mrs. Wyatt's preferences
- Apply standards of safety and promotion of client dignity

ATTITUDES

- Jeanette needs to be creative when adapting approaches to any self-care limitations that Mrs. Wyatt might have
- Jeanette needs to take responsibility for following standards of good hygiene practice

CHAPTER *38* *Critical Thinking Model for Nursing Care Plan for* Self-Care Deficit, Bathing/Hygiene (page 236).

KNOWLEDGE

- Cardiac and respiratory anatomy and physiology
- Cardiopulmonary pathophysiology
- Clinical signs and symptoms of altered oxygenation
- Developmental factors affecting oxygenation
- Impact on lifestyle
- Environmental impact

EXPERIENCE

- Caring for clients with impaired oxygenation, activity intolerance, and respiratory infections
- Observations of changes in client respiratory patterns made during poor air quality days
- Personal experience with how a change in altitudes or physical conditioning affects respiratory patterns
- Personal experience with respiratory infections or cardiopulmonary alterations

Assessment

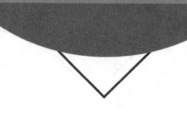

- Identify recurring and present signs and symptoms associated with Mr. Edwards impaired oxygenation
- Determine the presence of risk factors that apply to Mr. Edwards
- Ask Mr. Edwards about the use of medication
- Determine Mr. Edwards activity status
- Determine Mr. Edwards tolerance to activity

STANDARDS

- Apply intellectual standards of clarity, precision, specificity, and accuracy when obtaining a health history for a client with cardiopulmonary alterations

ATTITUDES

- Carry out the responsibility of obtaining correct information about Mr. Edwards and explaining risk factors, health promotion and disease prevention activities, and therapies for disease/symptom management
- Display confidence in assessing Mr. Edwards management of illness

CHAPTER *39* *Critical Thinking Model for Nursing Care Plan for* Ineffective Airway Clearance (page 251).

KNOWLEDGE

- Consider the other health care professionals caring for Mrs. Bottomley
- The impact of specific fluid regimens on the Mrs. Bottomley's fluid balance
- The impact of new medications on Mrs. Bottomley's fluid balance

EXPERIENCE

- Consider the previous clinical assignments you have had and how those clients responded to nursing therapies (what worked and what didn't?)

Planning

- Select nursing interventions to promote fluid, electrolyte, and acid-base balance
- Consult with pharmacists and nutritionists
- Involve Mrs. Bottomley and her family in designing the interventions

STANDARDS

- Therapies need to be individualized to Mrs. Bottomley's fluid balance and acid-base requirements

ATTITUDES

- Use creativity to plan interventions that will achieve an effective airway and integrate those into Mrs. Bottomley's activities of daily living
- Be responsible in planning nursing interventions consistent with the client's fluid balance and acid-base requirements

CHAPTER 40   *Critical Thinking Model for Ineffective Airway Clearance/Risk for* Fluid Volume Deficit (page 265).

Answers to Critical Thinking Models   541

KNOWLEDGE

- The characteristics of a desirable sleep pattern
- Basis for the expected outcomes in the plan of care

EXPERIENCE

- Previous client's responses to planned nursing interventions for promoting sleep
- Previous experience in adapting sleep therapies to personal needs

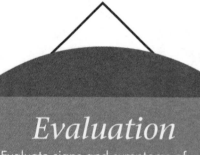

Evaluation

- Evaluate signs and symptoms of Julie's sleep disturbance
- Review Julie's sleep pattern
- Have sleep partner report Julie's response to therapies
- The expected outcomes developed during the plan of care serve as the standards to evaluate its success
- Ask client if expectations of care are being met

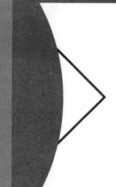

STANDARDS

- Use of established expected outcomes to evaluate Julie's plan of care (improved duration of sleep, fewer awakenings)

ATTITUDES

- Humility may apply if an intervention is unsuccessful; rethink the approach
- In the case of chronic sleep problems, perseverance is needed in staying with the plan of care or in trying new approaches

CHAPTER *41* *Critical Thinking Model for Nursing Care Plan for* Sleep Pattern Disturbance (page 274).

KNOWLEDGE

- Physiology of pain
- Factors that potentially increase or decrease responses to pain
- Pathophysiology of conditions causing pain
- Awareness of biases affecting pain assessment and treatment
- Cultural variations in how pain is expressed
- Knowledge of nonverbal communication

EXPERIENCE

- Caring for clients with acute, chronic, and cancer pain
- Caring for clients who experienced pain as a result of a health care therapy
- Personal experience with pain

Assessment

- Determine Mrs. May's perspective of pain including history of pain, its meaning, and physical emotional and social effects
- Objectively measure the characteristics of Mrs. May's pain
- Review potential factors affecting Mrs. May's pain

STANDARDS

- Refer to AHCPR guidelines for acute pain management
- Apply intellectual standards (clarity, specificity, accuracy, and completeness) when gathering assessment
- Apply relevance when letting Mrs. May's explore the pain experience

ATTITUDES

- Persevere in exploring causes and possible solutions for chronic pain
- Display confidence when assessing pain to relieve Mrs. May's anxiety
- Display integrity and fairness to prevent prejudice from affecting assessment

CHAPTER 42 *Critical Thinking Model for Nursing Care Plan for* Acute Pain (page 284).

Answers to Critical Thinking Models 543

KNOWLEDGE

- Roles of dietitians and nutritionists in caring for clients with altered nutrition
- Impact of community support groups and other resources in assisting clients to manage nutrition
- Impact of bad diets on client's overall nutritional status

EXPERIENCE

- Previous client responses to nursing interventions for altered nutrition
- Personal experiences with dietary change strategies (what worked and what didn't)

Planning

- Select nursing interventions to promote optimal nutrition
- Select nursing interventions consistent with therapeutic diets
- Consult with other health care professinonals (dietitians, nutritionists, physicians, pharmacists, and physical and occupational therapists) to adopt interventions that reflect Mrs. Cooper's needs
- Involve the family when designing interventions

STANDARDS

- Refer to AHCPR guidelines for acute pain management
- Apply intellectual standards (clarity, specificity, accuracy, and completeness) when gathering assessment
- Apply relevance when letting Mrs. May's explore the pain experience

ATTITUDES

- Persevere in exploring causes and possible solutions for chronic pain
- Display confidence when assessing pain to relieve Mrs. May's anxiety
- Display integrity and fairness to prevent prejudice from affecting assessment

CHAPTER *43*   *Critical Thinking Model for Nursing Care Plan for* Imbalanced Nutrition: Less Than Body Requirements (page 296).

KNOWLEDGE

- Physiology of fluid balance
- Anatomy and physiology of normal urine production and urination
- Pathophysiology of selected urinary alterations
- Factors affecting urination
- Principles of communication used to address issues related to self-concept and sexuality

EXPERIENCE

- Caring for clients with alterations in urinary elimination
- Caring for clients at risk for urinary infection
- Personal experience with changes in urinary elimination

Assessment

- Gather nursing history of the urination pattern, symptoms, and factors affecting urination
- Conduct a physical assessment of body systems potentially affected by urinary change
- Assess the characteristics of urine
- Assess perception of urinary problems as it affects self-concept and sexuality

STANDARDS

- Maintain privacy and dignity
- Apply intellectual standards to ensure history and assessment are complete and in depth
- Apply professional standards of care from professional organizations such as ANA and AHCPR

ATTITUDES

- Display humility in recognizing limitations in knowledge

CHAPTER 44 *Critical Thinking Model for Nursing Care Plan for* Functional Urinary Incontinence (page 307).

KNOWLEDGE

- Role of the other health care professionals in returning the client's bowel elimination pattern to normal
- Impact of specific therapeutic diets and medication on bowel elimination patterns
- Expected results of cathartics, laxatives, and enemas on bowel elimination

EXPERIENCE

- Previous client response to planned nursing therapies for improving bowel elimination (what worked and what didn't)

Planning

- Javier needs to select nursing interventions to promote normal bowel elimination
- Consult with nurtitionists and enteral stoma therapists
- Involve Larry and his family in designing nursing interventions

STANDARDS

- Individualize therapies to Larry's bowel elimination needs
- Select therapies consistent within wound and ostomy professional practice standards

ATTITUDES

- Javier needs to be creative when planning interventions for Larry to achieve normal bowel elimination patterns
- Display independence when integrating interventions from other disciplines in Larry's plan of care
- Act responsibly by ensuring that interventions are consistent within standards

CHAPTER *45* *Critical Thinking Model for Nursing Care Plan for* Constipation (page 317).

546   Answers to Critical Thinking Models

KNOWLEDGE

- Characteristics of improved mobility status on all physiological systems and the client's psychosocial and developmental status

EXPERIENCE

- Previous client responses to planned mobility interventions.

Evaluation

- Reassess Miss Adams for signs and symptoms of improved or decreasd mobility status
- Ask for Miss Adam's perception of mobility status after intervention
- Evaluate whether or not Miss Adam's expectations of care have been met

STANDARDS

- Use established expected outcomes for the Miss Adam's plan of care (lung fields remain clear) to evaluate her response to care

ATTITUDES

- Display humility when identifying those interventions that were not successful
- Use creativity when redesigning new interventions to improve Miss Adam's mobility status

CHAPTER *46* *Critical Thinking Model for Nursing Care Plan for* Impaired Mobility (page 328).

KNOWLEDGE

- Pathogenesis of pressure ulcers
- Factors contributing to pressure ulcer formation or poor wound healing
- Factors contributing to wound healing
- Impact of underlying disease process of skin integrity
- Impact of medication on skin integrity and wound healing

EXPERIENCE

- Caring for clients with impaired skin integrity or wounds
- Observation of normal wound healing

Assessment

- Identify the risk for developing impaired skin integrity
- Identify signs and symptoms associated with impaired skin integrity or poor wound healing
- Examine Mrs. Stein's skin for actual impairment in skin integrity

STANDARDS

- Apply intellectual standards of accuracy, relevance, completeness, and precision when obtaining health history regarding skin integrity and wound management
- Knowledge of AHCPR standards for prevention of pressure ulcers

ATTITUDES

- Use discipline to obtain complete and correct assessment data regarding Mrs. Stein's skin and or/wound integrity
- Demonstrate responsibility for collecting appropriate specimens for diagnostic and laboratory tests related to wound management

CHAPTER *47*   *Critical Thinking Model for Nursing Care Plan for* Impaired Skin Integrity (page 338).

KNOWLEDGE

- Understand how a sensory deficit can affect the client's functional status
- Role other health professionals might have in sensory function management
- Services of community resources
- Adult learning principles to apply when educating the client and family

EXPERIENCE

- Previous client responses to planned nursing interventions to promote sensory function

Planning

- Select strategies that assist Judy to remain functional in her home
- Adapt therapies based on short- or long-term sensory deficit
- Involve the family in helping Judy adjust to her limitations
- Refer Judy to appropriate health care professional and/or community agency

STANDARDS

- Individualize therapies that allow the client to adapt to sensory loss in any setting
- Apply standards of safety

ATTITUDES

- Use creativity to find interventions that help Judy adapt to the home environment

CHAPTER 48 *Critical Thinking Model for Nursing Care Plan for* Sensory Perceptual Alterations (page 346).

Answers to Critical Thinking Models 549

KNOWLEDGE

- Behaviors that demonstrate learning
- Characteristics of anxiety and/or fear
- Signs and symptoms or conditions that contraindicate surgery

EXPERIENCE

- Previous client responses to planned preoperative care
- Any personal experience Joe has had with surgery

Evaluation

- Evaluate Mrs. Cambana's knowledge of surgical procedure and planned postoperative care
- Have Mrs. Cambana demonstrate postoperative exercises
- Observe behaviors or nonverbal expressions of anxiety or fea
- Ask if client's expectation are being met

STANDARDS

- Use established expected outcomes to evaluate Mrs. Cambana's plan of care (ability to perform postoperative exercises)

ATTITUDES

- Demonstrate perseverance when Mrs. Cambana has difficulty performing postoperative exercises

CHAPTER *49*   *Critical Thinking Model for Nursing Care Plan for* Knowledge Deficit Regarding Perioperative Care (page 359).